Beauty around the World

Beauty around the World

A Cultural Encyclopedia

ERIN KENNY AND ELIZABETH
GACKSTETTER NICHOLS

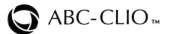

ABC-CLIO™

An Imprint of ABC-CLIO, LLC
Santa Barbara, California • Denver, Colorado

Copyright © 2017 by ABC-CLIO, LLC

All rights reserved. No part of this publication may be reproduced, stored in a
retrieval system, or transmitted, in any form or by any means, electronic, mechanical,
photocopying, recording, or otherwise, except for the inclusion of brief quotations in a
review, without prior permission in writing from the publisher.

Library of Congress Cataloging-in-Publication Data

Names: Kenny, Erin, 1969- author. | Nichols, Elizabeth Gackstetter, author.
Title: Beauty around the world : a cultural encyclopedia / Erin Kenny and
    Elizabeth Gackstetter Nichols.
Description: Santa Barbara, California : ABC-CLIO, [2017] | Includes bibliographical
    references and index.
Identifiers: LCCN 2016058358 (print) | LCCN 2017016328 (ebook) |
    ISBN 9781610699457 (ebook) | ISBN 9781610699440 (hardcopy : alk. paper)
Subjects: LCSH: Beauty, Personal—Cross-cultural studies.
Classification: LCC GT499 (ebook) | LCC GT499 .K46 2017 (print) |
    DDC 646.7/2—dc23
LC record available at https://lccn.loc.gov/2016058358

ISBN: 978-1-61069-944-0
EISBN: 978-1-61069-945-7

21 20 19 18 17   1 2 3 4 5

This book is also available as an eBook.

ABC-CLIO
An Imprint of ABC-CLIO, LLC

ABC-CLIO, LLC
130 Cremona Drive, P.O. Box 1911
Santa Barbara, California 93116-1911
www.abc-clio.com

This book is printed on acid-free paper ∞

Manufactured in the United States of America

Contents

List of Entries

Preface

Beauty is one of those notoriously difficult concepts to try to squeeze into mere words: we know it when we see it. Usually, beauty can elicit a response inside us, something that we are preconditioned to seek or desire. We need beauty to live because it draws us in, engages us, and touches our human experiences with awe and pleasure. It inspires us, gives us a sense of aspiration, taking us outside of ourselves and motivating us. According to some, beauty is essential to life and to happiness.

This text takes an interdisciplinary approach to the field of beauty studies. We try to provide historical and cultural context to the biological notion of "beauty." The prior research of the authors represents forays into thinking about beauty and bodies from the perspectives of the social sciences and the humanities. We are a cultural anthropologist with research experiences in both East and West Africa (Erin) and a cultural studies scholar specializing in cultures of Latin America (Elizabeth). We've both taught extensively on the topic of beauty and bodies in introductory classes to undergraduate students, where many of these entries were born.

We also both identify as feminist scholars. As such, we bring a critical lens to the ways that certain "natural" ideas about beauty have been socially constructed within patriarchal systems and the ways that these ideas have circulated throughout the postcolonial world. Using an intersectional framework, we are acutely aware of the ways that these notions may disproportionately affect women and people of color. We tried in this text to be very sensitive about issues of representation: we acknowledge and wish to never reproduce the symbolic violences done to marginalized peoples.

In this volume, we've listed 166 alphabetical entries that deal with some aspect of "beauty," understood as the aesthetic pleasure of visual appearance.

Of course, we found it difficult to be truly exhaustive in each entry, especially in the historical sense of chronicling all beauty patterns throughout time and space. In general, when a category is topped with the name of a nation, country, or tribal group, we have tried to provide the most vivid, iconic, or best-known version of that term or location.

This book will be most useful as a starting point for others looking for further reading or preparing for more serious interrogation into the issues of beauty. Each entry contains suggestions for additional sources that can be consulted. Readers should also be aware of the extensive bibliography of materials culled from books, popular magazines, scholarly articles, and the Internet, including several sources that we have translated ourselves from Spanish and French.

Acknowledgements

Erin would like to thank the many students in her ANTH 315 "Gender Sex and the Body" course over the last five years for all their enthusiasm and insights into ways of thinking about beauty, embodiment, and the roles these things continue to play in our lives. She would also like to thank her co-author, Elizabeth Gackstetter Nichols, for her generosity and practical approach to collaborative writing. Erin is extremely grateful for the friendship of the original group of "Rose's Writers" at Drury University from spring of 2015. The enduring friendship of Laura Burghart, the world's most beautiful cake maker and truth speaker, has enabled Erin to believe that she could do an amazing number of difficult things. Finally, she would like to thank Kiera, for always being a star: she's clever and patient and funny and everything Erin ever wanted in a daughter.

Elizabeth is first truly grateful to the brilliant and hilarious Erin Kenny. She'd also like to thank her CORE 201 "What Is Beauty" students for their willingness to think about and explore social norms of beauty and for introducing her to such gems as totalfratmove.com. Elizabeth is also very grateful to her Kira for the windows into cosplay and costuming, and for teaching her about crossplay, genderbending, and nonstandard beauty uses of sharpies. Elizabeth is grateful to Maria for reading every page of *Vogue* together; Rose's Writing group for tacos, tea time, and editing advice; Springfield Cosplay Group for inspiration and support; and her parents for their unflagging enthusiasm. Finally, Brad, thank you for being moral and tech support, for putting up with wigs in the bathroom, and for carrying all our stuff.

Introduction

In the United States, children are often taught "not to judge a book by its cover," and Israeli parents caution youth "not to look at the pitcher, rather look at what's inside." Yet paradoxically, societies around the world continue to make explicit the importance of physical appearance as a way to both ensure and gauge success. As the Arab proverb states, "beauty is power."

We've framed this introductory essay as both a celebration and a critique of beauty standards. Although the study of beauty around the world allows for a vibrant celebration of diversity and attractiveness, it also opens the possibility for an interrogation of beauty as a yardstick for personal achievement. We invite the reader to accept widely diverse notions of what constitutes "beauty" in different world cultures, but we also ask readers to go further and to be willing to think critically about the social expectations of race, class, and gender underlying culturally expected beauty practices. The reader may find it useful to ask the question, "Why is this particular appearance or standard of beauty preferred?" in order to begin to develop a more nuanced and critical understanding of beauty work and its many meanings.

Beauty Matters

In the 2016 U.S. presidential race, the issue of personal attractiveness came roaring to the forefront of national discourse. The heated conversations that followed revealed how social constructions of "beauty" underscore the complicated relationships between power, gender, control, and success within American politics. From the beginning of his campaign, Republican candidate Donald Trump was at the epicenter of enormous controversy about the significance of appearance. To begin, Trump criticized one of his primary opponents, the businesswoman Carly Fiorina, based on her appearance, memorably saying "'Look at that face! Would anyone vote for that? Can you imagine that, the face of our next president?!" (Estepa 2015).

Fiorina was not the only woman whose attractiveness was considered in the unusual and widely divisive campaign. The Democratic candidate, Hillary Clinton, had already been mocked and scrutinized for years by professional comics and late-night television hosts for her clothing choices, including a penchant for "masculine" pantsuits (Aylmer 2015). At the same time, Clinton was excoriated for showing even the slightest hint of cleavage. The standard challenge for Clinton's wardrobe was to find professional clothing that might "properly—which is to say, abashedly—disguise the fact that Clinton, a wife and a mother and a soon-to-be Madam Secretary [of State], was in possession of a pair of breasts" (Garber 2016). Later, as a candidate for president, Trump's supporters would circulate offensive buttons and

T-shirts lampooning Clinton for her "two fat thighs and two small breasts" (Schwab 2016).

In her campaign against Trump, Clinton further brought up the issue of beauty and appearance when she chastised her opponent for fat-shaming former Miss Universe Alicia Machado, sparking a wide debate. Trump, who owns the Miss Universe pageant, strongly chastised Machado after her win in 1996, when she put on weight. During that time, Trump publically discussed what he called Machado's "massive" weight gain, called Machado "Miss Piggy," and invited a crowd of media to supervise her workouts (Easley 2016, 9). Clinton made Trump's criticism of the beauty queen a campaign issue, accusing him of misogyny and bringing attention to Machado's claim that his treatment had led her to develop an eating disorder (Easley 2016). The national conversation that developed from this attention debated the issue of the importance of appearance, the duties of a beauty queen, and the social expectations for women in public as they are evaluated by society.

The unceasing evaluation of physical attractiveness was not limited to female participants in the 2016 election cycle, however. Trump himself was scrutinized and criticized for his appearance, in particular his hair and weight. Many articles were written exclusively on the candidate's hair, speculating whether it was a comb-over, or a wig, or even the product of scalp surgery. Trump himself remained vehemently defensive about his hair, insisting it was natural and not a toupee or wig, as many claimed. He even invited high-profile celebrities and fans to mess his hair up (Levine 2016). This attention to the candidate's hair highlighted how a full head of hair for men is a symbol of health, masculinity, and virility. The suggestion that Trump might be balding was an egregious slight to his strength and manhood.

Attention to Trump's hair, along with a series of unflattering statues of the candidate that emerged in cities such as New York, Los Angeles, and Seattle depicting him as naked, flabby, and overweight, pointed to how men, like women, are continually judged on their looks and how appearance can be symbolic of health and wealth (Hopper 2016).

Evolutionary psychologist Nancy Etcoff argues that for both men and women, beauty is essential to personal and professional advancement, as we perceive the inner worth of a person first through their external appearance. Etcoff (2000) cites a wide range of studies from psychology and sociology indicating that people judge others based on their appearance in less than a second. In that short amount of time we make snap decisions about wealth, class, race, health, and intelligence, all based on how a person looks.

Venezuelan fashion designer Carolina Herrera would agree with those studies, noting that "inner beauty, how we think, how we act, how we see things, is reflected in how we look" and therefore "looking good is very important because as much as they tell us that she shouldn't judge a book by its cover and that the habit doesn't make the monk, the truth is that everyone enters our perception through our eyes" (2009, 3–4).

Whereas many idealists would prefer to think that it is, indeed, "inner beauty" that matters most in the assessment of human value, the successes of celebrities and political figures emphasize the importance of an aesthetically pleasing outer shell that communicates desirability and recognition of social norms. When researchers interviewed more than 10,000 people from around the world about their evaluation of other people, physical attractiveness was one of the top ten most important things for everyone, from every country (Etcoff 2000). A study funded by the National Institutes of Health testing the straightforward hypothesis "beauty is good" demonstrated that people consistently attribute positive qualities to attractive people and negative qualities to those they find unattractive (Dion, Berscheid, and Walster 1972).

In short, beauty matters.

World Beauty: A Celebration

Beauty can be consoling, disturbing, sacred, profane; it can be exhilarating, appealing, inspiring, chilling. It can affect us in an unlimited variety of ways. Yet it is never viewed with indifference: beauty demands to be noticed; it speaks to us directly like the voice of an intimate friend. If there are people who are indifferent to beauty, then it is surely because they do not perceive it.

—Roger Scruton (2011, xi).

In 2013, Osmel Sousa, the self-proclaimed "International Beauty Czar" and head of the prestigious Miss Venezuela organization, gave an interview in which he confidently declared: "I say inner beauty doesn't exist. That's something that 'unpretty' women invented to justify themselves" (Neumann 2013). Many who read this opinion were upset and offended. Mr. Sousa, however, had put his finger on a fundamental idea that most agree with but few are willing to confront: physical attractiveness and beauty carry a resonance that matters powerfully to the opportunities, relationships, and experiences of most people.

Because of the central importance of "being beautiful" to the experience of being human, societies and individuals worldwide have invented, designed, adapted, and celebrated a wide variety of beauty ideals and beauty work that they have enacted throughout history and continue to practice on a daily basis. This volume seeks to give an overview of many of these aesthetics, beliefs, and practices and to also set them into a historical and cultural context.

Cultures around the world present a stunning variety of expressions of human beauty. Slim or round figures, muscular or delicate builds, simple or elaborate hairstyles, body modifications or expensive fitness regimes, and rustic or elegant jewelry are part of those different beauty norms. In an effort to contextualize "world" beauty, we made a conscious effort in this volume to discuss whether certain notions about beauty exist in their original (native, indigenous) context, or whether the practices were syncretic, foreign inspired, or foreign imposed, as part of a transnational global system. One of the expectations—or fears—of the era of globalization was that all vestiges of indigenous cultural preferences, tastes, and ideologies would be subsumed under a homogeneous standard of normalcy where everyone would want to look and act exactly the same way (Levitt 1983).

There are some obvious examples of cultural blending when it comes to global aesthetics. For example, blonde hair and a focus on breasts across Asia have become the unexpected new markers of female beauty (Miller 2006). In other parts of the world, like the Pacific Islands, slenderness has rather recently replaced a generous figure as the most appealing body type (Becker 1995). However, most anthropologists and ethnographers argue strongly that many aesthetic practices and preferences continue in their original cultural contexts. People in Brazil still celebrate the well-rounded bottom of women with fervor as in the past; appreciation for darkened or tattooed gums to make teeth look more noticeably bright continues in Senegal (Stewart 2013). Many anthropologists write about the ways that local standards of beauty are becoming syncretized; that is to say, global and local standards of beauty are undergoing a process of cultural blending, which allows for cultures to interpenetrate and for individuals to determine what the value of each aesthetic tradition lends to a newly emerging standard of personal beauty (Miller 2006). Inevitably, people all over the world are increasingly exposed to global standards of commercial advertising and a wide range of products designed to address beauty "defects" by hiding them, correcting them, or engaging in practices designed to combat them.

Although there are a notably wide range of expressions of beauty, overall, standards of beauty are composed of healthful bodies with clear skin and symmetrical features. Indeed, beauty in humans has been described for thousands of years as the perfect combination of "clarity, symmetry, harmony and vivid color" (Etcoff 2000, 15). Evolutionary psychologists, who seek to understand why we prefer what we prefer in our potential mates, would argue that all the items on this list are signals to the suitability of the person we are looking at as a mate. Symmetry and harmony of features signal strong and healthy DNA, clarity in skin is a mark of someone resistant to disease, and the bright color of lips and cheeks speaks to a healthy heart and good blood circulation. This may be the way we ensure the success of our species, by selecting mates that will bear us healthy children (Etcoff 2000).

Around the world, the personal and professional benefits of beauty from birth through childhood and into adulthood are well documented. Attractive children are better adjusted and enjoy greater popularity (Langlois et al. 2000). Among adults, those who are perceived as better looking are also judged to be more competent, better interpersonally, and more reliable (Ibid.). Attractive people are consistently treated better by others and enjoy more positive attention, as well as benefiting from the help and cooperation of others. In economic terms, it is possible to think about attractiveness as a form of "social capital." Social capital refers to the networks of relationships between people within a given culture. These networks facilitate effective functioning of the society. The benefits of social capital accrue to attractive people, finding that in general, they have greater confidence and higher levels of social skill (Gladstone and O'Connor 2013)

Other important factors to consider when assessing the effects of beauty include the relative stakes for conforming to standards of attractiveness, which may be very different for men than they are for women. Age, wealth, and racial identity may also be key factors in determining how crucial it is for any given individual to be perceived as attractive within any given social interaction. Beauty may not only consider the physical appearance of an individual within a static moment of time, but also, the way a person or a body moves through space. Poets around the world praise the beauty of a dancer or an athlete. They pause to comment upon the grace of motion of someone beloved. These musings about beauty open the field from what can be easily photographed in one frame and expand the idea of beauty to something that is linked to the passage of time.

As the famous saying goes, "Beauty is in the eye of the beholder." What is considered beautiful to some may not be universally acceptable as attractive to others. The notion of universal beauty standards is particularly true in the dehumanizing context of the colonizing era, when bodies of the "Other" were collected and displayed in order to entice, titillate, and legitimize racist systems of oppression (Karp and Lavine 1991).

Of course, differences between cultural conceptualizations of beauty are potentially intriguing and exciting, capable of inspiring curiosity and engagement with a larger world. The young lady on the cover of this book, happily posing with the stack of rings around her long, elegant

> "I always hear myself saying, 'She's a beauty! Or 'He's a beauty!' or 'What a beauty!' but I never know what I'm talking about."
>
> —ANDY WARHOL

neck, represents a different view of attractiveness than many Western readers may have encountered. Surprise and sudden or unexpected discovery of another way at seeing beauty offer the opportunity to learn, incorporate, and appreciate other cultures along with our own.

World Beauty: Three Critiques

An old, well-known piece of advice cautions, "Never judge a book by its cover." Although celebrating the beauty of people around the world promotes a positive appreciation of cultural difference, overvaluing physical appearance or collapsing cultural distinctions into stereotypes about how people look can be a dangerous social practice that causes misunderstandings. Several important cautions should be mentioned regarding responsible evaluations of human beauty.

Are Pretty Faces Worn by "Better" People?

Sensationalizing good looks may directly privilege the external appearance of a human being over their inner life, including their creativity, their experiences, their intelligence, their hopes, and their dreams. A biased orientation to reward "a pretty face" over another person who may be equally worthy of praise raises a number of important, sometimes uncomfortable, issues about the implicit value of "looking good." As many of the entries in this volume indicate, human beauty (and its perceived lack) can cause a great deal of pain, especially from the perspective of those who may not "measure up" to the standards of beauty.

Social stereotypes create realities that affect how we process cultural cues through a series of three social mechanisms in what is sometimes called "stranger-attribution behavior" by sociologists (Langlois et al. 2000). An individual, going about the daily business of life, encounters a stranger. First, the physical features of the individuals create a set of expectations for the behaviors and traits that the stranger will expect to see. Researchers argue that attractiveness is the most important influencing factor in the ways that this individual is immediately assessed or judged by the stranger. In other words, social expectations are created, in part, from physical cues and the ways that the stranger perceives these physical cues, fitting them into a cognitive framework about what is "beautiful."

Next, these expectations about the individual are acted upon by the stranger in the form of differential judgments and differential treatment. The type of treatment will be a measure of the degree to which the individual has been measured as either attractive or unattractive. There may be an invitation extended if the perception is positive, or in the event that the perception is not favorable, perhaps an opportunity is withdrawn. According to researchers, these perceptions take place at a subconscious, probably unacknowledged, level according to the social conditioning of the stranger. Factors in that conditioning include nearly infinite variables, including age, race, and gender, and more idiosyncratic factors about how physical beauty has been valued, personally experienced, and socially constructed by the stranger over the course of his or her life. Reactions to the attractiveness of the other person in the social setting can vary a great deal, but researchers do agree that within any given culture, there is a fairly narrow set of parameters that comprise "ideal" beauty.

Finally, as the original individual continues to process the reactions of the perceivers in his or her life, he or she internalizes these differential judgments and treatments, eventually developing behaviors and self-views that contribute to how the individual assumes his or her own physical appearance will affect others. Individuals may learn that their outward appearances predispose others to "like" them or give them the benefit of the doubt in social settings. Conversely, individuals may learn that their appearance fails to create any special response or possibly even elicits revulsion, fear, or pity. The individual internalizes this information and will adjust his or her approach to strangers based on that feedback in the future.

The consequences of not being considered "pretty enough" obviously vary from one individual to the next. Research from psychology suggests that the dominant tastes in terms of preferred complexion can limit the opportunities available for individuals who do not meet some arbitrary criteria. The notorious "paper bag" test was a widely used technique during the Jim Crow era in the United States, used to discriminate against those with a skin tone that was darker than that of a standard paper bag. Additionally, the standards of beauty associated with complexion may differ considerably between men and women. For example, skin tone ideal for women is lighter than the ideal for men (Baumann 2014). Research suggests that this bias is a "submerged" ideal that is not easily articulated (Ibid.). The 2011 documentary *Dark Girls* launches an emotional exploration of the biases and attitudes about standards of beauty and skin color bias in the contemporary United States to underscore how harmful standards of beauty can produce heartbreaking results about how individuals perceive their own attractiveness and self-worth.

In the words of the stunning pop star Beyoncé, "Pretty hurts."

Do Cultural Ideologies Offer Contradictory Messages about Beauty?

Beauty practices are often strikingly contradictory to cultural discourses about what the culture professes to value. Even though "beauty is only skin deep," the United States spends an estimated $62.46 billion per year on beauty products (Statista 2016). According to some, the price of pursuing social norms of beauty in time, money, and risks to health presents alarming evidence of damaging ideas and maladaptive practices for individuals. Whereas evolutionary biologists recognize and accept the theory that beauty preferences are nurtured by an evolutionary desire to continue the species, feminist scholars and social scientists may be critical of practices that seem to actually damage the health or well-being of individuals, the health of the environment, or the smooth functioning of a society.

For example, some argue that plastic surgery for teens is essential to stop bullying or establish the criteria needed for later professional successes in a young person's life. Others may criticize the parents of teens who endorse or finance expensive and dangerous procedures for their children "only" for vanity. However, a significant body of evidence indicates that beauty work and conforming to the social norms of beauty do indeed correlate with social acceptance, higher self-esteem, and overall success.

Attractiveness serves as an indirect form of power, especially for women, by increasing marriage proposals, social approval, job opportunities, or simply by expanding the range of social courtesies available. But cultural models of beauty may also be seen as evidence of other morally desirable traits, such as "goodness," effort, and discipline. In this way, it becomes possible to justify rewarding the "prettier" person because he or she is seen as more worthy. The legendary Greek poet Sappho wrote that to be beautiful is to be "good." The Polish-Australian cosmetics magnate Helena Rubenstein famously declared, "There are no ugly women, only lazy ones" suggesting that outward unattractiveness is a sign of moral failure (Stonehouse 2013).

With the rise of feminist thought, the somewhat narrow range of beauty options viewed within a backdrop of emerging beauty technologies caused scholars to wonder whether conformity to mass-mediated models of beauty rooted in patriarchal ideology outweighed the sense of individual self-image and self-confidence increasingly more accessible via beauty work options. One side viewed beauty work as a way of undermining women's tenuous economic power, squandering their resources on time-consuming and expensive products in a bid to heighten their appeal as objects within a male-dominated system that rewarded the "prettiest" girls with (potentially temporary) partnerships with males. The other side saw beauty work as an economic necessity and opportunity, allowing women to express their aesthetic urges and individuality in a system that oppressed them in other ways. Sixty years later, there is still no consensus on this fundamental split about the value of beauty for women (Bordo 1993; Kilbourne 1999; Pitts 2014). The fundamental question remains whether expectations of beauty and the creation of social norms of beauty represent more of a punishment or avenue to power for women, and perhaps men.

Those who criticize beauty work and social expectations of appearance for women frequently ignore evidence that beauty work is crucial for men as well. Signals of masculine attractiveness play a large role in establishing dominance hierarchies among men. In male-only situations, rank order develops quickly, frequently with the tallest, best-looking, or most athletic man at the top. In the military, as in business, studies have demonstrated how the man with the physical features that most conform to social norms of male beauty will climb to the highest rank or position (Etcoff 2000). Men then signal their power, wealth, and success to other men, as well as women, through their appearance, especially in their apparel, shoes, and accessories, like expensive watches or jewelry made of precious metals (Masi de Casanova 2015). The clothes may not "make the man," but a man signals that he has "made it" through his clothes.

Do Beauty Standards Force People to "Change"?

In an era of increasing globalization, many social theorists have suggested that the actual way people think about themselves is undergoing rapid change. Sociologist Anthony Giddens (1990) argued that modernity allows for the emergence of new expressions of the self in appearance and behavior, but that these new expressions are molded under conditions strongly influenced by the standardizing effects of commodity capitalism. The closer the appearance of the body comes to resembling the prevailing prototypes standardized by the culture, the higher the "exchange value" for the individual (Featherstone 1991, 177). That is to say that the prevailing way of thinking about the body as "a project" that requires attention, maintenance, and hard work to achieve a particular appearance creates new regimes of self-management and discipline that an individual must adhere to in order to be considered beautiful. Standards for bodies are predetermined according to prevailing models according to gender, class, and age (Miller 2006, 11).

Anthropologists are also interested in new and emerging subjectivities, especially among global youth, in an era of transnational visual imagery and rapid socioeconomic changes. Deeply contextualized studies like Brad Weiss's investigation of youth-oriented *kinyozi* (barbershops) in Tanzania (2009) or Bonnie Adrian's ethnography of emerging bridal practices in Taiwan (2003) demonstrates the complex cultural meanings and the emotional significance invested in culturally borrowed standards of attractiveness and beauty. Laura Miller's extraordinary study of new and emerging Japanese body aesthetics (2006) and Alexander Edmond's careful analysis of cosmetic surgery in Brazil (2010) are two other texts that offer close readings of how transnational beauty standards are reframing messages about personal identity, personal opportunity, and self-liberation. Often, these new modes of self-fashioning are at odds with "traditional" appearances and threaten to create intergenerational ruptures about national morality. New standards of beauty often challenge the old standards with expressly forbidden content, including independence, self-reliance, and alterative ideas about sexuality or marriage.

Hybrid versions of beauty may also appear to try to capitalize on the full range of menu options of beauty available to consumers. Many beauty practices, such as those practiced by body modification and tattoo devotees, may simultaneously incorporate "traditional" or "ancient" wisdom while also drawing on "cutting-edge technology." Sometimes these combinations of old and new beauty practices raise concerns about cultural appropriation as young people seek authenticity in their presentation of self. Examples of hybrid beauty styles include the widespread use of *mehendi* decorations and tattoos, as well as a refreshed interest in the so-called "lumbersexual" look, which incorporates enormous, well-groomed beards and is popular for young men in some urban areas.

Conclusion

The unwritten rules about relative attractiveness remain largely out of the control of individuals but exist as social norms. These standards of beauty have a direct impact on people's lives and the ways they respond to those norms. This volume provides a wide range of insights into beauty, beauty practices, and standards of beauty around the world. It is our hope that this context allows the reader to think critically about beauty and its many layers of meanings.

Further Reading

Adrian, Bonnie. 2003. *Framing the Bride: Globalizing Beauty and Romance in Taiwan's Bridal Industry.* Berkeley, CA: University of California Press.

Aylmer, Olivia. 2015. "The History of Pantsuits Shows Why We Care So Much about Female Politician's Style," *Quartz*, October 25. Accessed October 11, 2016. http://qz.com/525843/the-history-of-pantsuits-shows-why-we-care-so-much-about-female-politicians-style.

Baumann, Shyon. 2014. "The Moral Underpinnings of Beauty: A Meaning-Based Explanation of Light and Dark Complexions in Advertising." In: *The Politics of Women's Bodies: Sexuality, Appearance, and Behavior*, 4th ed., edited by Rose Weitz and Samantha Kwan, 258–76. New York: Oxford University Press.

Becker, Anne E. 1995. *Body, Self, and Society: The View from Fiji.* Philadelphia: University of Pennsylvania Press.

Berry, D. Channsin and Bill Duke. 2011. *Dark Girls.* Film. Directed by D. Channsin Berry and Bill Duke. Duke Media and Urban Winter Entertainment.

Beyoncé. 2013. "Pretty Hurts." Discrecording *Beyoncé* https://www.youtube.com/watch?v=LXXQLa-5n5w. Accessed January 29, 2017.

Bordo, Susan. 1993. *Unbearable Weight: Feminism, Western Culture, and the Body.* Berkeley, CA: University of California Press.

Dion, Karen, Ellen Berscheid, and Elaine Walster. 1972. "What Is Beautiful Is Good." *Journal of Personality and Social Psychology* 24, no. 3: 285–90.

Easley, Jonathan. 2016. "Ex-Miss Universe Becomes Surprise Sensation of Debate." *Hill*, September 28. Accessed October 11, 2016. http://thehill.com/blogs/ballot-box/presidential-races/298351-former-miss-universe-becomes-debate-surprise

Edmonds, Alexander. 2010. *Pretty Modern: Beauty, Sex, and Plastic Surgery in Brazil.* Durham, NC: Duke University Press.

Estepa, Jessica. 2015. "Donald Trump on Carly Fiorina: 'Look at that Face.'" Accessed October 11, 2016. http://www.usatoday.com/story/news/nation-now/2015/09/10/trump-fiorina-look-face/71992454/.

Etcoff, Nancy. 2000. *Survival of the Prettiest: The Science of Beauty.* New York: Anchor.

Featherstone, Mike. 1991. "The Body in Consumer Culture." In: *The Body, Social Process, and Cultural Theory*, edited by Mike Hepworth, Bryan S. Turner, and Mike Featherstone, 170–86. London: Sage.

Garber, Megan. 2016. "Why the Pantsuit?" Accessed October 11, 2016. http://www.theatlantic.com/entertainment/archive/2016/08/youre-fashionable-enough-hillary/493877/.

Giddens, Anthony. 1990. *The Consequences of Modernity*. Stanford, CA: Stanford University Press.

Gladstone, Eric and Kathleen O'Connor. 2013. "Sitting Pretty: Attractiveness, Social Capital, and Success." *Academy of Management Annual Meeting Proceedings* 2013, no. 1:17288. Accessed October 11, 2016. http://proceedings.aom.org/content/2013/1/17288.short/

Grogan, Sarah. 1999. *Body Image: Understanding Body Dissatisfaction in Men, Women, and Children*. New York: Routledge.

Herrera, Carolina. 2009. "Presentación." In: Titina Penzini *100% Chic: Como vestir bien Y tener un éxito seguro*." Caracas, Venezuela: Ediciones B.

Hopper, Nate. 2016. "Naked Donald Trump Statues Populate American Cities," *Time.Com*, p. 35, Accessed October 11, 2016. http://time.com/4458022/donald-trump-nude-statues/. MAS Ultra-School Edition, EBSCO*host*.

Karp, Ivan and Stephen D. Lavine. 1991. *Exhibiting Cultures*. Washington, D.C.: Smithsonian Press.

Kilbourne, Jean. 1999. *Deadly Persuasion: Why Women and Girls Must Fight the Addictive Power of Advertising*. New York: The Free Press.

Langlois, Judith H., Lisa Kalakanis, Adam J. Rubenstein, Andrea Larson, Monica Hallam, and Monica Smoot. 2000. "Maxims or Myths of Beauty? A Meta-Analytic and Theoretical Review." *Psychological Bulletin* 126, no. 3: 390–423.

Levine, Daniel. 2016. "Donald Trump's Hair: 5 Fast Facts You Need to Know." Accessed October 11, 2016. http://heavy.com/news/2016/05/donald-trump-hair-real-fake-natural -combover-hairpiece-wig-plugs/.

Levitt, Theodore. 1983. "The Globalization of Markets." Accessed January 29, 2017. Harvard Business Review. https://hbr.org/1983/05/the-globalization-of-markets.

Masi de Casanova, Erynn. 2015. *Buttoned Up: Clothing, Conformity and White-Collar Masculinity*. Ithaca, NY: Cornell University Press.

Miller, Laura. 2006. *Beauty Up: Exploring Contemporary Japanese Body Aesthetics*. Berkeley, CA: University of California Press.

Neumann, William. 2013. "Mannequins Give Shape to Venezuelan Fantasy." Accessed January 29, 2017. http://www.nytimes.com/2013/11/07/world/americas/mannequins-give -shape-to-venezuelan-fantasy.html. Pitts, Victoria. 2014. "Reclaiming the Female Body: Women Body Modifiers and Feminist Debates. In: *The Politics of Women's Bodies: Sexuality, Appearance, and Behavior*, 4th ed., edited by Rose Weitz and Samantha Kwan, 277–89. New York: Oxford University Press.

Schwab, Nikki. 2016. "Anti-Hillary Buttons Sold at Donald Trump rally Detail Her 'Fat Thighs' and 'Small Breasts' and Call Her a B****." Accessed October 11, 2016. http:// www.dailymail.co.uk/news/article-3571662/Anti-Hillary-buttons-Donald-Trump-rally -fat-thighs-small-breasts-call-b.html#ixzz4Mn5sVwW9.

Scruton, Roger. 2011. *Beauty: A Very Short Introduction*. Oxford, England: Oxford University Press.

Statista. 2016. "Revenue of the Cosmetic Industry in the United States from 2002 to 2016." Accessed October 11, 2016. http://www.statista.com/statistics/243742/revenue-of-the -cosmetic-industry-in-the-us.

Stewart, Dodai. 2013. "Meet the Women Who Tattoo Their Gums Black for a More Beautiful Smile," *Jezebel*, January 2. Accessed October 11, 2016. http://jezebel.com/5972634 /meet-the-women-who-tattoo-their-gums-black-for-a-more-beautiful-smile.

Stonehouse, Cheryl. 2013. "Helena Rubinstein, The Penniless Refugee Who Built a Cosmetics Empire." *Express.co.uk*, March 16. Accessed October 12, 2016. http://www.express .co.uk/life-style/style/384696/Helena-Rubinstein-the-penniless-refugee-who-built-a -cosmetics-empire.

Weiss, Brad. 2009. *Street Dreams and Hip Hop Barbershops: Global Fantasy in Urban Tanzania*. Bloomington, IN: Indiana University Press.

ACNE AND ACNE TREATMENTS

Smooth skin is a universally accepted beauty norm. Therefore, blemishes or pimples on the skin are also globally considered ugly and unappealing. Acne, the general term for these blemishes, is a source of concern and beauty work around the world. According to the American Academy of Dermatology (AAD), the general term "acne" refers to plugged pores, pimples, cysts, and nodules that can occur on the face, neck, chest, back, shoulders, upper arms, and/or upper legs (AAD 2016).

Acne is a skin condition common to all humans. Prevalent in adolescents and a continuing issue for adults as well, both men and women worldwide experience and seek to treat the pimples that appear on their skin. Caucasian skin is more likely than Asian or African skin to get acne, and acne is then more visible on pale skin (Etcoff 2000).

Eighty percent of all adolescents get pimples (Elsaie 2013). Adolescent boys are more likely to get acne than girls, and adult women are more likely to experience acne than adult men (Elsaie 2013). In general, females are much more likely to treat the blemishes with creams or concealers and are more likely to consult dermatologists (Etcoff 2000). Indeed, acne is the number-one reason why patients of both sexes consult skin doctors (Elsaie 2013).

Because of the emphasis placed on smooth skin as a worldwide indicator of beauty, the development of acne is potentially very damaging to a person's sense of self-esteem and self-worth. Any disease or condition of the skin is a psychological burden to a person, and acne has been shown to have significant mental repercussions for people who suffer from it. More than 30 percent of adolescents experience psychological problems associated with having acne, including embarrassment, social impairment, anxiety, frustration, anger, depression, and even suicidal thoughts (Elsaie 2013). Unfortunately, although acne causes anxiety, the anxiety itself can cause more acne, creating a vicious cycle.

Acne most commonly occurs on the face, but can appear on nearly any part of a person's skin. The condition is usually caused by the blockage of skin pores by dead skin cells, or the presence of bacteria known as *Propionibacterium acnes* (AAD 2016). Other causes of acne are smoking, premenstruation, stress, sleep deprivation, **cosmetics**, excessive sweating, and drugs such as steroids. Myths abound about the effect of different foods, such as chocolate or milk, on eruptions of acne, but no reliable link has been found between any specific food and skin blemishes (Hon and Leung 2010).

Dermatologists recognize several different forms of acne with different levels of severity. "Acne," or "*acne vulgaris*," is the general term used for the most common form of the condition (Hon and Leung 2010). Dermatologists also apply a graded scale when diagnosing acne, ranging from 1, for mild acne to 4, for severe acne. This more detailed level of categorization helps guide treatment (AAD 2016).

Because of the high importance cultures around the world place on smooth and healthy skin as a key indicator of beauty and worth, a wide range of treatments exist for acne problems in adolescents and adults. Mild acne may often be treated with over-the-counter products that don't require a prescription. Many of these products contain the chemicals benzoyl peroxide or salicylic acid (AAD 2016).

More severe acne is treated by dermatologists in a variety of ways. Topical products that are creams or ointments that can be applied directly to the skin are one option. These products usually contain a retinoid chemical, an antibiotic, or a stronger level of benzoyl peroxide or salicylic acid. Another option is a medicine or pill that a patient takes that works from the inside. Some examples of these are antibiotics, birth control pills, or a medicine called isotretinoin (AAD 2016).

There are also other treatments for acne that go beyond pharmaceutical products. Lasers can be used to reduce the amount of the *P. acnes* bacteria on the skin, for example. **Chemical peels**, a procedure where strong substances are applied to the skin to remove layers, are also an option if completed in the doctor's office. Finally, some dermatologists directly remove acne through a process called "drainage and extraction," especially for large pimples and cysts (AAD 2016).

See also: Bodybuilding; Chemical Peels and Fillers; Makeup and Cosmetics.

Further Reading

AAD. 2016. "Acne." Accessed August 2, 2016. https://www.aad.org/public/diseases/acne-and -rosacea/acne.

Elsaie, Mohamed L. 2013. *Acne: Etiology, Treatment Options and Social Effects*. New York: Nova Science Publishers, Inc.

Etcoff, Nancy. 2000. *Survival of the Prettiest: The Science of Beauty*. New York: Anchor.

Hon, K. L. E., and Alexander K. C. Leung. 2010. *Acne: Causes, Treatment, and Myths*. New York: Nova Science Publishers, Inc.

ADVERTISING

People are surrounded on a daily basis by billboards, bumper stickers, radio, television, mailings, e-mails, and sidebars on almost any Web site. Each of these is filled with messages from advertisers aimed at selling us something. The goal of advertising is to make people feel that they need a specific product, and then, that they want one particular brand over all other brands. Advertisements typically feature messages that are targeted at specific audiences and are designed to create or shape desires. These messages are tailored specifically to tap into the power of emotions and frequently play on the anxieties, fears, or concerns of their target audience. The advertiser consciously selects and transmits messages through attractive, healthy, happy, and secure-looking spokespeople, the kind of people who present an ideal image (Common Sense Media 2016).

The way these images are used can have a profound influence on establishing or reinforcing gender and sexual norms about beauty. Advertising messages are often

explicitly gendered to appeal specifically to either men or women
by playing upon vanity and a
shared desire to be considered
attractive.

Commercials became more
commonplace with rise of indus-

"Most women are dissatisfied with their appearance—it's the stuff that fuels the beauty and fashion industries."

—ANNIE LENNOX

trialism in the late 19th century, and one of the first audiences for direct advertising
was women, taking up the role as domestic consumers in a growing industrialized
economy. Technological advancements led to "ready-to-wear" clothes (replacing
custom-made garments), and advertising was key in establishing a market for
buyers. The clothing industry designed the first department stores to be inviting
to fashionable women, eager to make the "right" choices about their consumption.
Women's magazines also began to appear, with fashion spreads to create desires and
influence tastes about what might be considered beautiful (Mierau 2000).

The main goal of advertising is to sell more products, which are imagined to fit
within the social values of the time and the place. During World War II, American
women were recruited to work outside the home in factory jobs, but were still
encouraged to use the right products to keep their hands lovely and feminine by
using special creams and skin-care products. In the post-WWII era, women as the
primary homeowners became the main target of advertisers, who sought to promote "labor-saving devices" for women within the household, including electric
appliances, fancy cleaning products, and prepackaged foods (Mierau 2000). Advertisers also targeted women within the home. These campaigns stoked an increased
desire for products that promoted more allegedly healthful behaviors, including
germ-free products, personal hygiene products designed to be used in **bathing and
showering**, and an emphasis on "fitness."

Advertisements carefully cultivate the maintenance and preservation of traditional roles, while also creating new products that reflect the ambitions of industry
to push into new directions to increase sales volume. As the popular television program *Mad Men* demonstrated, advertising quickly became more technical and even
scientific in its approach to court the business of consumers, relying on the insights
of psychology. A study of the content of advertisements in popular magazines from
the 1950s to the 1980s portrayed women as the primary consumers of beauty
products. Advertisements also show a world that is not necessarily representative
of reality: images of women are frequently young, beautiful, and thin (Busby and
Leichty 2013). A wide variety of products became available to women to enhance,
improve, or change their appearance.

Critics have often pointed out that in their efforts to transmit images of individualistic consumers who are in dire need of a particular product to make them
feel healthier, more attractive, happier, or more secure, advertisers often resort to
tactics that reinscribe differences in **class** and race, including economic access to
these products (Common Sense Media 2016). The portrayal of expertise and authority in advertising is frequently male and white, though some advertising campaigns
have emphasized the rise in women's economic and social autonomy, including

the now-infamous Virginia Slims "You've Come a Long Way, Baby" campaign, which attempted to convince women to become smokers.

Jean Kilbourne is one of the most influential critics of advertising's effects on women. Her 1979 film, *Killing Us Softly: Advertising's Image of Women*, is widely used around the world. In the film, she deconstructs print advertisements to illustrate the ways in which women's and men's bodies are dismembered, packaged, and "used to sell everything from chain saws to chewing gum" (Kilbourne 1999, 27). She argues that most viewers, especially women, internalize the powerful message that their bodies are objects that must be appealing in order to be valued. With increasing technological and photographic techniques to "perfect" the illusion of idealized beauty, the standard to maintain a beautiful self is both punishingly high and ultimately unattainable, affecting the self-esteem of young women and contributing to other social factors that increase rates of eating disorders, self-loathing, and potential suicides among youth. Kilbourne says, "Advertising encourages us not only to objectify each other but also to feel that our most significant relationships are with the products that we buy" (Kilbourne 1999: 26–77).

Elena Rossi's 2015 documentary *The Illusionists* examined the spread of Western media messages to other parts of the world. One commentator in the film states, "The selling of Westernized images has become the badge of modernity . . . The notion of how you join globalized culture is the taking of a Western body" (Rossini 2015). Many young people attempt to capitalize on access to the external power of "globalization" by appropriating Western standards of beauty.

See also: Bathing and Showering; Class.

Further Reading

Busby, Linda J. and Greg Leichty. 2013. "Feminism and Advertising in Traditional and Nontraditional Women's Magazines 1950s–1980s." *Journalism Quarterly* 70: 247–64.

Common Sense Media. "What Is the Impact of Advertising on Teens?" Accessed October 12, 2016. https://www.commonsensemedia.org/marketing-to-kids/what-is-the-impact-of-advertising-on-teens.

Kilbourne, Jean. 1979. *Killing Us Softly: Advertising's Image of Women*. DVD. Directed by Margaret Lazarus and Renner Wunderlich. Boston: Media Education Foundation.

Kilbourne, Jean. 1999. *Deadly Persuasion: Why Women and Girls Must Fight the Addictive Power of Advertising*. New York: The Free Press.

Mierau, Christina. 2000. *Accept No Substitutes*. New York: Lerner: 66.

Rossini, Elena. 2015. *The Illusionists: A Film about the Globalization of Beauty*. DVD. Directed by Elena Rossini. Boston: Media Education Foundation, 2015.

AIRBRUSHING

Airbrushing refers to the technique of "retouching" photos that can add or remove objects or people, erase blemishes, or alter the shape or size of a body. In the early days of photography, a wide variety of retouching, or airbrushing, techniques were especially useful for consumers who paid professional studios to create flattering images.

In the 19th century, hand brushing with ink or paint was the most common technique for altering photographs to create higher-quality images. This process often left visible brush strokes within the photographs. In the 1890s, "airbrushes" were invented, which allowed for smoother edits to remove photos with moles, scars, or other imperfections. At the turn of the 20th century, people also liked to add a color wash to photos taken in studios. The colorized photographs were so popular that processing factories expanded to offer more extensive alterations of photographs. Continued improvements in photographic technology, including the invention of the Kodak Brownie, reduced the need for professional airbrushing, although many photographs could still be retouched. Today, digital photography allows images to be manipulated more easily with computers through programs like Photoshop (Xue 2015).

Retouching photographs within **advertising** campaigns often has the distinct goal of improving the look of the spokesmodel in order to improve her or his appearance to perfection. In the last decade, a number of critics have charged that such manipulation of images is misleading and manipulative. They argue that in promoting distortions of beauty or beauty products, they create unrealistic and even damaging expectations on the part of the potential customer (McDermott 2015).

Dove's "Real Beauty" campaign produced a commercial video demonstrating the degree to which a model's appearance was altered following the photo shoot. Many recognize that some women may be suffering from poor self-esteem because of the degree to which airbrushing techniques portray a kind of "unattainable perfection" that may never be achieved in reality. To address the reported dissatisfaction "real" women felt about

> "Beauty is the greatest seducer of man."
> —PAULO COEHLO

altered images of beauty, Dove worked with computer programmers to create a digital application. The app, called "Beautify Action," was made available to art directors, graphic designers, and photo retouchers to "undo" airbrushing and Photoshopping (Wasserman 2013). Several celebrities have announced that they will no longer allow their images to be airbrushed, a stipulation included by Kate Winslet in her 2015 contract with Lancôme's parent company, L'Oreal (McDermott 2015).

Airbrushing also refers to a makeup technique designed to even out skin tone or to enhance the effect of **cosmetics**. The airbrush is used in lieu of sponges, brushes, or manual application of the makeup directly to the skin. Airbrushing equipment is available commercially and favored for rapid, even distribution of sunless tanning products over a large area of the skin. Additionally, makeup artists who work in theatrical venues make use of airbrushing for some dramatic effects, especially in productions that require nonhuman or extra-human appearances, such as science fiction "alien" characters, or with the use of prosthetic makeup (Xue 2015).

Airbrushing lends itself well to the technique known as "contouring" (also called "shading," which uses two different hues of strategically applied and thoroughly blended face makeup to highlight the bone structure, making the nose appear smaller, cheekbones sharper, the jaw more angular, the forehead smaller, and the eyes bigger) and its spin-offs: tontouring (a contouring technique that substitutes self-tanner for a wider palette of cosmetics) and strobing (a technique of adding cosmetic "highlights" to points on the face that should catch light, including the tops of the cheekbone, the inner brow bone just above the brow, the outer brow bone below the tapered end of the brow, the inner corners of the eye, the bridge of the nose, the cupid's bow above the top of the lip, and the apple of the chin) (Xue 2015). Finally, with the advent of high-definition video in film and television, more and more makeup artists are trading in their conventional sponges and brushes for the airbrushing technique, which can deliver a quicker, "flawless" skin tone to an actor's appearance.

See also: Advertising; Dove Campaign for Real Beauty; Makeup and Cosmetics.

Further Reading

McDermott, Maeve. 2015. "Kate Winslet Won't Let Her Ads Be Airbrushed." *USA Today*. October 22. Accessed May 16, 2016. http://www.usatoday.com/story/life/entertainthis/2015/10/22/kate-winslet-wont-allow-airbrushing-her-beauty-ads/74378740.

Wasserman, Todd. 2013. "Dove's 'Beautify' Photoshop Action Un-Airbrushes Images of Models." Mashable. March 6. Accessed May 16, 2016. http://mashable.com/2013/03/06/dove-photoshop- action/#Y_WV03O_KOqb.

Xue, Faith. 2015. "From 1500 to 2015: The Fascinating History of Contouring. Byrdie. November 13. Accessed July 14 2016. http://www.byrdie.com/history-of-contouring.

APATANI TRIBE, INDIA

The Apatani, also called the Tani, are one among twenty-six tribal groups in northeastern **India**'s Arunachal Pradesh. The region borders China, Bhutan, and Myanmar. The tribal groups in this region share a Tibeto-Mongoloid language and comprise an ethnic minority in contemporary India. Numbering about 60,000, the Apatani practice wet rice cultivation in elaborately designed paddies that make sustainable use of local ecological richness to irrigate and produce impressive yields. Though the heavy labor is done without farm animals or machines, the rice paddies also stock fish, which improves the nutritional options of the group.

Today, Buddhism is the predominant religion in the region, but the Apatani also practice a unique blended (or syncretic) faith called Donyi-Poloism (also Danyi-Piilo), which emphasizes indigenous beliefs based in nature and highlights the unique identity and worldview of this isolated group. The Apatani believe that a divine being called Sedi is the originator of the universe. They believe that all things are a part of Sedi: the bones of this creator became the mountains and rocks of the world, his tears became the rain and the water, and his hair provides the plants humans need to survive. Sedi's two eyes are the sun (Donyi) and the moon (Polo). These two principles of sun and moon are marked in Apatani cosmology as being distinctive of male and female aspects of existence. The ethical system of this creation ideology insists that these eyes in the sky focus light and enable humans to become aware of goodness, which can be measured by beauty, purity, and simplicity. It is the responsibility of individuals to promote aesthetic beauty and goodness in their appearance and their dress.

Historically, women of the group distinguished themselves from other tribes through long, straight facial **tattoos** along the bridge of the nose and

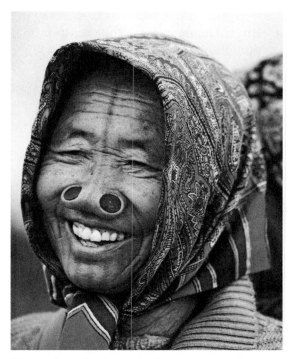

Woman from the Apatani tribe, with nose plugs and facial tattoo. The Apatani are a tribal group of people living in the Ziro valley in Arunachal Pradesh, India. For young women, the practice has largely disappeared. (David Evison/Dreamstime.com)

the distinctive-looking *yapinghule* (sometimes called *yapping hullo,* or *y'apiñ hullo*), nose plugs inserted into the flesh of the outer nose on both sides. The effect serves to emphasize large holes in the sides of the nose which reveal the plug. These nose plugs are made by burning bamboo or cane and then rubbing it against a hard surface until it is flattened and smooth. The process of wearing the plugs begins during girlhood, and the size of the plug is increased incrementally as the skin of the outer nose stretches to accommodate the plug (Wyke 2015).

While no one is really certain how the practice of nose plugs for women started, the commonly accepted story is that villages throughout Arunachal Pradesh used to practice extensive raiding among neighboring tribes. Some speculate that the striking traditional nose plugs were designed to protect the young women of the tribe by making them appear less attractive to raiders, especially the Nishi, who lived in the highlands above the Apatani villages (Wyke 2015). Though the area is very peaceful today under nationalist pressures, it remains remote, and the history of regional conflict reportedly prompted this extreme measure for women's appearance (Chaudhuri 2013).

Apatani women also wear prominent facial **tattoos** and practice perforation of the upper earlobes for wearing *rutting yarang,* flat brass rings of about three to four inches in diameter that are fitted through the hole in the ear. The facial tattoos bisect the face laterally, with a long dark line running from the middle of the brow to the tip of the nose. Chins are also tattooed in a series of five vertical stripes that stretch from the bottom of the lip to the underside of the chin. Women typically wear their long **hair** gathered in a bun at the top of the head. Brass rods are sometimes used to enhance the hairstyle.

Apatani men also wear large brass earrings and dark facial tattoos in the shape of a "T" on their chins. Men, especially young men, also grow their hair long and wear it in a prominent knot at the center of their forehead, called a *pwdiñ*. The gathered hair is held in place with a brass rod.

The practice of wearing nose plugs in the traditional way is fading out today as part of lifestyle changes influenced by globalization. *Yapinghule* are no longer worn by young women, and according to most reports, this custom has been falling out of favor with young people since the early 1970s as an increasing tourist trade to the region brings outside influences to the culture (Wyke 2015).

See also: Body Modification; Hair; India; Jewelry; Tattoos.

Further Reading

Chaudhuri, Sarit Kumar. 2013. "The Institutionalization of Tribal Religion: Recasting the Donyo-Polo Movement in Arunachal Pradesh." *Asian Ethnology* 72, no. 2: 259–77.

Sarma, Rashmirekha. 2012. "Intangible Cultural Heritage of Arunchal Pradesh." *Antrocom Online Journal of Anthropology* 8, no. 2: 512.

von Fürer-Haimendorf, Christopher. 1962. *The Apa Tanis and Their Neighbors*. New York, The Free Press.

Wyke, Tom. 2015. "The Worst Place in the World to Catch a Cold: The Indian Tribe Where the Woman Must Have 'Nose Plugs' Fitted as Rite of Passage." July 16. Accessed October 12, 2016. http://www.dailymail.co.uk/news/article-3164012/The-worst-place-world-catch-cold-Indian-tribe-woman-nose-plugs-fitted-mark-adults.html#ixzz4MsrEkWJW.

ARGENTINA

Standards of beauty and appearance in many Latin American nations are the product of a diverse mix of cultural and historical influences. Some countries across the region, such as Mexico, have large populations of indigenous peoples, who held their own ideals of beauty and developed their own beauty practices long before the arrival of European colonizers. Other nations in Latin America, such as Brazil, experienced an influx of African ideals of beauty through the importation of slaves and the continuing presence of people of African descent. In the case of Argentina, however, where the small indigenous population was mostly wiped out by European colonizers, and the agricultural needs of the nation did not include the manual labor required by slaves, norms of beauty and appearance are still tied to European ideals of appearance and hard work.

Latin American nations such as Argentina gained their independence from Spanish and Portuguese colonial control in the 1800s and then began the hard process of building a national identity for themselves in their new republics. For most Latin American intellectuals, that meant finding a way to both claim the new territory through continued colonization, the founding of new farms and ranches, and the production of more citizens to take control of the area (Sommer 1991). For European-descended men setting public policies on issues such as immigration and marital law, the clear preference was to promote the reproduction of more—and whiter—citizens (Stepan 1991).

Following the ideology of eugenics (the concept of the racial superiority of some races over others), the Argentine government sought to improve the overall health, intelligence, and moral worth of the citizens of their nation through a program of selective breeding and sterilization, based on the idea that white DNA was more valuable to create strong, healthy, intelligent, and hard-working people to populate the new nation (Rodriguez 2011).

What this has meant for beauty norms in Argentina over the several hundred years since independence is a continuing preference for Euro-descended elements of appearance: wavy blond **hair**; light skin and **eyes**; and a tall, slim form. Beyond those basic elements, however, Argentina continues to promote and reward a style of beauty that communicates hard work and personal discipline along with a strong sense of maternal care and concern. Beauty in Argentina is often understood as a beautifully made-up and hard-working mother figure who represents the ideals of virtue and self-control (Nichols 2014).

In the early 20th century, Argentina rewarded women for their beauty in terms of their work ethic. From the 1930s to the 1970s, Argentina's main system of **beauty pageants** crowned the "prettiest little worker" in each region, from vineyard workers to women working in factories. The winners were selected to represent "the perfect combination of worker and beautiful woman . . . a female worker who was first and foremost a mother" (Lobato 2005, 83). These local and regional avatars of hard work, motherhood, and beauty then went to Buenos Aires, where the "Queen of Work" was crowned in a national pageant on May 1 (International Worker's Day) (Lobato 2005).

Initially, First Lady Eva Perón was charged with the honor of selecting Argentina's Queen of Work and Beauty. Perón (commonly known as "Evita") herself was the embodiment of those values: an image of beauty, virtue, and self-sacrifice in Argentina, honored in film, novels, and a myriad of displays of public art. Argentina's later female president, Cristina Fernandez de Kirchner, representing ultra-feminine beauty and power, often gave speeches in front of an image of Evita and commissioned a string of public monuments to the former first lady (Bellotta 2012).

Both Evita and Cristina are famous for their work ethic; their status as "mothers" of the nation; and their careful attention to fashion, style, **cosmetics**, and hair care. Evita is perhaps most famous for her controlled blond hair, swept back in a chignon, her preference for French clothing designers, and her extensive collection of **jewelry**. In her public image, Evita was a fairy princess and avatar of European style. What's more, Evita was a poor, illegitimate girl who, through hard work (as an actress and radio personality) and a good marriage, rose to fame and fortune. In this way, she was not only the fairy godmother, but Cinderella to many Argentinians.

Fernandez de Kirchner, first lady of Argentina from 2003–2007 and president of the republic from 2007–2016, is also both a symbol of beauty and hard work. Known popularly in Argentina as "Cristina," the president is known and admired for both her work to increase the standard of living for the poorest Argentines and her personal style, which combines careful and liberal application of makeup, elaborate **manicures**, and voluminous and catwalk-ready hairstyles. Cristina is famous for her passion for clothes and beauty work as political tools and asserts the perfect image of "a woman politician with every right to assume her femininity and combativeness" (Donot 2013).

See also: Class; Hair; Makeup and Cosmetics; Manicures; Mexico; Pageants—International, National, and Local Contests.

Further Reading

Bellotta, Araceli. 2012. *Eva y Cristina: La razón de sus vidas*. Vergara: Buenos Aires.

Donot, Morgan. 2013 "Cristina Fernández de Kirchner, de 'una reina' a la encarnación del pueblo de la Argentina." *Ensemble: Revista electrónica de la Casa Argentina en Paris*. 5, no. 6. Accessed February 4, 2013. http://ensemble.educ.ar/.

Lobato, Mirta Zaida, ed. 2005. *Cuando las mujeres reinaban: Belleza, virtud y poder en la Argentina del siglo xx*. Buenos Aires: Biblos.

Nichols, Elizabeth Gackstetter. 2014. "Ultra-Feminine Women of Power: Beauty and the State in Argentina" In: *Women in Politics and Media: Perspectives from Nations in Transition,* edited by Maria Raicheva-Stover and Elza Ibroscheva. London: Bloomsbury.

Rodriguez, Julia. 2011. "A Complex Fabric: Intersecting Histories of Race, Gender, and Science in Latin America." *Hispanic American Historical Review* 91, no. 3: 409–19.

Sommer, Doris. 1991. *Foundational Fictions: The National Romances of Latin America*. Berkeley, CA: University of California Press.

Stepan, Nancy Leys. 1991. *The Hour of Eugenics: Race, Gender and Nation in Latin America*. Ithaca, NY: Cornell University Press.

BALDNESS

Because **hair** is such a socially significant indicator of health and beauty, its converse, baldness, is most commonly understood around the globe as ugly—a sign of infirmity, old age, or disease. While hair loss and baldness happen for a variety of reasons, from genetic predisposition to illness, baldness, and the beauty work and treatments associated with hair loss, are most often associated with men.

Women may suffer from hair loss due to cancer treatments or less common conditions such as alopecia. Men, however, are widely predisposed genetically to lose their hair. Indeed, more than half of all men lose some hair by the age of 50. By the age of 70, that number jumps to 80 percent. Baldness in men is most commonly associated with a genetic condition called androgenic alopecia, commonly referred to as male pattern baldness (Foster and Malia 2016).

Baldness has been undesirable since at least BCE 4000, when cures for baldness included rubbing the head vigorously with dog paws, dates, or asses' hooves (Etcoff 2000). The Christian Bible tells of men applying bear grease to their heads when humiliated by others for their lack of hair, and in the 1700s, scholars thought baldness was a sign of thinking too hard (Silver 2013). Although in the 21st century, we do not associate baldness with intellectual or moral failure, modern science does give some credence to the idea that baldness is a sign of weaker health. One study found that balding at the top of the head in men was significantly associated with a higher risk of heart attacks (Etcoff 2000).

In the 20th and 21st centuries, baldness has continued to be seen as less attractive, leading to a wide-ranging and ever-evolving list of treatments for baldness, mostly aimed at men. Toupees, or small wigs to cover bald spots, were introduced and popularized in the 1940s, and hair plugs, or grafts of hair from one hairy area of a man's body to his bald scalp, were invented in the 1950s (Silver 2013). In the 1980s, a drug originally designed to treat high blood pressure, minoxidil, was found to regrow hair and has been widely used for that purpose, often under the brand name Rogaine (Etcoff 2000). A host of other, less medically grounded treatments have come and gone over the years. A few notable types of beauty work and products designed to combat baldness in the late 20th century included skull tattooing and "hair in a can"—a spray-on **cosmetic** that allowed men to color their scalps the same color as their remaining hair.

By 2016, a wide array of treatments and products were in development, from stem cell implantation to new types of hair transplants with microbots (miniature robots) (Foster and Malia 2016). The International Society of Aesthetic and **Plastic Surgery** recommends either the grafting of hair follicles from the back of a man's head to the balding areas or "strip grafts" in which a whole strip of the patient's own skin, including the hair follicles, is grafted on to the balding area (ISAPS 2016b). In 2014, more than 100,000 patients worldwide underwent hair restoration surgery, with the highest number of recipients in Brazil, South Korea, and the United States. Of these hair restoration patients, 20 percent were women and 80 percent were men (ISAPS 2016a). All of this activity points to and emphasizes the widespread desire among men to keep or restore their hair after suffering hair loss.

Finally, although many products and treatments exist and are being continually developed to minimize balding, some men choose to address the issue through hair-styling. One common way some men seek to hide a bald scalp is through the "comb-over," a technique in which the remaining hair is grown long enough to style over the bald area, hiding the hair loss.

While thick, full hair is traditionally associated with attractiveness in both women and men, style and fashion can also turn the tables and create a trend in head shaving, especially for men. Athletes like Michael Jordan or actors such as Vin Diesel and Dwayne Johnson choose baldness as a symbol of strength and success (Etcoff 2000).

See also: Hair; Hair Extensions and Weaves; Plastic Surgery.

Further Reading

Etcoff, Nancy. 2000. *Survival of the Prettiest: The Science of Beauty*. New York: Anchor.
Foster, Dan and Michelle Malia. 2016. "The Cure for Baldness (Yes, It's Finally on Its Way)." *Men's Health* 31, no. 2: 65.
ISAPS. (2016a). "Global Statistics." Accessed July 11, 2016. http://www.isaps.org/Media /Default/global-statistics/2015%20ISAPS%20Results.pdf.
ISAPS. (2016b). "Hair Restoration." Accessed July 11, 2016. http://www.isaps.org/procedures /hair-restoration.
Silver, Marc. 2013. "New Baldness Cure Joins History of Hair-Loss Fixes." *National Geographic*. Accessed July 1, 2016. http://news.nationalgeographic.com/news/2013/10/131022-bald -cure-hair-toupee.

BARBERSHOP

In ancient times, the barbershop was a one-stop shop for men's grooming, styling, and wellness needs. Removal of **facial hair** is a resource-intensive activity. Whereas the very wealthy could afford to retain a personal barber, trained barbers with the necessary tools of the trade (including small knives in a variety of shapes, razors, a comb, mirror, and cloth to wrap around the customer's face) made a good living providing hair removal services to the general public in the ancient cities of Mesopotamia, Greece, and Egypt.

Early shaving blades were made from copper, gold, and sharpened obsidian glass. Shaving was time consuming, requiring water and a hot towel to soften the stubble and a razor that required constant sharpening. Barbers also trimmed nails, provided delousing services, and extracted teeth. Hair removal improved hygiene and was typically done outside. Roman barbers, called *tonsors*, worked in the public baths or established open-air barbershops, called *tonstrina*. Bronze Age shaving kits were part of the military equipment distributed to Roman centurions for times when they were not able to find the services of a professional (Comitatus 2015).

In medieval Europe, "barber surgeons" were called upon to provide grooming services with their expensive and sharp razor blades. Monks of the age were required to maintain a distinctive hairstyle called a *tonsure*, which included **baldness** at the top of the head for sanitary reasons. Because of their unique tools and setup, barber surgeons also addressed illness through bloodletting, usually with the use of leeches. The sharp straight razors of barber surgeons also allowed them to perform amputations when necessary. The traditional red-and-white pole associated with barbershops is believed to represent the bandages and blood common to the profession.

During the 19th century, Victorian barbershops were significant spaces for men in Europe and the United States to enjoy a shave from a professional wielding a double-edged razor and the rich lather of shaving soap. The fictional murdering barber known as Sweeney Todd, probably an urban myth that was popularized in the penny dreadful novels of the Victorian age, provides a grisly cautionary tale about the very real danger of shaving with a straight razor. Barbers were typically well-trusted members of the community, and barbershops often served ale or other refreshments for men who gathered there. The aptly named "barbershop quartet," an *a capella* singing ensemble typically made up of four men, emerged during this time, but really became popular during the neo-Victorian movement of the 1920s which saw the rise of vaudeville in both amateur and commercial venues and encouraged the presence of male fraternal organizations and nondomestic social spaces (Amateur-Casual 2015).

In 1901, an American traveling salesman named King C. Gillette improved the so-called "safety razor." Gillette's design allowed consumers to invest in a relatively high-priced handle and then to buy replaceable, disposable razor blades, which were designed to be used only a few times. This revolution in **hair removal** technology allowed consumers to purchase razors and to take care of their grooming at home much more safely and efficiently than the previously available blades that required sharpening and extreme care. The invention also contributed to the decline of the **masculine** social spaces of the barbershop. In the 1960s, Gillette introduced stainless steel blades that lasted longer and resisted rust, and rival Bic introduced the first totally disposable razor.

Like **salons**, barbershops are community hubs of same-sex interaction. Today, ethnographic research on barbershops in contemporary urban communities in the United States demonstrates that barbershops are not merely places for people to come for hair care services; they also act as important discursive spaces for black community members to come together to participate in day-to-day activities, to talk frankly about pressing issues, and to exchange information that helps the community maintain its distinctive identity and strength (Alexander 2003).

The popular *Barbershop* series of films starring Ice Cube, studio releases from 2002 featuring all-black casts and directed by young African American filmmakers, continue into the "post-soul" era of the 21st century, highlighting spaces for the urban poor to grapple with the political and economic transformations of the

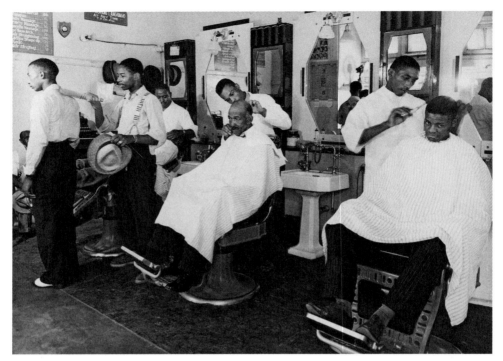

A barbershop in Washington, D.C., 1942. Today, barbershops are still hubs of same-sex inter-action, especially in African American communities. (Corbis via Getty Images)

age and the significant challenges posed to young men of color who are expected to achieve and consume within a culture that provides them with little opportu-nity to reach their goals (Mukherjee 2006).

Young men in urban Tanzania also spend a great deal of time interacting with other members of the community at or around barbershops, called *kinyozi*. The local barbershop advertises the latest in fashion and lifestyles imported from around the world, often within a male-only setting where music is played and underemployed young men are encouraged to socialize. The haircuts available at these barbershops are often elaborately shaved designs, which require a good deal of maintenance. These young men often take looking stylish very seriously. Because they may also find themselves marginalized, many find temporary solace in the company of other men who are also grappling with potential blows to their masculinity within an indifferent global economy (Weiss 2009).

See also: Facial Hair; Hair Removal; Masculinity; Salons.

Further Reading

Alexander, Bryant Keith. 2003. "Fading, Twisting, and Weaving: An Interpretive Ethnogra-phy of the Black Barbershop as Cultural Space." *Qualitative Inquiry* 9, no. 1: 105–28.

Amateur-Casual. 2015. "How Did Victorian Gentlemen Shave in the 19th Century?" Accessed November 24, 2015. http://sharpologist.com/2011/11/how-did-gentlemen-shave-in-the-nineteenth-century.html.

Comitatus. 2015. "Roman Shaving." Accessed November 24, 2015. http://www.comitatus
.net/romanshaving.html.

Mukherjee, Roopali. 2006. "The Ghetto Fabulous Aesthetic in Contemporary Black Culture: Class and Consumption in the Barbershop Films." *Cultural Studies* 20: 599–629.

Picker, Randy. 2010. "Gillette's Strange History with the Razor and Blade Strategy," September 23. Accessed November 24, 2015. *Harvard Business Review.* https://hbr.org/2010/09
/gillettes-strange-history-with

Weiss, Brad. 2009. *Street Dreams and Hip Hop Barbershops: Global Fantasy in Urban Tanzania.*
Bloomington, IN: Indiana University Press.

BARBIE

Cleverly reconciling contradictory desires and moral concerns about women's sexuality, Barbie was launched during the Cold War era when American-made commodities and the model suburban home were turned into key symbols and
safeguards of democracy and freedom. Originally designed as a novelty toy named
"Lili" for U.S. soldiers during World War II, Barbie was presented as a good girl
who was sexy, but didn't have sex.

The iconic doll was first introduced in 1959 and has sold more than any other
toy in history once the Mattel Corporation started marketing her to children. Barbie dolls were originally crafted from a durable plastic mold created by the same military weap-
ons design team that developed
"Hawk and Sparrow" missiles for
the Raytheon Company. Mattel
estimates that over 95 percent of
females in the United States have owned at least one Barbie between the ages of
three and eleven (Urla and Swedlund 1995, 278).

> "Beauty is the bait which with delight allures man to enlarge his kind."
> —SOCRATES

Barbie was presented to the public as a "teenage" fashion doll, and her rise in
popularity was likely linked to the mid-century creation of a distinctive teenage
lifestyle. Marketed with a wide range of frilly and fashionable clothing, accessories,
and housing items, Barbie dolls were designed to help create the ultimate linkage between late capitalist femininity, which pairs endless consumption, with the
achievement of an "appropriately gendered" body (Urla and Swedlund 1995).
"Little girls learn, among other things, about the crucial importance of their appearance to their personal happiness and to the ability to gain favor with their friends"
(Urla and Swedlund 1995, 281). In short, Barbie exemplifies the way in which
gender and "being feminine" in the late 20th century became a commodity that could
be negotiated and bought in order to conform with cultural standards of beauty.

Over time, Barbie's somewhat "cool" facial features, with arched brows and
pursed red lips, gave way to a more youthful, straight-haired teenage look, with an
exaggerated, wide-eyed smile (Urla and Swedlund 1995). However, Barbie's body
dimensions remained the same, with distinctly impossible physical proportions.
In scaling Barbie to life-size proportions, if she were to be 5'10" (the height of a
fashion model), she would have a 35-inch chest, with a 20-inch waist and a hip
circumference of 32.5 inches, making her clinically anorectic (Urla and Swedlund 1995).

In 1991, Mattel introduced a new line of "ethnically correct" fashion dolls with slightly more generous proportions, named Shani, Asha, and Nichelle. These dolls came available in light, medium, and dark skin tones and had newly sculpted facial features "based on real African American faces" and also reportedly had changes to their bodies to be more in keeping with a more diverse population (Chin 1999). International versions of the doll soon followed, though the "excessive slenderness" of her proportions remained consistent (Garber 2016).

Frequently cited as a standard of ideal female beauty, especially American beauty, in recent years, some parents have expressed reluctance to allow their children to play with the three-dimensional fashion doll, as her dramatic **hourglass** body type may cause their daughters (and sons) to internalize unrealistic expectations about beauty and promote feelings of dissatisfaction, depression, or self-loathing, potentially leading to **body dysmorphia** or **eating disorders**.

As the women's movement gained strength in the 1970s, there was a growing self-consciousness about the sexist imagery of women (Urla and Swedlund 1995). As a fashion model, Barbie continually created a new identity rooted in cultural fantasy with every outfit, but despite efforts to diversify "Bride Barbie" into "Animal Rights Activist Barbie," parents were not sold on the supposed social conscience and expansion of gender roles that Mattel tried to offer in the doll.

Parents were wary with some reason. Psychological researchers place importance on the interactive relationship between children and their playthings, noting that children learn what is important and what is expected of them through the toys they are presented with (Chin 1999, 306). Analyses of the Barbie phenomenon suggest that the doll does not look like a real woman, but rather like someone who has undergone extensive plastic surgery, creating unrealistic expectations about women's bodies for those who come in contact with the toy.

In her study of Barbie dolls around the world, M. G. Lord cites Simone de Beauvoir in *The Second Sex* to note that even before the invention Barbie, a "doll" can refer to a female adult, and "to doll up" means to dress up in fussy, feminine clothes. De Beauvoir felt that this is more than a linguistic coincidence, but underscores the ways that men objectify women and women, in turn, learn to objectify themselves.

Recent research indicates that girl children are not the only ones susceptible to strong feelings associated with self-image and toys: a study by Pope et al. (1999) found that over a thirty-year period, boys' action toys transformed to display more muscular forms than their predecessors, with many boys' toys displaying levels of **progressive muscularity** far exceeding the outer limits of what humans can actually achieve. Given that the boys' action toy market accounted for $949 million in 1994 alone, these transformations in male body expectation reach a large number of impressionable children.

Regardless, many women (and men) have personal interactions with a Barbie doll dating back to childhood that have irrevocably shaped their thinking about gendered identity. Adults' recollections of their own childhoods are not the equivalent of children's interactions with the toy, but many writers and theorists have highlighted the ways that the Barbie toy was instrumental for individuals to bend, twist, or flip the apparently natural or accepted **social construction** of gender during childhood to create alternative narratives about the possibilities of appearance and gendered identity (Rand 1995). This "queer" play creates a fundamental tension between the commodity packaged by Mattel and the consumers who put their own meanings into representations of Barbie in ways that often transgress the carefully managed profile of the corporate doll.

At forty, Barbie got a makeover. In 1997, a new version of the doll was introduced to the public, revamped in order to achieve more realistic proportions, including a wider waist, slimmer hips, and a reduction of her bustline.

See also: Blondes and Blonde Hair; Body Dysmorphic Disorder; Breasts; Eating Disorders; Hourglass Shape; Progressive Muscularity; Social Construction of Beauty.

Further Reading

Caldwell, Christina. 2016. "Check Out Barbie's Brand New Body (Or Should We Say 'Bodies'?)" *Twenty-two Words*. Accessed October 12, 2016. http://twentytwowords.com/check-out-barbies-brand-new-body-or-should-we-say-bodies.

Chin, Elizabeth. 1999. "Ethnically Correct Dolls: Toying with the Race Industry." *American Anthropologist* 101, no. 2: 305–21.

Garber, Megan. 2016. "Barbie's Hips Don't Lie." *The Atlantic*. January 28. Accessed October 13, 2016. http://www.theatlantic.com/entertainment/archive/2016/01/barbies-hips-dont-lie/432741.

Lord, M. G. 1994. *Forever Barbie: The Unauthorized Biography of a Real Doll*. New York: William Morrow and Company.

Pope, Harrison G., Roberto Olivardia, Amanda Gruber and John Borowiecki. 1999. "Evolving Ideals of Male Body Image as Seen Through Action Toys." *International Journal of Eating Disorders* 26, no. 1:65–72.

Rand, Erica. 1995. *Barbie's Queer Accessories*. Durham, NC: Duke University Press.

Urla, Jacqueline and Alan C. Swedlund. 1995. "The Anthropometry of Barbie: Unsettling Ideals of Feminine Beauty in Popular Culture." In: *Deviant Bodies: Critical Perspectives on Difference in Science and Popular Culture,* edited by Jennifer Terry and Jacqueline Urla. Bloomington, IN: Indiana University Press, 277–313.

BATHING AND SHOWERING

Throughout much of the world, the notion of proper hygiene and cleanliness is paramount for being beautiful. Bathing is not only considered part of a beauty regimen, but may also be associated with purification or cleansing the body in order to prepare for rituals or ceremonies.

Washing and bathing can take place in lakes, rivers, and streams and is especially important in the Indian and Hebrew cultural traditions. Into the 21st century, across India, there are many *ghats*, which are steps leading down to a river, especially a holy river, where people can bathe, perform ritual ablutions (washing), or even do laundry.

In the Hebrew tradition, ritual immersion, or *mikveh*, signifies ritual purity and the ability to wash away things that are considered unclean. Those who convert to Judaism must undergo a *mikveh* in "living water," or a pool of natural water that flows freely sometimes connected to springs or underground wells. Women are also required to immerse in a bath after menstrual periods or childbirth in order to resume sexual relations with their partners. Additionally, ritual purity is required to enter the temple.

In the ancient world of Mesopotamia, Anatolia, **India**, **Egypt**, Rome, and **Greece**, bathing was a communal activity that often took place in specially built indoor public baths. Archaeologists have excavated a 4,000-year old public bath at Mohenjo-Daro, in present-day Pakistan. Egyptian baths date back 3,000 years. In India, people developed steam rooms to combine bathing and massage.

Throughout the Far East, bathing traditions have endured since ancient times. Bathing practices continue to be used to cultivate beauty, to cleanse the body, and to enhance relaxation. In **China**, indoor bathrooms date to the T'ang Empire (between 600 and 900 CE). In **Japan**, public bathing is central to community life and is featured in Japanese creation legends. Though predated by rituals of Buddhism, the public baths introduced during the Edo period (1609–1868) are known as *sento*. The Japanese term *yudedako*—or "boiled octopus"—refers to the pleasant relaxation enjoyed by the body after a long soak in hot water.

In ancient Rome, *thermae* were large, imperial facilities used for public bathing. The range of amenities available varied, of course, by the location and fashionability of the establishment. While some Roman leaders furnished the people with free baths and oil, typically an entrance fee was charged to bathers. Roman baths represented significant innovations in the architecture of the day, as the bath was fed by water from nearby rivers or streams using aqueducts, which could heat the water before channeling it into the pool used for bathing. Before entering the baths, some bathers first disrobed, were anointed with oil, and then exercised in the open courtyards to work up a slight sweat, likely a variation adopted from the Greek tradition of public *gymnasia*. Bathers entered the bath via the atrium, which sometimes included indoor water closets called *latrina*. Massages were optional, as was a process known as strigiling, which involves scraping the skin with specially designed instruments to remove oil, sweat, and dirt. Bathers were also invited to enjoy steam baths and submerge themselves in water. The pools were known as *frigidarium* (a cold "plunge-bath"), the highly decorated *tepidarium* (a warm bath with heated water and air), and the *caldarium*, usually floored with a mosaic and with basins for pouring cold water on the bather's head at the conclusion of the session (Fagan 1999).

Most Roman cities had at least one *thermae* (or *balneae*, a smaller version of the larger bath) that was used not only for bathing, but also for socializing. Baths were places where Romans gathered daily in large numbers in intimate proximity to enjoy meals, entertainment, business, and pleasure. Evidence from Pompeii shows that even those who were able to afford private baths in their homes used the public facilities for some occasions (Fagan 1999). The poet Horace confirms that baths were a daily part of a writer's routine and even served as meeting spaces for furtive lovers, where a young woman's chaperone could be left outside and a couple could find some privacy. Most baths, though, had gendered segregated spaces or allowed men and women to bathe at different times (Fagan 1999).

In the Islamic world, daily ablutions are required of the faithful. The *hammam*, or Turkish bath, is a method of cleansing that begins with relaxing in a heated room, like a sauna, followed by a wash in cool water. The architecture of the Turkish buildings was heavily influenced by the Roman baths, but Muslim baths favored running water. *Hammams* were common during the Ottoman Empire and spread to include most parts of the Islamic world. During the Victorian era, these public baths were enjoyed by colonial Europeans, who frequently painted distorted and racist fantasies of women's baths as overtly sexual spaces of lascivious, naked foreign women. Nevertheless, it's likely that the so-called "Orientalist" obsession of the **other** also helped to kick off a resurgence of hygienic practices within Europe, as public baths opened in Manchester in 1848 and in London in 1860 (Leigh 1995).

Early Christians rejected baths (and many other Roman customs) as both immodest and vain. Ideas about wellness in the medieval period were influenced by efforts to balance the four "humors" and that exposure to excessive amounts of water would dilute the ability of the individual to remain healthy. The spread of the Black Plague discouraged many from participating in public bathing, and bath houses further deteriorated in Europe, becoming synonymous with brothels of the age. Medieval Christians espoused a doctrine of *alousia* (going unwashed) in order to prove the dominance of a righteous soul over the weakness of the body.

Between 1890 and 1940, America's culture of consumption took off and the modern bathroom emerged as a newly equipped space for administering bodily care alongside new ideals of bodily hygiene (Lupton and Miller 1992). At the end of the 19th century, Western consumers turned away from the intricate and plush interiors of the Victorian era with a new awareness of its potential as a breeding ground for germs and dust. More streamlined interior bathrooms began to appear in affluent homes made up of fixtures including nonporous materials, flush surfaces, and rounded edges. Porcelain enamel was preferred, with white, washable surfaces that reflected contemporary theories of hygiene. Cleanliness was medicalized as "hygiene," which also translated to the maintenance of an attractive appearance to others. Initially, the shower was linked to male use and athleticism, referred to as the "morning bracer."

Showering indoors with hot water first became possible in 1883 in Germany when the "rainbath" was introduced at the Berlin Hygiene Exhibition. Showers became popular in England, a bathing modification borrowed from the tropical regions where colonial officials had been stationed. An 1895 catalogue for

---

Matis

The culture of the Matis people of the Amazonian basin in Brazil is highly endangered. Numbering fewer than 200 people, the women of this small group of foragers goes to the river each morning to bathe. Men, menstruating women, and wives of peccary hunters are excluded from the communal bathing area, though men bathe individually in waters upstream from the women. The Matis practice facial tattooing and they wear disklike ear gauges made of shell and wood. Unlike most Amazonian peoples, the Matis appreciate body hair, especially around the mouth, and regard it as a sign of maturity. To emphasize facial hair, the Matis ornament their lips with disks and sticks to signal a man's entry into adulthood. Palm thorns are also placed along the outer edges of the noses of elder men in order to more closely resemble the mighty jaguar. Chiefs sometimes wear peccary tusks through their nostrils to emphasize their prestige.

Montgomery Ward features a "shower bath ring," which allowed a bather to stand in the center of a porcelain tub to fit the ring around his neck and enjoy a self-contained rainstorm to wash away dirt and provide a feeling of refreshed rejuvenation (Lupton and Miller 1992).

By the 1920s, most American homes were constructed with prefabricated bath and shower ensembles built into recessed nooks of the family bathroom for more frequent showering. In the 20th century, advertising and access to a growing array of beauty products transformed individual hygiene standards to include the notion that adults could and should shower daily and wash their hair much more frequently.

See also: China; Egypt; Greece; India; Japan; The "Other"; Wudu.

Further Reading

Fagan, Garrett G. 1999. *Bathing in Public in the Roman World*. Ann Arbor, MI: University of Michigan Press.

Leigh, Michelle Dominique. 1995. *The New Beauty: East-West Teaching in the Beauty of Body and Soul*. Tokyo: Kodansha American.

Lupton, Ellen and J. Abbott Miller. 1992. *The Bathroom, The Kitchen, and the Aesthetics of Waste: A Process of Elimination*. Cambridge, MA: MIT List Visual Arts Center.

Nova Online. 2000. "A Day at the Baths." Secrets of Lost Empires. Accessed November 15, 2015. http://www.pbs.org/wgbh/nova/lostempires/roman/day.html.

Said, Edward. 1978. *Orientalism*. New York, Vintage Books.

Sherrow, Victoria. 2001. *For Appearance' Sake: The Historical Encyclopedia of Good Looks, Beauty, and Grooming*. Westport, CT: Oryx Publishing.

BBW (BIG, BEAUTIFUL WOMAN)

The acronym BBW, for "big, beautiful woman," likely first emerged in the 1970s as a shorthand reference for a **fetish** common in some pornography. Later, the term was also used on dating Web sites that featured so-called "plus size" women, which typically is understood to reference women from about 180 to 500+ pounds (Jones 2015).

Of course, standards of female beauty change according to culture and by the era. Several hundred years ago, fleshy, round Rubenesque bodies were preferred. Today, however, the overwhelming standard for female beauty includes slim, toned, and athletic bodies. Despite the current preferences, some men admit that the bodies they find most beautiful are larger and more generous than the conventional standards of beauty. When Sir Mix-a-Lot joyfully announced in 1992 "I like big **butts** and I cannot lie," he opened a conversation about women's ideal size that touched on issues of race and size that continues today. Black men often describe a body ideal that can be referred to as "thick," with more generous curves and proportions, usually conforming to an "**hourglass**" shape (Dodero 2011). The BBW does not always conform to those proportions, however, and can sometimes be described as having a pear, apple, or melon shape.

In the 21st century, the term has come to be embraced by body-positive and fat-activist women who are working on the larger social goal of size inclusivity. The standards of any society for what is considered to be most attractive for women are intimately tied up with the values of the time and the **social construction of beauty**. Most American women in the contemporary era have been raised in a culture where thin is good and fat is bad, and most women live in fear of being labeled "fat" because it devalues them as women. Like the Rebel Wilson character in the popular *Pitch Perfect* films who introduces herself "Fat Amy" before any of the other women in the group can label her as "the fat one" behind her back, women of the BBW movement are intent on reclaiming the word "fat" to challenge the pervasive idea that the term can only hold negative connotations. Rather than choosing euphemistic labels like "chubby" or "plump," which can be unintentionally demeaning, fat activists claim they are refusing to allow fatness to be demonized. In so doing, they liberate themselves and open a space to be considered beautiful in an alternative way that challenges the standard narrative of female beauty in the culture. In 2016, JCPenney became among the first major department store chains to advertise directly to BBW with its critically acclaimed campaign, "Here I Am" (Mazziota 2016).

BBW tags are often used to indicate a **fetish** or sexual preference for fat women on dating sites. There are fat appreciators (people who see beauty in fatness, sometimes referred to as "chubby chasers," especially in the gay community), gainers (those who find sexual satisfaction in gaining weight), feeders (those who find sexual pleasure in having a partner who is actively gaining weight), and feedees (those who find sexual pleasure in gaining weight, often through the help of a partner) (Ospina 2015). There are also negative connotations to these categories of feedism, including controlling and abusive men who force women to gain weight for their own pleasure, as in the Australian film *Feed* (2005), about an investigator tracking a man suspected of force-feeding women to death (XOJane 2015). There are similarities, but also important differences, to the phenomenon sometimes referred to as **wife fattening** that occurs in some regions of the world.

See also: Body Positivity; Butts and Booty; Fetish; Hourglass Shape; Social Construction of Beauty; Wife Fattening.

Further Reading

Dodero, Camille. 2011. "Guys Who Like Fat Chicks," May 4. The Village Voice. Accessed November 23, 2015. http://www.villagevoice.com/news/guys-who-like-fat-chicks-6433916.

Jones, Georgina. 2015. *Bustle*. "Is There a Size Limit to Reclaiming the Word Fat?," September 27. Accessed November 23, 2015. http://www.bustle.com/articles/98664-is-there-a-size-limit-to-reclaiming-the-word-fat.

Mazziota, Julie. 2016. "JCPenney Promotes Body Positivity in New Ad Campaign that Says 'Fat Girls Can Do Whatever They Want'," June 20. *People*. Accessed June 21, 2016. http://www.people.com/article/jc-penney-body-positivity-ad-campaign.

Ospina, Marie Southard. 2015. "7 Things You Didn't Know About the Term BBW," November 2, 2015. *Bustle*. Accessed November 23, 2015. http://www.bustle.com/articles/121011-7-things-you-didnt-know-about-the-term-bbw?utm_source=facebook&utm_medium=owned&utm_campaign=bustle.

XOJane. 2015. "It Happened to Me: I Have a Sexual Fetish for Being Fed and Gaining Weight." Accessed November 23, 2015. http://www.xojane.com/sex/weird-controversial-sexual-fetish-known-as-feedism.

BEARDS. *See* Facial Hair.

BINDI

The small, bright dot worn on the forehead just above the brow line in South Asian countries, known as a bindi (or *tilak*), is worn by both men and women for religious, social, and aesthetic reasons. Married women usually wear a red bindi, but may also wear other colors, a rhinestone, or a commercially available sticker. A black dot worn in the same place is known as a *pottu* and is sometimes placed on young unmarried women as a protection against the evil eye.

Historically, within the caste system, Brahmins, who were priests or academicians, wore a bindi of white sandalwood to signify purity; the Khatriyas, who became the kings, warriors, and administrators, wore red bindis to signify valor; the Vaishya businessmen wore yellow bindis to signify prosperity; and the Sudra wore black bindis to signify their service to the other castes (Das 2015).

The placement of the bindi is meant to assist in the maintenance of energy and to improve concentration. It signifies awareness of a third eye, or the seat of concealed wisdom possible to all human beings in an awakened state of consciousness. The placement corresponds to *Ajna*, the sixth chakra recognized by Hinduism, Buddhism, and Jainism, and indicates the physical point around which a symbolic mandala representing the universe is created. This spot is also frequently represented in Hindu iconography as a sacred lotus (Das 2015).

Placement of a bindi over the Ajna chakra is a reminder to oneself and to society to see through the mind's eye a bigger picture of the "Universe as One." Within the Ayurvedic tradition of holistic medicine, the location of the bindi corresponds to the location of the pineal gland and was marked with yellow and red sandalwood, yellow and red turmeric, saffron, flowers, ash, and zinc oxide, all of which are thought to have cooling properties that soothe the nerves and conserve energy.

In addition to the rich religious tradition surrounding the practice, a bright red bindi is seen to enhance beauty. Historically,

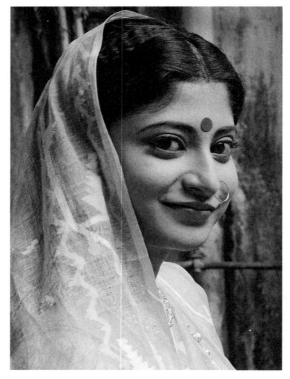

An Indian woman wearing a bindi, Kolkata, India. Bindis are not only aesthetically pleasing; they also signify spiritual purity. (Dreamstime.com)

a bindi could be applied with a skillful pinch of vermilion powder about the size and shape of a fingertip. Other materials to create a paste for dispensing bindis include sandal, *kumkum* (made from red turmeric), and *sindoor* (made from zinc oxide and dye).

As part of the Hindu marriage ceremony, a groom painted a red mark on the part of his bride's hair. Following marriage, women were expected to always wear a bindi in public, sometimes also enhanced with a bright red mark of vermilion paste made in the part above their hair to signify a commitment to the long life and well-being of their husbands. Following the death of her husband, a widow usually stops wearing a bindi, though she may reapply her bindi during puja (prayers) or religious festivals.

In the contemporary marketplace, a much wider range of ornamental bindis in various shapes, sizes, and colors are available. Scarlet-colored resin secreted by some insects is commonly used to make reuseable bindis in Bangladesh, Myanmar, Thailand, Laos, and Vietnam. Self-adhesive bindis are also sold in a variety of materials, including felt or thin metal. Colorful and sparkly sticker bindis come in ready-to-wear packets with a variety of sizes, colors, designs, and materials, especially to coordinate with special clothing as a decorative component of an outfit, regardless of religious affiliation (Antony 2010).

Today, it is also possible to see many celebrities and other people who are not South Asians wearing bindis as a fashion statement, which raises concerns about the cultural appropriation and **exoticizing** of the beauty standards of **other** cultures. Madonna, Gwen Stefani, Katy Perry, Lady Gaga, and Selena Gomez have all been criticized for their efforts to incorporate this religious symbol into their "exotic" fashion looks (Aran 2014).

See also: Exoticizing; India; Jewelry; Makeup and Cosmetics; The "Other."

Further Reading

Antony, Mary Grace. 2010. "On the Spot: Seeking Acceptance and Expressing Resistance through the Bindi." *Journal of International and Intercultural Communication* 3, no. 4: 346–68.

Aran, Isha. 2014. "Take that Dot Off Your Forehead and Quit Trying to Make Bindis Happen." Accessed November 20, 2015. Jezebel. http://jezebel.com/take-that-dot-off-your-forehead-and-quit-trying-to-make-1563531208.

Das, Subhamoy. 2015. "Bindi: The Great Indian Forehead Art." Accessed November 20, 2015. About Religion. http://hinduism.about.com/od/bindis/a/bindi_2.htm.

"BLACK IS BEAUTIFUL MOVEMENT," OR BLACK POWER

Beauty can be understood as a representation of idealized cultural values; the form and appearance of beauty is often highly politicized. The rise and embrace of the "black is beautiful" movement sought to overturn centuries of teachings that described black bodies as savage, uncivilized, and diseased.

The colonial era in Africa focused heavily on a culturally divisive notion of the potentially violent and contagious black body as compared to the sanitized, white

European body (Comaroff and Comaroff 1992). White bodies were not only considered better in and of themselves, but also, during this time, represented a whole array of **disciplinary practices** that included a number of restrictive, repressed consumption habits, teaching people to control their bodies by telling them what they could not do.

Missionaries in the mid-19th century concerned themselves with imposing methods of sanitation on Africans in an effort to reform and "civilize" African bodies and established a standard of beauty that excluded dark skin. Stereotypical ideas about the appearance of **the Other** were, and still are, often used to support discriminatory practices and exclusionary policies.

Overwhelmingly, beauty standards in the United States were based on white women's features until the early 1960s. With a few notable exceptions, including singers Josephine Baker and Lena Horne or actress Dorothy Dandridge, few black women were celebrated at a national level for their beauty. Black women were encouraged to straighten their naturally curly hair using a variety of processing and heat options in order for it to appear more like white women's hair.

The "black is beautiful movement" began in earnest in the 1960s, with the rising Civil Rights Movement in the United States. During this time, black activists worked to reclaim an alternative standard to white beauty that had been imposed upon them during the era of colonialism and slavery and thus marginalized their appearance. It critiqued black popular culture and dramatically demonstrated how the lives of black subjects in the West had been marked by the slave trade and the dehumanizing effects of racism (Dash 2006, 31).

The movement also highlighted the necessity for black subjects to learn about history, acknowledge the complex power relations that characterized the spread of African people around the world, and recognize their own ability to take action in reclaiming their own voices to name oppression. Spurred by the political energy of "Black Power," visible in movements like the Nation of Islam and the Black Panthers, African American communities across the United States demanded a new standard of female beauty.

Robyn Gregory made news in 1966 when she became Howard University's first Afro-wearing homecoming queen, where it was estimated that only about 300 of the university's 11,000 students wore their hair naturally (Walker 2007). In 1970, an Afro-wearing woman became the first black Cherry Blossom Festival Princess in Washington, D.C., and darker-skinned, Afro-wearing beauty contestants found greater success in beauty **pageants**. Cheryl Browne, Miss Iowa 1970, became the first African American Miss America contestant (Walker 2007), though the first African American winner of the Miss America contest was Vanessa Williams, in 1983.

In an effort to eradicate widespread exclusionary and discriminatory practices, African Americans rejected the ideas that the standards of "white" beauty should be the measure of all bodies. In an influential 1962 essay, American writer and political activist Eldridge Cleaver declared that black liberation would not be possible unless African Americans could claim their "crinkly" hair as their own (Walker 2007, 187). Following this movement, both men and women began to embrace "natural" hair that was not straightened or processed, including braiding, hair wrapping, hair twisting, and cornrows (small tight braids worn close to the scalp). Cornrows are also sometimes called "canerows" or "track braids."

Probably the most iconic look of the "natural" hair aesthetic was the so-called "Afro" style, which allowed hair to grow long and then be picked out into a loose style that surrounded the head. The style celebrated qualities intrinsic to African hair, including its coil and capacity to grow into a thick mass (Dash 2006).

> "I want to talk about natural black hair, and how it's not just hair. I mean, I'm interested in hair in sort of a very aesthetic way, just the beauty of hair, but also in a political way: what it says, what it means."
>
> —CHIMAMANDA NGOZI ADICHIE

Unprocessed hair was seen as a challenge to the traditional standards of grooming and styling central to established images of black femininity in the United States. The hairstyle came to represent youthful, urban identity and skepticism of authority, and was a crucial part of demonstrating solidarity and appreciation of one's cultural heritage. The Afro was widely viewed as time saving, empowering, and most of all, "natural."

In 1966, Stokely Carmichael declared "black is beautiful," and African Americans rallied to this powerful political message about racial pride and political commitment to black consciousness. This can be seen in a 1969 *Newsweek* poll of black Americans that revealed strong support for and acceptance of the Afro though people were more inclined to wear the hairstyle in urban areas and the northeastern states (Walker 2007). Women typically created larger Afro styles than men, often paired with large dangling earrings. The more "feminine" Afros for women typically required more maintenance than the male styles, and women were encouraged to cultivate the glamour of a large Afro style.

Writer Michelle Wallace noted that blackness notwithstanding, black men still did not prefer women with short hair. Despite claims that it was an effortless style, the full Afro of feminine black consciousness still required a great deal of hard work and money to maintain (Wallace 2007). Hair in the 21st century continues to carry profound social significance and meaning for some black women who may choose particular hairstyles (including a full Afro, dreadlocks, or braids) as a symbol of their resistance to racial and gendered beauty norms (Wingfield 2008).

Interestingly, African writers commented that the Afro as a symbol of heritage was a uniquely American invention. A complex history exists within the interplay of African influences on the fashions of Americans, and vice versa (Nyamnjoh, Durham, and Fokwang 2002). Tanzanian writer Kadji Konde pointed out that East African women traditionally wore their hair in closely cropped or elaborately braided styles, avoiding "wild oiled bushes on the skull" (Walker 2007, 188). Cultural critic Kobena Mercer also noted that the Afro was neither African nor natural, but rather a carefully cultivated revisionist notion of cultural identity, which could also be co-opted and marketed to individuals who wanted to appear to be young, hip, or trendy. When women renounced hair-straightening products in favor of the Afro, some beauty entrepreneurs feared the loss in product sales (Wingfield 2007).

However, the Afro ultimately became incorporated into the world of commercial beauty as "sheen" products emerged to treat the dryness, breakage, and scalp ailments of hair that was left to do its own thing. The "Afro Queen" became a new category at hair trade show contests. A new market of Afro hair care products began to appear, shelved side by side with products designed for straightening hair (Walker 2007). A very popular market also opened for Afro wigs.

The "black is beautiful" movement also led the way to a new, more cosmopolitan moment in the fashion industry, highlighting African-print dashikis, vivid colors, and large beaded necklaces and earrings. Beauty product advertising of the era illustrates the commodification of "soul" during the late 1960s and early 1970s (Walker 2007, 174). African American–owned companies led the way in this energy, but they were joined by white-owned companies hoping to appeal to a larger audience.

Caroline Jones at the Aziza cosmetics company developed a line of Bronze Beauty cosmetics that specifically targeted dark-skinned consumers who had rejected makeup in earlier years for the insufficient range of colors available to them (Walker 2007). The central theme for much of this targeted marketing was the idea of "freedom," including the ability to wear natural hairstyles, separate from endless visits to the salon, and to develop independent beauty standards that did not rely on imitation of the narrow choices offered through white beauty products and advertising. In 1968, *Ebony* magazine ran a full-page ad for the product Nadinola featuring a full-face close-up of a black woman with an Afro with the simple caption, "Black is beautiful." Ironically, the starkly striking and influential advertisement was for a **skin-bleaching** cream (Walker 2007).

An early high-profile icon of the "black is beautiful" movement in the United States was activist Angela Davis, noted for her large, natural hairstyle. An outspoken advocate for the Black Panthers, Davis inspired many with her uncompromising politics and her natural glamour. A pop-culture crossover of the look was on the 1960s cult show, *Star Trek*, with Nichelle Nichols cast as Lieutenant Uhuru (which means

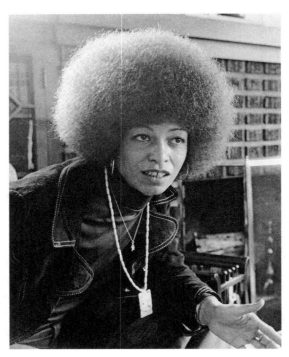

Black Power activist Angela Davis is seen at home in East Oakland, California, on September 9, 1974. She wears two chains representing her commitment to struggle—one is gold, with the hammer and sickle of the Communist Party; the other is ivory with a dragon, an ancient symbol of strength and harbinger of revolution. (AP Photo)

"freedom" in Swahili) holding down the communications station on the bridge of the USS *Enterprise*. Sporting knee boots, massive hair, and a short miniskirt uniform, Nichols' character Uhuru was also one half of the first on-screen interracial kiss in 1968.

Another "natural" hairstyle that gained popularity in part due to its political symbolism in the United States is known as "**dreadlocks**." The style, initially associated with the pan-African spirit of the Rastafarian movement and popularized by reggae superstar Bob Marley, emerged from the Caribbean and was adopted by African Americans beginning in the late 1970s.

See also: Disciplinary Practices/Disciplinary Power; Dreadlocks; Hair; Hair Straightening; The "Other"; Pageants—International, National, and Local Contests; Skin Whitening.

Further Reading

Bailey, Eric. J. 2008. *Black America, Body Beautiful: How the African American Image Is Changing Fashion, Fitness, and Other Industries*. Westport, CT: Praeger.

Comaroff, James and Jane Comaroff. 1992. *Ethnography and the Historical Imagination*. Boulder, CO: Westview Press.

Dash, Paul. 2006. "Black Hair Culture, Politics, and Change." *International Journal of Inclusive Education* 10, no. 1: 27–37.

Hobson, Janell. 2005. *Venus in the Dark: Blackness and Beauty in Popular Culture*. New York: Routledge.

Leeds, Maxine. 1994. "Young African-American Women and the Language of Beauty." In: *Ideals of Feminine Beauty: Philosophical, Social, and Cultural Dimensions*, edited by Karen A. Callaghan. Westport, CT: Greenwood Press, 147–59.

Leeds Craig, Maxine. 2002. *Ain't I a Beauty Queen? Black Women, Beauty, and the Politics of Race*. New York: Oxford University Press.

Nyamnjoh, Francis B., Deborah Durham and Jude D. Fokwang. 2002. "The Domestication of Hair and Modernised Consciousness in Cameroon: A Critique of the Context of Globalization." *Identity, Culture and Politics* 3, no. 2: 98–124.

Walker, Susannah. 2007. *Style and Status: Selling Beauty to African American Women, 1920–1975*. Lexington, KY: University of Kentucky Press.

Wingfield, Adia Harvey. 2008. *Doing Business With Beauty; Black Women, Hair Salons, and the Racial Enclave Economy*. Lanham, MD: Rowman and Littlefield.

BLONDES AND BLONDE HAIR

Only 2 percent of the world's population is born blonde, making naturally blonde hair a very rare commodity. Blonde hair has been, and internationally continues to be, an aspirational element of beauty. More than a third of all the hair dye sold in the United States in 2006 was to make hair blonde. In South Korea, national statistics indicate that more than 80 percent of youth in their twenties lighten their hair (Pak 2007).

Hair color has been used as a visual symbol of moral and intellectual worth for centuries. Ancient Greek actors wore blonde wigs when portraying heroes and black wigs when portraying villains. Historically, angels, princesses, saints, and fairy godmothers are overwhelmingly portrayed as blonde (Rich and Cash 1993). Blonde hair has figured as a symbol of beauty and eroticism for many years. Beginning in the 17th century, the biblical figure of Eve in John Milton's *Paradise Lost* was noted for her blonde hair as an indicator of her wanton feminine sexuality (Rich and Cash 1994).

In the 20th century, blonde hair for both men and women continued to be used frequently to communicate goodness and purity, beauty, and attractiveness. In silent film era, blonde women were most often cast in the roles of innocent and gentle characters, with brunettes being selected for erotic or violent figures (Nunez 2010).

As the 20th century progressed, beauty icons such as Marilyn Monroe and Jane Mansfield widened the portrayal of blonde women in film to include sexualized and sensually attractive women. This trend was then played out in print publication such as the pornographic periodical *Playboy,* which in the 1960s and 1970s featured more blonde women as centerfolds than it did brunettes of redheads (Rich and Cash 1994).

One indicator of the popularity and power of blonde hair is the prevalence of that hair shade in hair-coloring products. In the year 2000, across all hair-coloring manufacturers, there were five hundred different shades of blonde hair color to choose from (Etcoff 2000). The Western preference for blonde women over time is also evident in the number of English expressions alluding to the desirability of being blonde, among them "blond bombshell," "blondes have more fun," and "gentlemen prefer blondes." This perception of increased opportunities and advantages for blonde women is also present outside English-speaking nations in areas such as Latin America and Europe. In her 2014 memoir, Venezuelan supermodel Patricia Velásquez, a Wayuu Indian woman, recounts her struggle to make a mark in the international modeling industry as an effort to "fight my way through the blonde standard" (Velásquez 2014).

The "blonde standard" notwithstanding, an international preference for blonde beauty is not monolithic or without exception. By the late 1980s, the Miss Universe pageant, for example, had been won by a series of dark-haired women from around the globe (Jones 2008).

The generally perceived preference for blondes as symbols of beauty is also tied to notions of blonde hair as an indicator of not just innocence, but also simple-mindedness and stupidity. In English, the prevalence of the "blonde joke" assumes the generally held belief that blondes are not as intelligent as other people (Thomas 1997). When people are asked to describe people who they only see in photographs, they tend to assume that blondes are weaker, more submissive, and less experienced (Etcoff 2000).

Today, in the wake of a proliferation of technologies and global styles that transcend borders, a wide variety of people of color also dye their hair shades of blonde as part of "a palette of styling techniques" (Dash 2006, 34) that allow them a wider range of self-expression.

See also: Brunettes and Black Hair; Exoticize; Hair; Supermodels; Venezuela.

Further Reading

Dash, Paul. 2006. "Black Hair Culture, Politics, and Change." *International Journal of Inclusive Education* 10, no. 1: 27–37.

Etcoff, Nancy. 2000. *Survival of the Prettiest: The Science of Beauty.* New York: Anchor.

Jones, Geoffery. 2008. "Blonde and Blue-Eyed? Globalizing Beauty, c. 1945–c. 1980." *The Economic History Review.* 6, no. 1: 125–54.

Nunez, Rocio. 2010. "Chick Flicks Prefer Blondes: What Chick Flicks Reflect About the American Woman's Beauty Ideal." *Conference Papers—International Communication Association 2010. Communication & Mass Media Complete.* Accessed September 1, 2015.

Pak, Suchin. 2007."Erasing Ethnicity." *Marie Claire (US Edition)* 14, no. 10: 56.

Rich, Melissa K. and Thomas F. Cash. 1993."The American Image of Beauty: Media Representations of Hair Color for Four Decades." *Sex Roles* 29, no. 1/2: 113–24.

Thomas, Jeannie B. 1997. "Dumb Blondes, Dan Quayle, and Hillary Clinton: Gender, Sexuality, and Stupidity in Jokes." *The Journal of American Folklore* 110, no. 437: 277–313.

Velásquez, Patricia. 2014. *Straight Walk: A Supermodel's Journey to Finding Her Truth.* Franklin, TN: Post Hill Press.

BODYBUILDING

Bodybuilding, the practice of strengthening and enlarging the muscles through exercise and weightlifting, is a sport and activity practiced all over the globe. Normally associated with men, but in the 21st century also engaged in by women, bodybuilding allows people to seek an ideal of muscular definition for their bodies through lowering their levels of body fat and forming large, symmetrical muscles.

The overall goal of those who engage in bodybuilding either professionally or as a hobby is to become "shredded," a term that describes, simultaneously, the size of muscles and muscle groups, the symmetry of those muscles from one side of the body to the other, and the definition of those muscles as they are visible under the skin. Someone who is "shredded" has extremely low body fat and a high level of muscle separation, with individual muscles obviously visible.

As early as the 16th century, bodybuilding, or the development of muscles and muscle groups through lifting weights, was widespread and popular in India, where stone dumbbell weights known as *nals* were used (Robson 2016). Creating muscle and strength by lifting stone was the most common form of bodybuilding worldwide until the late 1800s. In the 19th century, bodybuilding became popular in the United States and Great Britain through the work of the famous German strongman Eugene Sandow, who popularized the idea of perfecting the body through exercise and such activities as cart pulling and lifting animals in the late 1800s.

Sandow began his career as a sideshow and vaudeville strongman, lifting large weights and challenging audience members to copy his feats of strength (Daley 2003). Later, Sandow leveraged this career into an empire based on his views on body improvement, opening gymnasiums, inventing exercise equipment, and publishing a magazine called *Physical Culture* that featured him posing, showing off his muscles in very skimpy attire. Today these photos are very similar to the poses of competing body builders (Daley 2003).

By the early 20th century, bodybuilding competitions were popular, with participants from around the world posing and showing off their musculature for prize money. The "Mr. America" competition was held in 1940, and the international "Mr. Universe" contest for body builders was first held in 1950. By the 1960s, bodybuilding, especially in California at places such as "Muscle Beach," attracted large crowds. Hollywood noticed the winners, founding acting careers for such Mr. Universe and Mr. Olympia champions as Steve Reeves, Frank Zane, and Dave Draper (Robson 2016).

In bodybuilding competitions, participants go onstage to pose for a panel of judges for approximately 30 minutes in order to have their bodies, muscles, and physical appearance judged. Each competitor traditionally aims for a **skin tone** of "body builder bronze," a skin color that is often achieved by the use of spray-on tan products. In competition, participants often oil their bodies to give them a sheen and highlight their muscles. Wearing very small bathing suits, competitors are then judged on the symmetry of their muscles, as well as the mass, definition, and proportion (WNBF 2016).

Beauty norms around the world have traditionally preferred noticeable and large muscles for men rather than women. Indeed, studies show that women with

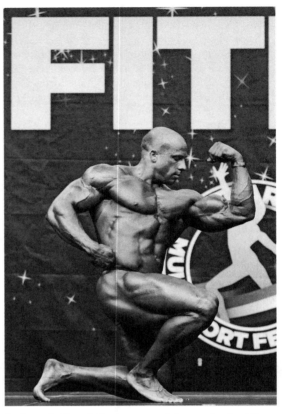

Szalma Attila of Hungary participates in the Fitparade Bodybuilding Championships in Budapest, Hungary, October 17, 2010. Many body builders continue to participate in international competitions. (István Csák/Dreamstime.com)

larger-than-average muscles and a stronger appearance are often stereotyped as "too masculine" or other socially undesirable personality traits (Ryckman et al. 1992). Despite these findings, women since the 1980s have increasingly become interested in bodybuilding, and the international organizations that set standards have responded by including women in their competitions and judging (IFBB 2016).

In the late 20th and early 21st centuries, many body builders continue to participate in internationally judged competitions. The main international organization that plans and executes such events is the IFBB, or International Federation of Bodybuilding and Fitness. The IFBB holds more than 2,000 local, regional, national, and international competitions for men and women each year in events such as classic bodybuilding, women's bikini, children's fitness, and wheelchair bodybuilding (IFBB 2016).

Some of the most famous bodybuilding athletes have moved beyond success in the arena of building muscle and have moved on to acting careers. The Austrian

Arnold Schwarzenegger, the U.S. television star Lou Ferrigno, Indian Bollywood star Varinder Singh, and Egyptian movie star El-Shahat Mabrouk all began their careers as body builders competing in international competitions (IFBB 2016).

While bodybuilding is seen by many as a way to improve health and muscle tone, exaggerated or obsessive participation in bodybuilding can be dangerous to participants' health, leading to obsessive behaviors such as eating disorders or **body dysmorphia**, a condition in which people become overly preoccupied with a physical defect or lack that only

Manohar Aich, The Indian "Pocket Hercules"

Continuing a centuries-long tradition of bodybuilding in India, Manohar Aich, at four feet, eleven inches tall, was the first Indian man after independence to be crowned Mr. Universe. At the age of 15, Aich began supporting his family by displaying his body at fairs and festivals across India. Soon after, he was hired by the British military as a fitness instructor. He worked until 1941, when he slapped an officer for insulting India. After his court-martial, he dedicated his time in jail to bodybuilding, emerging even more muscular than before. In 1954 he won the Mr. Universe competition in London at the age of 40. Aich dedicated the rest of his life to training Indian body builders until his death in 2016 at the age of 104.

they can see. With bodybuilding, participants can become convinced that they are never big or muscular enough, despite the opinion and observation of others (Thompson 2016). This type of preoccupation can lead participants in bodybuilding to the use of problematic substances such as anabolic steroids.

Body builders and other athletes routinely use such doping agents as steroids, human growth hormone, or insulin to increase muscle mass, a practice that, despite health warnings, is steadily increasing (Baker and Grace 2012). This practice, often known as "juicing," has some known risks, such as loss of impulse control (also known as 'roid rage) and the development of masculine physical attributes such as body hair for women (CBSNews 2007). Much of the long-term effect of the use of doping agents, however, is inconclusive. Steroids and other enhancements have been blamed for everything from cancer to heart disease. While there is evidence to support those claims, most researchers do not believe that there is enough evidence to conclude that these are scientifically proven (Baker and Grace 2012).

See also: Eating Disorders; Masculinity; Progressive Muscularity; Skin Tone; Tanning; Weight.

Further Reading

Baker, Julien and Fergal Grace. 2012. *Perspectives on Anabolic Androgenic Steroids (AAS) and Doping in Sport and Health*. New York: Nova Science Publishers, Inc.
CBSNews. 2007. "Facts and Myths about 'Roid Rage." Accessed June 10, 2016. http://www.cbsnews.com/news/facts-and-myths-about-roid-rage/.
Daley, Caroline. 2003. *Leisure & Pleasure: Reshaping & Revealing the New Zealand Body 1900–1960*. Aukland, NZ: Aukland University Press.
IFBB. 2016. "About the IFBB." Accessed June 9, 2016. http://www.ifbb.com/about-the-ifbb.
Plummer, John. 2016." Ryan Terry: Fit and Functional." *Muscle & Fitness* 77, no. 3: 108–17.

Robson, David. 2016. "A History Lesson in Bodybuilding." *Bodybuilding*. Accessed June 9, 2016. http://www.bodybuilding.com/fun/drobson61.htm.

Ryckman, Richard M., et al. 1992. "Social Perceptions of Male and Female Extreme Mesomorphs." *Journal of Social Psychology* 132, no. 5: 615.

Thompson, J. Kevin. 2016. "Body Image, Body Building and Cultural Ideals of Muscularity." Accessed June 9, 2016. http://thinkmuscle.com/articles/thompson/body-image-and-bodybuilding.htm.

WNBF. 2016. "2015 WNBF Bodybuilding Judging Criteria." Accessed June 10, 2016. http://www.worldnaturalbb.com/wp-content/uploads/2015/05/2015-Juding-Criteria-BODYBUILDING.2.pdf.

BODY DYSMORPHIC DISORDER

Body dysmorphic disorder (BDD) was identified as a distinct psychiatric disorder and listed by the American Psychiatric Association in the DSM-III in 1987 (Brewster 2011). Those diagnosed with the disorder suffer from a distressing or impairing preoccupation with perceived defects in their appearance. Prior to 1987, medical literature included descriptions of patients who suffered from "dysmorphophobia," an obsession with their own "ugliness," even though their appearance was objectively normal to others (Brewster 2011).

In order to be diagnosed with BDD, the preoccupation must be significant enough to cause debilitating distress in the individual's life. These exaggerated fears of unattractiveness are frequently accompanied by maladaptive behaviors, as BDD sufferers are compelled to act on their desire to change their appearance through **plastic surgery, cosmetic dentistry**, or dermatology and to develop potentially life-threatening **eating disorders**. BDD is increasingly recognized by practitioners as a somatoform disorder, which means that it can cause bodily symptoms, including pain. BDD is clinically distinct, but occurs in conjunction with a range of disorders that exist as part of obsessive-compulsive behaviors, eating disorders, and depression (Hunt, Theinhaus, and Elwood 2008).

> "By plucking her petals, you do not gather the beauty of the flower."
>
> —RABINDRANATH TAGORE

Both men and women suffer from anxiety and depression associated with BDD. They fear that they are marked by deformity, thought to be permanently inadequate, and continually judged by others. Sufferers may engage in extreme levels and frequencies of mirror gazing, picture taking, grooming, makeup application, hairstyle changes, clothing changes, exercising, dieting, and grasping of the body. Women are reported to be obsessed with their weight and the size of their hips. They also pick at their skin and camouflage it with makeup and cosmetics. Women also display high rates of an eating disorder called bulimia nervosa. Men were more likely to be preoccupied with the build of their body, size of genitalia, and hair thinning. Men suffering from BDD are prone to alcoholism and obsessive **bodybuilding** behaviors (Phillips and Diaz 1997).

Clinicians speculate that BDD may be caused by a combination of unrealistic societal standards and expectations, parental pressure, poor self-esteem, and neurobiological imbalances. In particular, researchers note that the cultural emphasis on physical beauty promotes beauty-based psychological disorders like BDD and eating disorder. Young people are continually exposed to images of beauty through television, the Internet, and the media, which may induce increased internal pressure aimed at attaining similar features or initiate feelings of self-doubt and inadequacy when such features cannot be attained. The symptoms and behaviors associated with the disorder may be triggered by some event during adolescence that includes genetic, cultural, and/or psychological factors. BDD is found worldwide; however, the types of bodily concerns of those affected vary according to culture. It is more common, for example, to find complaints of **eyelids** in Japan and Korea than in other parts of the world.

BDD may be addressed with cognitive behavioral therapy consisting of elements such as exposure, response prevention, and cognitive restructuring. Some treatment also includes prescriptions for certain types of psychotropic drug regimens, especially those with selective serotonin reuptake inhibitors (SSRIs).

See also: Bodybuilding; Eating Disorders; Eyelid Surgery; Makeup and Cosmetics.

Further Reading

Brewster, Keith. 2011. Body Dysmorphic Disorder in Adolescence: Imagined Ugliness." *The School Psychologist*. Accessed November 24, 2015. http://www.apadivisions.org/division -16/publications/newsletters/school-psychologist/2011/07/adolescent-dysmorphic -disorder.aspx.

Hunt, Thomas J, Olie Theinhaus and Amy Ellwood. 2008. "The Mirror Lies: Body Dysmorphic Disorder." *American Family Physician* 78, no. 2: 217–22.

Phillips, K. A., and S. F. Diaz. 1997. "Gender Differences in Body Dysmorphic Disorder." *Journal of Nervous Mental Disorders* 185, no. 9: 570–77.

BODY MODIFICATION

Humans are likely the only creatures in the world that refuse to allow nature to dictate how they look. Our capacity for self-modification and adornment is an important characteristic of what it is to be human. Humans may alter their bodies for a variety of reasons, including to register participation in a social group, to claim an identity in opposition to a group, to signal a significant change in status or identity (for example, a rite of passage), or to attain a cultural standard of beauty (Reischer and Koo 2004). Forms of body modification may include **tattooing**, piercing, cutting, elongating, scarification, branding, footbinding, corsetry, and surgical insertion of subdermal implants. Body modification may also include cosmetic surgery.

In non-Western cultures, body modification often accompanies a rite of passage that marks a change in status from one social identity to another. In 1909, Dutch anthropologist Arnold van Gennep identified three stages of a rite of passage designed to accompany the transformation of an individual from one stage to another. Rites of passage are often characterized by physical suffering, discomfort, or pain, which is symbolically meaningful for the initiate and the larger social group. In the first stage, the individual is separated from the group and undergoes a metaphorical "death," stripped of their previous social status. In the second stage, the "liminal," or transitional, stage, the individual is confronted with a clearly defined challenge or act that they must endure with stoicism or culturally appropriate indifference. Most ritual body modification happens in this second stage, where the individual who is transitioning to a new status is physically marked through some ordeal, including branding, tattooing, or cutting. In the final stage, the individual is reincorporated into the social group with a newly bestowed status (Pitts 2003).

In the contemporary West, rites of passage are rarely marked by ritual pain. Body modification that causes physical harm has often been viewed as a form of self-mutilation and is often negatively framed as repulsive, repugnant, dangerous, "crazy," and pathological. Perhaps paradoxically, body modification can also appear fascinating, salacious, **exotic**, and forbidden (Pitts 2003).

In many Western cities, body modification subcultures have emerged, especially around tattooing. Piercing, branding, or heavy tattooing may be seen as an elimination of conventional beauty ideals, but may also be intentionally enacted as a subversive technique to challenge traditional feminine standards to create a new form of beauty (DeMello 2000).

Tattooing is one way in which people rebel against traditional beauty norms. Tattoos are often seen as markers of criminality or poverty, and the stigmatization of the tattoo has allowed it to also be a way for groups who desired the opportunity to stage symbolic rebellion and to create a subculture that tolerated and embraced personal and political body art (Pitts 2003). Tattoos can be rejections of a male-controlled society, medical narratives about health, or traditional religions.

However, body modification also importantly allows the individual the chance to transform themselves through the act of modifying the body in order for it to be more empowered and authentically his or her own (Wojcik 1995). Through deliberate body modification, the individual body itself may be viewed as a key transformative space for exploring identity, experiencing pleasure, and establishing community with others. Contemporary Western body modification advocates see the practice as empowering and liberating.

California activist Fakir Musafar is usually credited as being the "father" of the modern primitive movement since his performance at the 1977 International Tattoo Convention in Reno, Nevada. He advocated the notion that body modification went beyond the aesthetic and could include a dimension of profound spiritual exploration and creation of community that went beyond "shallow" practices of personal adornment. His message was well received by a hungry community of what is sometimes called neotribals, eager to reconnect with their physical bodies in a disaffected global age. Musafar suggested that body modification and also "body play" (which combines extreme pain with ceremonial trance through such acts as suspension by hooks or the passage of skewers through the chest or limbs in order to experience transcendent pleasure or other affective experiences) allowed an individual to demonstrate symbolic control over their own bodies by experiencing or adorning them in ways that were normally discouraged or even prohibited by Western culture (Favazza 1987). These contributions also added to the rise and popularization of bondage, discipline, dominance, and submission (BDSM) and fetish communities at the end of the 20th and beginning of the 21st centuries.

The message of self-control over one's own body resonated deeply with many alternative communities, especially feminists and the gay community. Despite big changes in the norms of society, many contemporary women, in particular, rarely feel in control of their own sexuality, health, and bodily safety (Pitts 2003). Beginning in the early 1990s, many cultural studies experts noted what they called a "tattoo renaissance" to refer to the rise in tattoo parlors across the United States and the rising interest in tattoos among the middle class, especially women. Body art became a normalized option even for those people who did not consider themselves to be part of the underground tattoo community, allowing individuals to embrace rituals and markings of indigenous groups or to invent their own. A study of articles on body modification in 12 major U.S. newspapers between the years 1995 and 2000 found that aside from tattoos, however, body modification was still viewed as "mutilation" in about half of the accounts and that gender complicated the tendency of reports to suggest that those who chose body modifications were "sick" (Pitts 2003).

Additionally, contemporary forms of body modification may explore ancient or non-Western practices as alternatives to alienating Western culture, which is seen as numbed or unresponsive to elemental desires or needs, in a quasi-spiritual effort to reconnect with the body's spiritual, sexual, or communal potentials (Vale and Juno 1989). Called "neotribal" or "modern primitive," the contemporary practices of some body modification techniques call upon a shared colonial legacy that somehow views the "Other" as more deeply embodied and authentic. "Indigenous bodies have been framed as simultaneously abject and appealing, wholly **Others** and more desiring and desired" (Pitts 2003, 120).

For young people in the 21st century, a proliferation of magazines, Web sites, exhibitions, and books detailing and celebrating body modification have dovetailed with the increased number of studios and venues to allow for an explosion in the styles and expressions of body modifications that are possible and deemed attractive. The increase in interest and practitioners has also allowed body modification to take on the dimension of technological invention.

Biomedical and information technology allow neotribals, cyberpunks, and other body modifiers to create new body styles, including the use of subdermal implants or laser-created brands. Phoenix, Arizona–based artist and body modification practitioner Steve Haworth pioneered the use of subdermal implants, which allow clients to screw and unscrew ornamental objects into their bodies. Though the procedures are extreme and involve opening the flesh to accommodate the implants, Haworth is not a doctor and does not use anesthesia. He learned most of his craft from his first career as a designer and manufacturer of medical equipment for plastic surgery. Since 1986, his business, Haworth Tech Company, has attracted an almost cult-like following of extreme body modification aficionados who seek out his unique form of body modifications. Haworth also advocates the intensely painful practice of flesh hook suspension popularized by Fakir Musafar through his online community, *Life Suspended* (Life Suspended 2016). The person may choose to be hung by the back, chest, or chest and stomach, and the duration of the suspension varies. For initiates, suspensions are described as an important way to overcome fear and achieve personal transformation, often in the company of trusted partners or friends.

New age subdermal implants have also found a wider set of applications in the neotraditional process of "pearling," or "genital beading," which includes the permanent insertion of small beads beneath the skin of the genitals, including the labia or the shaft or foreskin of the penis. Today, the beads are made of Teflon, silicone, surgical steel, titanium, or some other metal, but historically, pearls were used for this purpose, which appears to have started among Filipino sailors prior to the 16th century. The purpose of this form of body modification is said to enhance the sexual pleasure of one's partner during intercourse (Wojcik 1995).

See also: Exoticize; Jewelry; The "Other"; Scarification; Tattoos.

Further Reading

DeMello, Margo. 2000. *Bodies of Inscription: A Cultural History of the Modern Tattoo Community*. Durham, NC: Duke University Press.

Favazza, Amando. 1987. *Bodies Under Siege: Self-Mutilation in Culture and Psychiatry*. Baltimore: The Johns Hopkins University Press.

Life Suspended. 2016. Accessed September 10, 2016. http://www.lifesuspended.org.

Pitts, Victoria. 2003. *In the Flesh: The Cultural Politics of Body Modification*. New York: Palgrave Macmillan.

Reischer, Erica and Kathryn Koo. 2004. "The Body Beautiful: Symbolism and Agency in the Social World." *Annual Review of Anthropology* 33: 297–317.

Silverman, Larry. 2007. *Flesh and Blood: A Documentary about Body Modification*. Film. Directed by Larry Silverman. GRB Entertainment. http://fleshandbloodmovie.com.

Thompson, Rosemarie Garland. 2009. *Freakery: Cultural Spectacles of the Extraordinary Body*. New York: New York University Press.

Vale, Vivian and Andrea Juno, editors. 1989. *Modern Primitives: Investigation of Contemporary Adornment Rituals*. San Francisco: Re/Search.

Wojcik, Daniel. 1995. *Punk and Neo-Tribal Body Art*. Jackson, MI: University of Mississippi Press.

BODY POSITIVITY

Bodies of individuals around the world are increasingly judged by nearly impossible standards. In many cultures, body shape ideals form a tangible symbol of wealth and status where standards of beauty are formed through the lens of economics and globalization (Savacool 2009). The "fantasy body" in the United States, for example, stands 5 feet 9 inches and weighs 115 pounds with generous C-cup breasts. Very few women can achieve this type of body without genetic predispositions and/or surgical enhancement. Indeed, as Nancy Etcoff notes, women with these measurements are "genetic freaks" (2000).

Research indicates that preferred body images vary among cultures as well as within cultures across groups and time (Bailey 2008). Within the United States, comparative sociological research finds that the ideal body image for the self was roughly the same for African American men and white men with low socioeconomic status. However, African American women enjoyed a significantly greater ideal body image compared to white women. More than 25 percent of the white women surveyed were satisfied with their body, whereas more than half of

> "The beauty of a woman is not in the clothes she wears, the figure that she carries, or the way she combs her hair."
>
> —Audrey Hepburn

the African American women in the study were satisfied with their current self-image (Becker et al. 1999). The issue of social **class** may play a role in these findings.

Many young people, especially teenage girls, report feeling anxious, stressed, or discouraged after exposure to thirty minutes of advertising (Martin and Gentry 1997). Researchers speculate that a young woman's self-perceived body image can change after watching a half-hour of television programming and advertising. There is some controversy about whether these feelings occur for all teens or only for young people who already struggle with low self-esteem (Posavac, Posavac and Posavac 1998).

Rising in part due to the increasing attention paid to negative experiences around "fat shaming" or "body shaming" (which can be defined as the practice of making critical, judgmental, and potentially humiliating comments about a person's body, especially their weight or their size), a number of organizations affiliated with youth health began speaking out about the ways that body shaming culture, and its tools of bullying and self-objectification, can ruin lives. Some reports also indicate that body shaming specific to young men has been on the rise in the new millennium, with the increased insistence of a validation cycle stemming from an omnipresent social media stoking hyperconsciousness of personal appearance for both the famous and the nonfamous alike (Brodeur 2015).

In May 2016, *Buzzfeed*, the Internet's largest aggregator of news, launched "Body Positivity" week. Writers and commentators were invited to weigh in on body issues including illness and disability, body dysmorphia and eating disorders, self-expression, media representations, and misconceptions about bodies perpetuated by the dominant culture. "By amplifying so many diverse voices, we hope to represent people often left out of mainstream media narratives, and to provide resources for readers as they move through their respective body image journeys" (Gerstein 2016).

Started in 1996, *The Body Positive* is a Web site devoted to "creating a world in which people are liberated from self-hatred, value their beauty and identity, and use their energy and intellect to make positive changes in their own lives and in their communities" (The Body Positive 2016). The program is designed to provide people of "all ages, sizes, sexual orientations, gender, ethnicities, abilities and socioeconomic levels with a whole-person, non-shaming approach to the mystery and miracle of living in a human body." Aiming to reimagine beauty, the "Be Body Positive" model is composed of five course competencies, or skills, that should be practiced daily to live peacefully and healthfully with body positivity. These competencies include reclaiming health, practicing intuitive self-care, cultivating self-love, declaring one's own authentic beauty, and building community.

See also: BBW; Body Dysmorphic Disorder; Class.

Further Reading

Bailey, Eric. 2008. *Black America, Body Beautiful: How the African American Image Is Changing Fashion, Fitness and Other Industries.* Westport, CT: Praeger.
Becker, Diane M., Lisa R. Yanek, Dyann Matson Koffman and Yvonne C. Bronner. 1999. "Body Image Preferences among Urban African Americans and Whites from Low-income Communities." *Ethnicity and Disease* 9, no. 3: 377–86.
The Body Positive. 2016. Accessed October 13, 2016. www.thebodypositive.org.
Brodeur, Michael Andor. 2015. "Why Male Body Shaming Is on the Rise in the Media." The Boston Globe. March 8. Accessed October 13, 2016. https://www.bostonglobe.com /lifestyle/2015/03/08/manshaming/F4IOidjmYSzlbTvMGua0sJ/story.html.
Etcoff, Nancy. 2000. *Survival of the Prettiest: The Science of Beauty.* New York: Anchor.
Gerstein, Julie. 2016. "Welcome to Body Positivity Week." Buzzfeed. May 9. Accessed May 16, 2016. https://www.buzzfeed.com/juliegerstein/this-is-why-were-doing-body -positivity-week?utm_term=.klJpbVBaq#.gsAdzvRAE.
Martin, Mary C. and James W. Gentry. 1997. "Stuck in the Model Trap: The Effects of Beautiful Models on Female Pre-Adolescents and Adolescents." *The Journal of Advertising* 26, no. 2: 19–34.
Posavac, Heidi D., Steven S. Posavac and Emil J. Posavac. 1998. "Exposure to Media Images of Female Attractiveness and Concern with Body Weight Among Young Women." *Sex Roles* 38, no. 3/4: 187–201.
Savacool, Julia. 2009. *The World Has Curves.* New York: Rodale.

BOTOX

The popular cosmetic injection of botulinum toxin, popularly known as "Botox" is often used as a nonsurgical cosmetic procedure for those seeking smoother skin. According to the International Society of Aesthetic and Plastic Surgeons this procedure uses botulinum toxin type A, injected under the skin, to "to correct annoying expression lines in the face," reversing the effect of years of facial expressions such as squinting and frowning (ISAPS 2015a). "Botox" is the brand name of the most commonly used version of the botulinum toxin, which also comes marketed under the brand names Dysport and Xeomin.

Botulinum is a toxin associated with a type of foodborne illness known as botulism. The neurotoxin, if ingested and left untreated, will cause paralysis of the body's muscles and can cause death due to respiratory failure. That paralytic effect, however, is the reason that the toxin can be successfully used as an aesthetic treatment to smooth wrinkles. The correction occurs because botulinum toxin temporarily paralyzes the muscles responsible for lines on the face and the associated wrinkles (IASPS 2015a).

The injection of botulinum as a beauty treatment is a relatively recent invention, beginning in the 1990s in the United States through the practice of one Los Angeles physician. By 2002, the brand Botox had been introduced and had received approval by the U.S. Food and Drug Administration (FDA) as a cosmetic product

(Mello 2012). By 2014 the IASPS reported almost 5 million botulinum toxin injection procedures worldwide (IASPS 2015b).

The brand "Botox" and associated branded botulinum toxins are credited by some as completely changing the face of cosmetic and aesthetic medicine (Mello 2012). The noninvasive, cheaper, and relatively quick application of the toxin has made it, and other injections, more popular than older remedies for facial wrinkles such as facelifts.

While the principal recommended and approved use of botulinum toxin is for the reduction of facial wrinkles through limited paralysis of facial muscles, many other therapeutic and cosmetic applications have been tried and approved. The neurotoxin has been proven to provide relief to those suffering from some uncontrolled muscle contractions and excessive underarm sweating. The injection has also been tried, if not approved, for a range of cosmetic issues from breast plumping to widening of the eyes (Mello 2012).

A normal Botox injection series is conducted as an outpatient procedure that lasts less than thirty minutes. There are few side effects, but some may include visible pinpricks, light bruising, or a slight headache for the first week after the treatment. Because of the paralyzing effect of the toxin, a few individuals who receive botulinum toxin injections experience a drooping of one or both eyelids after the procedure, but this corrects itself after a few days (ISAPS 2015a).

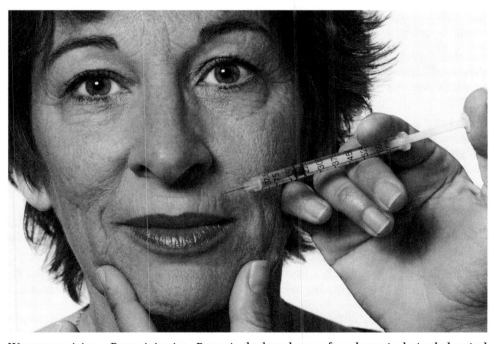

Woman receiving a Botox injection. Botox is the brand name for a bacteria-derived chemical that smoothes wrinkles by preventing muscle contractions. The practice was popularized in the 1990s. (Laurin Rinder/Dreamstime.com)

See also: Advertising; Facelifts; Wrinkles.

Further Reading

ISAPS. (2015a). "Botulinum Toxin." Accessed November 17, 2015. http://www.isaps.org/procedures/botox.

ISAPS. (2015b). "Global Statistics." Accessed November 17, 2015. http://www.isaps.org/Media/Default/global-tatistics/2015%20ISAPS%20Results.pdf.

Mello, Susan. 2012. "Selling a Super Cosmeceutical: Contextualising Risk in Direct-to-Consumer Advertising of BOTOX® Cosmetic." *Health, Risk & Society* 14, no. 4 (June): 385–98.

BRAZIL

The huge South American nation of Brazil has a worldwide reputation for beauty. The home of some of the world's most powerful and successful supermodels, fashion designers, and plastic surgeons, Brazil has come, in many ways, to represent beauty and beauty work on the international stage.

Part of what many observers credit for the recognized beauty of the Brazilian people is the unique racial and ethnic mix of citizens living in the nation. The product of several centuries of intermarriage and mixing among three groups: indigenous peoples, the descendants of African slaves, and white European colonizers, modern Brazil is proud of its *meztiço,* or mixed, multiracial identity (Edmonds 2010). Although scholars may differ on the overall effectiveness of the extent to which racial equality has been achieved, the Brazilian state has, for decades, promoted the ideal of Brazil as a "racial democracy" (Edmonds 2010).

One place in Brazilian society where racial identities combine and compete is in the area of physical beauty, especially for women. Whereas in some nations such as India, light skin is specifically idealized, in Brazil, "brown is beautiful" and a warm, tanned complexion is prized as an ideal of beauty (Edmonds 2010). While this beauty ideal that combines ethnic heritages is true, other elements of appearance linked to racial identities compete to define beauty in Brazil. The traditional preference for small **breasts** has, in the 21st century, begun to lose out to a preference for the larger breasts associated with European and North American beauty standards.

What remains relevant, however, is a well-shaped and sizeable rear end. This ideal for the bottom in Brazil, known through a wide variety of euphemisms such as "***bunda***," is so common and widespread that specific national pageants exist to showcase solely women's **butts**. One such pageant, an event called "Miss BumBum" is so popular that the online voting for the winner topped more than 2 million votes in 2014 (Miss BumBum 2015). The ideal shape presented by the contestants includes much wider, thicker, and shapelier legs and buttocks than may often be associated with the European ideal as demonstrated in a pageant such as Miss Universe.

Competing and coexisting preferences for larger or smaller breasts, larger and more rounded buttocks, and smaller or more "defined" European-style noses are one of the reasons that Brazil is a world leader in the development, study, and practice of **plastic surgery**. Considered by many in Brazil to be an essential way for both men and women to increase their self-confidence and self-esteem, plastic surgery is a common and commonly accepted beauty practice (Edmonds 2010). In 2014, the International Society of Aesthetic and Plastic Surgeons (ISAPS) reported that Brazil was second only to the United States in a number of indicators of the prevalence of cosmetic surgery and led the United States in many other categories, such as the number of procedures performed in buttocks augmentation, **nose jobs**, and eyelid surgeries. Indeed, according to the ISAPS, Brazil was number one in the world in the number of total face and head procedures and surgeries on the body and extremities (ISAPS 2015).

In Brazil, plastic surgery is free, if subject to a long waiting list, in government-run hospitals and clinics (Edmonds 2010). This policy reflects the notion that beauty work and plastic surgery are methods for advancement and gains in self-esteem and mirrors the work and research of Brazil's most famous plastic surgeon, Ivo Pitanguy. Pitanguy, a pioneer of plastic surgery for women of all social classes, believes that all citizens, including the poor, have the "right to be beautiful" (Edmonds 2010, 14). For Pitanguy, a plastic surgeon is a "psychologist with a scalpel," able to help men and women overcome shyness, self-doubt, and other suffering through operations to improve their appearance (Edmonds 2010, 51).

The most common plastic surgeries performed in Brazil again reveal the competing and combined ideals of racial and ethnic beauty. Thousands of buttocks augmentation surgeries are performed every year in Brazil to allow women, especially, to gain the prized *bunda* that many point to as an element of Afro-Brazilian beauty. At the same time, Brazil is also the world leader in the number of rhinoplasties, as many Brazilians, both men and women, seek a surgery called the "correction of the negroid nose," a procedure that identifies the nose associated with African heritage as a deformity (Edmonds 2010, 109).

Other common beauty practices that have become embraced and widespread even outside the nation of Brazil include those related to **hair**, both hair management and removal. One study suggests that Brazilian women find hair work, products, and salon visits to be essential to their professional and personal success (Ferreira 2016). Those who seek an ideal of beauty that includes long, straight, and flowing hair, for example, seek a procedure known as the "Brazilian blowout." A blowout is a process designed for those with the curly hair often associated with African heritage. In a "Brazilian blowout" the hair is treated with a keratin solution and then flat-ironed. The resulting straightening lasts several months, through repeated washings (McIntyre, Carter, and Huang 2009).

Given the historically high degree of racial intermixing in Brazil, hair also denotes a key marker of racial difference (Caldwell 2004). Most Brazilians are acutely aware of the social and racial significance of slight differences in hair texture. Hair texture is widely commented upon, even in the lyrics of popular songs, including an awareness of what is referred to as *cabelo ruim*, or "bad hair." Awareness of textural gradations of hair types can be used as a standard for categorizing individuals into racial and color groups.

For black women in Brazil, hair texture takes on added significance according to racialized constructions of femininity and female beauty, which may serve to marginalize women of particular descent groups. Afro-Brazilian women, especially those of the younger generation, also participate in creating styles that celebrate *negras assumidas* ("racially conscious black women"), including *cabelo arame* ("wire hair"), by proudly appropriating symbols of the black diaspora, such as jewelry and clothing choices that reflect an African heritage (Ibid.). As seen in the **black is beautiful movement** in the United States, the perception of "beauty" and the associated political significance of hair and particular hairstyles are subject to change and contestation.

Another common procedure related to hair that originates in Brazil and has become famous and common worldwide is the practice of body waxing for **hair removal** (Nichols and Robbins 2015). For both men and women who find body hair unattractive, a "Brazilian" often refers to a waxing of either part or all of a person's body. The practice originated, and is still widely practiced, in the coastal Brazilian city of Rio de Janeiro, famous for the small size of the bathing suits that its citizens wear. In order to eliminate public hair considered unsightly, Brazilians began the practice of using hot wax spread on body parts for hair removal. The hot wax is spread on the parts of the body where hair is to be removed, and as the wax cools, it is removed, bringing the hair with it (Keyishian 2000). While this practice originated in the pubic area for women, the practice has also been used to accommodate very small bikinis for men, and is also used to remove hair from men's chests and backs. This process, performed worldwide, is often known in English-speaking nations as a "manzilian" (Paddy 2008).

Finally, Brazil is known worldwide for both its internationally famous supermodels and its fashion designers. Brazil is the world's fifth-largest textile producer in the world and the fourth-largest producer of clothing, and fashion plays a key role in the national pride in and understanding of beauty (*Courier Mail* 2012). Brazil has produced a series of internationally successful fashion designers such as Francisco Costa. Costa began his career working in his family's clothing factory and worked his way up to the position of creative director for Calvin Klein, where he continues to design fashion that speaks to his Brazilian roots. In 2012 the Macy's chain of department stores chose Costa to create a line of Calvin Klein dresses called "Brazil, A Magical Journey" campaign (Nichols and Robbins 2015).

Costa's and other designers' collections are regularly shown at Sao Paolo fashion week, Latin America's biggest fashion event. The shows take place in Sao Paolo, Brazil, in October and November and are both a showcase for Brazilian fashion and a springboard for Brazil's growing collection of **supermodels**. The internationally renowned model Gisele Bündchen, for example, got her start at Sao Paolo fashion week and moved on to be, by 2013, the world's highest-paid fashion model (Blasberg 2013).

See also: "Black Is Beautiful Movement," or Black Power; Bunda; Butts and Beauty; Hair; Hair Removal; International Pageant; Nose Jobs; Plastic Surgery; Supermodels.

Further Reading

Blasberg, Derek. 2013. "Gisele Bündchen's Model Life." *WSJ* (November 7): 28.

Caldwell, Kia Lilly. 2004. " 'Look at Her Hair': The Body Politics of Black Womanhood in Brazil." *Transforming Anthropology* 11, no. 2: 18–29.

Courier Mail. 2012. "Colourful Creations Abound as Brazil Unveils Fresh Take on Winter Fashion." October 31. Accessed October 14, 2016. https://www.pressreader.com/australia /the-courier-mail/20121031/textview.

Dávila, Jerry. 2014. "Brazilian Race Relations in the Shadow of Apartheid." *Radical History Review* no. 119: 122–145.

Edmonds, Alexander. 2010. *Pretty Modern: Beauty, Sex and Plastic Surgery in Brazil*. Durham, NC: Duke University Press.

Ferreira, Daniel. 2016. "Brazil Dominates Hair Care in Latin America." Accessed February 11, 2016. http://www.happi.com/issues/2014-01-01/view_latin-america-news/brazil -dominates-hair-care-in-latin-america/.

ISAPS. 2015. "ISAPS International Survey on Aesthetic/Cosmetic Procedures Performed in 2014." Accessed November 10, 2015. http://www.isaps.org/Media/Default/globalstatistics /2015%20ISAPS%20Results.Pdf.

Keyishian, Amy. 2000. "The Brazilian Bikini Wax: All the Facts." *Cosmopolitan* 229, no. 2: 158.

McIntyre, Samantha, Holly Carter and Joyce Huang. 2009. "Star Treatment: The Brazilian Blowout." *People* 72, no. 1: 124.

Miss BumBum. 2015. "*Com destaque para Miss Bumbum Evangélica, imprensa internacional noticia chegada de fim da competição e a marca de 2 milhões de votos.*" Accessed November 10, 2015. http://missbumbumbrasil.com.br/com-destaque-para-miss-bumbum-evangelica -imprensa-internacional-noticia-chegada-de-fim-da-competicao-e-a-marca-de-2-milhoes -de-votos/.

Nichols, Elizabeth Gackstetter and Timothy Robbins. 2015. *Pop Culture in Latin America and the Caribbean*. Santa Barbara, CA: ABC-CLIO.

Paddy, Hintz. 2008. "Men Spend to Put a Beautiful Skin on Beast Within." August 24. *Courier Mail, The (Brisbane)*. Accessed October 14, 2016. *Newspaper Source*, EBSCOhost.

BREAST AUGMENTATION AND REDUCTION SURGERIES

The International Society for Aesthetic Plastic Surgery (ISAPS) defines "breast augmentation" as a procedure designed to "improve the size and appearance of the breasts by implanting saline or silicone **breast** implants either under or over the chest muscle, thus producing a cosmetic enhancement" (ISAPS 2015a). This procedure, also commonly known in English as "breast enlargement" or colloquially, a "boob job," is one of the most common aesthetic **plastic surgeries** performed in the world. Women seeking breast augmentation surgery generally fall into three groups: those seeking to reconstruct breasts after mastectomy or lumpectomy, those seeking to cosmetically enhance the shape and size of their breasts for aesthetic reasons, and those persons born male seeking to transition to female.

The practice of augmenting the size and shape of the female breast has been recorded in international history dating back to the year BCE 3000. Invasive surgical practices related to breast modification, however, date internationally from the 18th century. During that period, early experimentation into augmentation saw materials such as ivory, metal, glass, and rubber surgically implanted into women's breasts (Sarwer, Nordmann and Herbert 2000).

Early experiments in surgical augmentation in the 19th century led to more widespread research into the different procedures and substances that could be used to increase breast size. In 1890s Germany, Dr. Robert Gersuny pioneered the use of injections of paraffin wax into women's breasts. This procedure, however, soon revealed serious side effects and complications for patients, including the development of cysts and tumors known as parrifnoma. While this procedure continued to be used worldwide through the early 20th century, most European and U.S. surgeons had abandoned the practice by the 1920s (Erguvan-Dogan and Yang 2006).

During the 1920s, many nations, including the United States, developed a preference for a boyish shape that deemphasized the female breast. In the early 20th century, women regularly took to wearing foundation garments aimed at breast reduction (Sarwer, Nordmann and Herbert 2000). After this period, however, the generalized preference for large breasts, particularly attributable to such international beauty icons as Marilyn Monroe and Jane Russell, saw a resurgence, and experimentation with substances and procedures used to increase breast size continued through the early and mid-20th centuries (Haiken 1999). In the United States, liquid silicone and fat from a woman's own body were often injected, and some experimentation occurred with fat, muscle, and skin grafts to women's breasts (Sarwer, Nordmann and Herbert 2000).

While researchers note that international preferences for slim and boyish figures or more voluptuously curvy silhouettes have come and gone in Western-centered international media over the last century, by the late 1900s, the globalized norm of beauty presented the ideal of a lean, athletic body shape with large and full breasts (Sarwer, Nordmann and Herbert 2000). This thin but full-breasted body ideal then spurred new ideas and procedures designed to enhance women's bust size.

In the late 20th and 21st centuries, the international community of aesthetic plastic surgeons used mainly breast implants filled with silicone or saline to achieve the desired improvement in breast size and shape (IASPS 2015a). Whereas early versions of the silicone breast implant experienced problems with ruptures, causing serious health issues for the women receiving them, by the 21st century, reformulations of the implants meant that both silicone-filled and saline-filled devices were regularly implanted into women seeking breast enlargement (Breast 2010).

For those seeking breast augmentation, the choice between silicone and saline implants is generally informed by the "feel" of the implant. Silicone reportedly feels more "natural," but carries a higher potential for scarring. Saline implants generally leave less of a scar, but have a higher risk for potential leakage than either silicone gel or saline fluid (Breast 2010). Recently, an additional option has emerged: fat transfer for breast augmentation, a technique that uses **liposuction** to remove fat from one area of a person's body in order to transfer it to the breasts. This option produces a less obvious increase in breast size, but is sometimes preferred by women seeking a more "natural" method of breast enhancement (Leopardi et al. 2014).

While such procedures as paraffin or silicone **injections** for breast augmentation may carry dangerous consequences, these procedures are still offered in many nations to those without the financial or social access to licensed practitioners. Poor women in some Asian nations, for example, still seek "back-alley" paraffin injections for breast augmentation, in part because the procedure is quick, cheap, and relatively painless in the moment, while providing an initially attractive result (Erguvan-Dogan and Yang 2006). In nations such as Brazil, transgender women, whose societal marginality keeps them from access to licensed clinics, also often seek silicone injections to increase their breast size (Edmonds 2010).

In 2015, the ISAPS reported that more than 1.3 million breast augmentation surgeries had been performed worldwide in 2014. The majority of these procedures were performed in the United States (297,297 surgeries) and Brazil (185,042). The next most-common nations in which the most breast enlargement surgeries had been performed were Germany, Mexico, France, Colombia, and South Korea (ISAPS 2015b).

Although breast augmentation surgery is one of the most commonly performed aesthetic surgeries for women, breast reduction procedures are also performed worldwide for reasons of both health and aesthetics. Breast reduction surgery for women often aims to reduce the size and improve the shape of the breasts and is most commonly performed in order to relieve back, shoulder, or neck pain. Breast reduction surgery in men, known as gynecomasty, is more common for men seeking aesthetic changes. The procedure for men seeks to "reduce overly developed male breasts and nipples to provide a masculine chest appearance" (ISAPS 2015c). In 2014, the ISAPS reported that more than 172,000 men had a gynecomastic procedure, making it the fourth most-common aesthetic surgery for men, behind eyelid opening, liposuction, and rhinoplasty (ISAPS 2015b).

See also: Breast Binding (Chest Binding); Breasts; Corsets, Shapewear, and Waist Trainers; Injections; Liposuction; Plastic Surgery.

Further Reading

Breast. 2010. "The 'Breast' Choice." *Dermatology Times*. Winter: 12–13.

Edmonds, Alexander. 2010. *Pretty Modern: Beauty, Sex and Plastic Surgery in Brazil*. Durham, NC: Duke University Press.

Erguvan-Dogan, Basak and Wei T. Yang. 2006. "Direct Injection of Paraffin into the Breast: Mammographic, Sonographic, and MRI Features of Early Complications." *American Journal of Roentgenology* 186, no. 3: 888–94.

Haiken Elizabeth. 1999. *Venus Envy: A History of Cosmetic Surgery*. Baltimore: Johns Hopkins University Press.

ISAPS. 2015a. "Breast Augmentation." Accessed August 20, 2015. http://www.isaps.org /procedures/breast-augmentation.

ISAPS. 2015b. "ISAPS International Survey on Aesthetic/Cosmetic Procedures Performed in 2014." Accessed August 20, 2015. http://www.isaps.org/Media/Default/globalstatistics /2015%20ISAPS%20Results.pdf.

ISAPS. 2015c. "Male Breast Reduction." Accessed August 20, 2015. http://www.isaps.org /procedures/male-breast-Reduction.

Leopardi, Deanne, et al. 2014. "Autologous Fat Transfer for Breast Augmentation: A Systematic Review." *ANZ Journal of Surgery* 84, no. 4: 225–30.

Sarwer, David B., Jodi E. Nordmann and James D. Herbert. 2000. "Cosmetic Breast Augmentation Surgery: A Critical Overview." *Journal of Women's Health & Gender-Based Medicine* 9, no. 8: 843–56.

BREAST BINDING (CHEST BINDING)

Breasts may be bound by certain foundation garments designed to flatten and deemphasize the bustline in some cultural contexts, or during some historical eras, to present a more "boyish" figure that might be considered more attractive in women than the bombshell **hourglass shape** often referenced in contemporary cultures.

Classic standards of Chinese beauty preferred flat-chested women and practiced *shu xiong*, or breast binding. Chinese women during the early years of the Republic of **China** (1912–1949) wore tightly fitted vests with a line of tight buttons under their outer garments in an effort to minimize the appearance of **breasts** and avoid a feeling of shame. Small breasts were associated with virtue, chastity, and innocence and were encouraged for women who wanted to become dutiful wives and loving mothers. A popular saying from Guangdong of the era stated, "Men with large chests become Prime Minister, women with large chests are shrew mothers." Like with **footbinding**, the practice was eventually abandoned over health concerns.

Japanese fashions were also designed to create a "pillar shape" by flattening the breasts close to the body to minimize the swollen look of a "pigeon chest" (*hatomune desshiri*). A specially designed undergarment called a *datemaki* was meant to be worn under the traditional Japanese kimono. This garment was made of gauze and padding and wrapped around the torso from the chest to the waist. Any appearance of breasts was further depressed with an outside sash around the kimono called an *obi*. The placement of the obi could also indicate the social status of the woman wearing the kimono. An *obi* tied high up over the bust indicated an innocent, unmarried woman who was a virgin, whereas an *obi* tied low over the breasts denoted a more mature woman (Miller 2006). Traditional **geisha** typically tied the *obi* in the lowest position possible, highlighting the more eroticized nape of the neck. Today, few Japanese women bind their breasts on a daily basis, adopting aesthetic looks that highlight **breasts** instead.

American "flappers" of the roaring 1920s also frequently bound their breasts to make them appear less prominent and to give the body a younger, more androgynous look considered attractive in the day. The 1920s were a particularly important decade for women as the United States entered the modern era with the combination of social changes that included the vote and fast-paced technologies, including electricity, the radio, the automobile, and aviation. Women aspired to look like icons of the era, including Clara Bow, Zelda Fitzgerald, and Josephine Baker. Women's dresses were purposely shaped to hide women's curves with a knee-length, dropped waist and sleeveless or V-shaped in the front and the back. Women limited the amount of skin they showed and preferred a flat-chested "unibust" look without cleavage. They also cut off their long tresses from earlier eras and went with a bobbed style, ideally a razor-sharp cut that fell to the chin line or slicked back behind the ears and tucked up into a close-fitting cloche hat.

As in many African cultures, girls (*surbaajo*) among the **Wodaabe** Fulani people of Niger pass through a number of stages that are marked by rites of passage in order to become adult women (*yarijo*). Between childhood and adolescence, Wodaabe girls are forbidden to wear their brightly colored clothing and jewelry. Instead, they dress in all black and are socially isolated and known as "*boofiido*." These adolescent girls undergo a period of training that prepares them to become wives and mothers. During this time, their breasts are bound tightly in order to induce sagging, which is thought to both minimize sexual desirability and to improve her capacity for breastfeeding. This painful process may last for many months and can create sores and blisters on the skin of the young woman. The process is endured because it transforms a sexually attractive physical feature into a more culturally appropriate, mature, maternal shape, which some argue is more highly valued by the nomadic Wodaabe.

In some historical contexts, breast binding is associated with appropriate feminine **modesty** and piety. Until this century, Catholic nuns were also encouraged to bind their breasts under their severe habits in order to minimize the creation of desire in men around them (Karlan 2016).

The most common material for binding breasts is a cloth strip or sash. Today, compression materials like Spandex are widely available, as well as compression sports bras or swimming suits. Some binding materials can cause physical risk or harm when binding is not done carefully. People with asthma or spine deformities may be especially at risk for further harm, especially if binding with Ace bandages, duct tape, or similar products. Breasts that are bound too tightly or for too long can lead to breathing trouble, back pain, and rashes or yeast infections under the breasts.

Increasingly, chest binding is practiced today by transgender men or gender-nonconforming individuals in an effort to create a flatter chest and to give a more desired illusion. YouTube offers a wide variety of do-it-yourself ideas for transgender men to customize garments designed to reduce the appearance of breasts. More and more attractive products are appearing on the market to serve this purpose, easily found and ordered on the Internet. T-shirt–style binders made of Spandex-like fabric are now commercially available, as well as a variety of sports bras and other garments, which may be layered to mechanically compress the breasts. Some of these designs now feature embellishments, like lace and ribbons (Chapin 2015). Health officials warn that it is not safe to wear these binders for too many hours in a row, as they may cause skin irritations or difficulty breathing. Sleeping in a binder is definitely not recommended. Designers who make this new generation of binders argue that in a climate of potential hostility or violence directed toward transgendered people, binders are more than affirming or empowering: they may actually be lifesaving.

Breasts may also be bound using similar techniques for athletics or for accelerated recovery. The goal in these instances is not aesthetic, but rather to reduce breast movement during vigorous sports or following an injury or surgery.

See also: Breasts; China; Geisha; Hourglass Shape; Japan; Wodaabe.

Further Reading

Chapin, Angelina. 2015. "Underwear for Transgender People." September 24. *The Guardian*. Accessed May 18, 2016. http://www.theguardian.com/lifeandstyle/2015/sep/24/underwear-for-transgender-people-shapewear

"From Breast Binding to Bikinis." 2016. Cultural China. Accessed May 18 2016. http://traditions.cultural-china.com/en/15Traditions12412.html

Karlan, Sarah. 2016. "All the Questions You Had About Chest Binding, But Were Afraid to Ask." BuzzFeed LGBT. Accessed May 18, 2016. http://www.buzzfeed.com/skarlan/all -the- questions-you-had-about-chest-binding-but-were-afrai#.ybEOLO7MLM.

Loftsdóttir, Kristín. 2008. *The Bush Is Sweet: Identity, Power, and Development among WoDaaBe Fulani in Niger.* Uppsala: Nordiska Afrikainstitutet.

Lubitz, Rachel. 2015. "These May Look Like Normal Shirts—But for Trans People, They Can Be Life-Changing." December 29. Style.Mic. Accessed May 18, 2016. https://mic .com/articles/131271/binders-may-look-like-normal-shirts-but-for-some-trans-people -they-can-be-life-changing#.ijHtkzhmS.

Miller, Laura. 2006. *Beauty Up: Exploring Contemporary Japanese Body Aesthetics.* Berkeley, CA: University of California Press.

BREAST IRONING

Breast ironing (also called "breast flattening") is a form of **body modification** practiced in Cameroon as a technique to inhibit the development of a young girl's breasts, either to make them grow more slowly or to make them disappear completely (Tchoukou 2014). The practice has also been reported in the West African nations of Benin, Ivory Coast, Guinea, Togo, and Guinea-Bissau. The painful technique involves pressing heated objects against the developing breast tissue of a young girl from about age eight on in order to suppress maturity of the breasts. A wide range of heated or boiled objects are used to accomplish the ironing, including metal or wooden spatulas, stones, coconut shells, pestles, brooms, and hot seeds of black fruits. Breast bands are also sometimes worn to bind the breasts low and tight to the chest.

A study in 2006 found that about one-quarter of all Cameroonian girls and women had experienced some form of breast ironing, sometimes called "breast sweeping" in South Africa, in their lives, usually performed by a mother, nurse or caretaker, aunt, older sister, grandmother, or the girl herself (Ndonko and Ngo'o 2006). In a much rarer set of occasions, the study found that breast ironing was completed by a traditional healer, father, brother, cousin, friend, or neighbor. Burns are common, and the practice can cause permanent damage to the milk ducts, infection, dissymmetry of the breasts, and tissue damage including marks and black spots that never heal.

Breast ironing is believed to have been revived or even to have begun in its current form in recent years. Traditionally, adult women in all Cameroonian ethnic societies practiced breast massage, often with heated objects, in order to induce the flow of breast milk for a new mother or to reduce the sensation of pressure common during weaning (Tchoukou 2014). Frequently taught to younger women by older women as a way to relieve discomfort, the primary intention of earlier breast ironing practices was not to crush the mammary gland, but rather to warm and massage the breast in order to control the flow of breast milk.

In recent years, it appears that the advice of older women has been revived in response to increased rates of sexual violence against girls and women in urban areas, including a way to protect girls from sexual harassment and rape; preventing or delaying early pregnancy by removing signs of puberty; and allowing a girl to

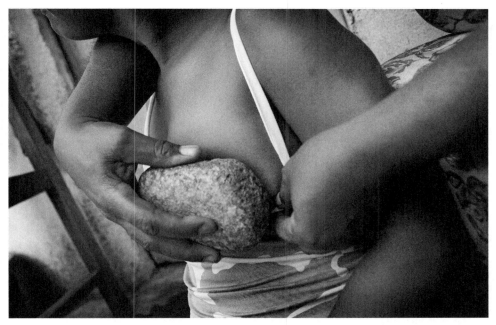

Breast ironing with a hot stone in Douala, Cameroon. The practice of "breast ironing" involves pounding and massaging the developing breasts of young girls with hot objects. The practice is often carried out by mothers to delay the sexual development of their daughters. (Aurora Photos/Alamy Stock Photo)

pursue her education instead of being promised to another family for an early marriage (Bawe 2011).

Unlike most practices in this volume, which describe body modifications as an enhancement for beauty, this practice appears to be more concerned with minimizing the beauty of young girls and women that make them vulnerable to sexual predation and violence. In many ways, this practice is an effort to make girls and women invisible to men so that they do not draw unwanted sexual attention. Over the last fifty years, improved nutritional standards, including higher percentages of fat in the diet, have increased the onset of early puberty (Tapscott 2012).

In general, breast ironing is conducted exclusively by women, especially mothers and grandmothers, on girls. The practice sometimes falls under the category of "family violence" as defined by the United Nations High Commission on Human Rights (Bawe 2011). Cameroonian women often lack control over their sexual or reproductive rights, and discussions or education about sexuality is culturally taboo, making it difficult for parents to educate their children about sexuality or contraception (Tchoukou 2014). Older women fear the possibility that their daughters may become "ruined" or "spoiled" if they succumb to early sexuality. They also fear that their daughters will be victims of sexual predators, as boys and men in Cameroon are generally not held accountable for sexual activity or rape.

Current cultural assumptions always place blame for sexual assault on the female victim, who drew the attention of the male and incited his desire. Despite a wide variety of social changes that accompany globalization and urbanizations, mothers are keenly aware of the continuing traditional social expectation to raise "pious" daughters as an important symbol of the family's integrity and reputation. Many mothers and grandmothers see breast ironing as a way of addressing early pregnancy. They believe that their efforts enhance and promote a girl child's future successes and those of her family, prolonging her possibilities for education and finding a better marriage. While the practice is undoubtedly painful and potentially harmful, the motivations of the family members who continue these practices remain an investment in rendering these girls unattractive, or at least to disguise their sexual maturity to the **male gaze**, in order to protect them from sexual predation.

Efforts are currently underway in a few government legislatures to curtail breast ironing by making it illegal. Fewer efforts, however, concentrate on addressing or eliminating male violence against women.

See also: Body Modification; Breast Augmentation and Reduction Surgeries; Breast Binding (Chest Binding); Male Gaze.

Further Reading

Bawe, Roasline Ngunshi. 2011. "Breast Ironing: A Harmful Practice that Has Been Silenced for Too Long." Gender Empowerment and Development. Office of the High Commission on Human Rights 2011. Accessed October 1, 2016. http://www.ohchr.org/Documents /HRBodies/CEDAW/HarmfulPractices/GenderEmpowermentandDevelopment.pdf.

Tchouckou, Julie Ada. 2014. "Introducing the Practice of Breast Ironing as a Human Rights Issue in Cameroon." *Journal of Civil and Legal Services* 3, no. 21: 121. Accessed October 1, 2016. http://www.omicsgroup.org/journals/introducing-the-practice-of-breast -ironing-as-a-human-rights-issue-in-cameroon-2169-0170.1000121.php?aid=26082.

Ndonko, Favien and Germaine Ngo'o. 2006. "*Etude sur le Modelage des Seins auCameroun.*" GTZ National Study. Accessed October 1, 2016. www.cameroon-today.com/support-files /en- fgm-countries-cameroon.pdf.

Tapscott, Rebecca. 2012. "Understanding Breast Ironing: A Study of the Methods, Motivations, and Outcomes of Breast Flattening Practices in Cameroon." Feinstein International Center of Tufts University. Accessed October 1, 2016. fic.tufts.edu/assets/Understanding -breast-flattening.pdf.

BREASTS

As a key secondary sexual characteristic, breasts are among the most visible sign of women's femininity and sexual maturity. Breasts are highlighted in standards of women's beauty around the world. The dimensions of the breasts balance hips and buttocks to create a bust–waist–hip ratio that many cultures determine to be an ideal **hourglass shape**. A buxom hourglass shape has been highly sought in the sexual fantasy of the United States since at least the post-war era, exemplified by sexy "bombshells" like **Marilyn Monroe**.

In the contemporary **United States**, breasts are **fetishized**; like the phallus, or penis, they represent a unique measure and symbol of desire—in many cases, they are the way that the totality of a woman's sexuality is measured. The relationship between men's penises and women's breasts is argued by some scholars, who note that the "best" breasts are just like the phallus: high, hard, and pointy like those of **Barbie** (Young 1992).

This emphasis on the importance of the breasts as a way to evaluate women means that female people must choose to either refuse or accept the critique. Women often respond to the continual evaluation of their chests by hunching, wearing baggy clothes, or alternately, by throwing back the shoulders and welcoming the **male gaze** and its assessment of her worth. What matters most is how the breast looks and how it measures up to the normalizing standards of the culture (Young 1992).

Western women's fashion sometimes hints suggestively at the covered breast in order to pique the interest of the viewer through strategic uses of cleavage or **décolletage**. During the reign of Louis XIV in France, fashionable ladies adopted the habit of entertaining in their dressing rooms and promoting the *en dishabille* style, leaving the stays of petticoats undone to show ample amounts of their breasts (Downing 2012, 19). Exposed skin was dusted with whitening cosmetics (often containing lead), and the pertness of the bosom was highlighted with a tracery of blue veins drawn on the breasts. This suggestive revealing of parts of the breast continues into the 21st century as "underboob" (the glimpse of the underneath of the breast) and "sideboob" (a view of the side of the breast), two other variations allowed by modern fashion (Walker 2016).

Breast augmentation is the most common form of surgical body modification in the United States, with some estimates suggesting that nearly 5 percent of all American women have undergone breast augmentation (PHPS 2012). Typical characteristics of "natural-style" breasts that are promoted by breast augmentation specialists include an areola smaller than 40 mm in diameter and a breast size that is pert and proportionate to the chest width, waist size, and height of the woman. The nipple should form an equilateral triangle with the notch above the sternum— that is to say that the distance between the nipples and from each nipple to the notch should be about the same. Breasts should appear pert and full.

In Western cultures, women's breasts are almost always expected to be controlled through the use of bras or **shapewear.** Unbound breasts do not remain the firm and stable objects desired by the beauty standards of the culture. Perhaps more dramatically, breasts that are unbound display the nipples, which are considered indecent, because nipples are reminders of how the breasts are related to sexual pleasure. As some note, it is nipples that designate the breasts as "active and independent zones of sensitivity and eroticism" (Young 1992), a reality not lost on the activist organizers of scores of "Free the Nipple" demonstrations and rallies across the United States since the release of Lina Esco's 2014 film.

Despite the intense sensitivity of breasts, male-centered culture tends not to think about breasts as belonging to women themselves. Rather, a woman's breasts, the coverage of them, the appearance of them, and the uses of them are often seen as belonging to others, including her lover, her husband, or her baby (Young 1992). Society also weighs in on what women can and cannot do with their breasts, many times insisting that even the partial sight of a woman's breast while she is feeding a baby is inappropriate and offensive (Acker 2009).

Of course, the cultural attractiveness of large breasts is by no means universal, and preferences for size and shape vary worldwide. In Japan, for example, large breasts are a source of embarrassment. Japanese aesthetics value straight, clean, geometric lines, such as are best suited to wearing kimonos (Miller 2006). Breasts that are too large or too prominent are often referred to negatively as "pigeon's breast."

Young Mende girls in West Africa are proud of their developing breasts and traditionally display them prominently. The word for breast, *nyini*, means "bite of sweetness," referring to both the sustenance-giving capacity of a lactating breast and to the erotic bites given to the breast by a lover. Breasts, which are frequently uncovered during adolescence, may be openly evaluated, touched, and fondled admiringly. As a girl is growing up, the community observes her to see "if the breast has come," and the development of breasts in girls is considered noteworthy and important to the overall well-being of the group (Boone 1986). Once a girl's breasts bud and *wuli* ("stand up"), she is considered to be sexually mature and ready to enter into adult life.

This period marks the beginning of instruction and training from the Sande society, a culturally significant group for the Mende people, within which women administer rites of passage to young girls over the course of several years. The Mende expression *nyini hu vandango* praises breasts, declaring "the breast is fully ripe." Later, as women become mothers, they may still reveal their breasts in public spaces in order to nurse infants, sometimes up to three years. A full, firm, wide breast is the preferred ideal: it should be more rounded and heavy at the bottom, thick, and secure to the body with minimal jiggle or shake when a girl dances (Boone 1986). The Mende compare the breast to a calabash (tawa) in order to judge ideal size, shape, hardness, and function. Breasts should be wide enough to cover the entire surface of the chests, and erect, rounded breasts shaped like globes that are fully visible with no underside are considered the most beautiful. Most consider the breasts to be the most beautiful in women nursing their first or second child, before the breast has "fallen" or become flabby.

For the Mende, nipples are also an important signifier of beauty for the breast itself. The compound word for nipple, *nyini la wonde*, contains references to three other body parts: the breast itself, the term for mouth or opening where milk escapes, and the term for male foreskin, thereby designating the capacity of the nipple to become turgid and erect during sexual arousal as an analogue to the penis (Boone 1986). Another more poetic term for the nipple is *nyini la bowa*, which compares the "mouth of the breast" to the petals of a flower.

In north central Australia, in order to promote the growth of girls' breasts, aboriginal men have assembled and sung chants in order to charm the breasts to grow as part of a coming-of-age ceremony (Spencer and Gillen 1899). In the morning, the girl would appear before the men with her mother, and her body would be rubbed with fat and straight lines painted with red ochre down her back and the center of her chest and stomach. She would be anointed with certain necklets and head-rings in order to activate the magic charged with assisting her body into puberty (Spencer and Gillen 1899).

See also: Barbie; Body Modification; Corsets, Shapewear, and Waist Trainers; Décolletage; Fetish; Hourglass Shape; Japan; Male Gaze; Monroe, Marilyn; Sexy; United States.

Further Reading

Acker, Michele. 2009. "Breast Is Best . . . But Not Everywhere: Ambivalent Sexism and Attitudes Toward Private and Public Breastfeeding." *Sex Roles* 61, no. 7–8: 476–90.

Boone, Sylvia Arden. 1986. *Radiance from the Waters*. New Haven, CT: Yale University Press.

Downing, Sarah Jane. 2012. *Beauty and Cosmetics 1550–1950*. Oxford, England: Shire Publications.

Esco, Lina. 2014. *Free the Nipple*. Film. Directed by Lina Esco. Bethsabée Mucho/Disruptive Films/Emotion Pictures. http://freethenipple.com.

Miller, Laura. 2006. *Beauty Up. Exploring Contemporary Japanese Body Aesthetics*. Berkeley, CA: University of California Press.

Pacific Heights Plastic Surgery (PHPS). 2012. "Swimming in Breast Implants." Accessed October 3, 2016. https://www.pacificheightsplasticsurgery.com/breast-implant-statistics.

Spencer, Baldwin and F. J. Gillen. 1899. *The Native Tribes of North Central Australia*. Accessed September 15, 2016. http://www.sacred-texts.com/aus/ntca/ntca14.htm.

Walker, Harriet. 2016. "Grown-up Gowns Are Back Who Got It Right at the Globes." January 13. *Times, The (United Kingdom)*. Accessed October 14, 2016. *Newspaper Source*, EBSCOhost.

Young, Iris Marion. 1992. "Breasted Experience." In: *The Body in Medical Thought and Practice*, edited by Drew Leder, Boston: Kluwer, 215–30.

BRUNETTES AND BLACK HAIR

Combined, brown and black are the most two most common **hair** colors in the world. The color results from the degree of eumelanin in the chemical composition of the hair, responsible for the absorption of ultraviolet radiation from the sun. Less eumelanin in the hair shaft yields lighter-colored hair, common to those whose ancestors historically may have lived farther from the equator. Typically, people with brown hair are described as "brunette." Brunette hair can range from dark brown to light ash brown, with several shades in between. As with blonde hair, around the world there are differing values associated with brown or black hair and different cultural preferences for the shade and texture of people's locks.

For the Mende of West Africa, a woman's hair must always appear clean, smooth, shiny, well-groomed, and braided into a flattering style. Only a deep black color is acceptable to Mende aesthetics; for hair to appear brownish is thought to look dusty or dirty (Boone 1986). Because of this preference, both men and women of the Mende traditionally dye their hair a deep black using indigo dye obtained from the *njaa* plant (*Indigofera tinctoria*), although today commercial hair dye is also popular.

Women of the Indian subcontinent still practice beauty routines established centuries ago to maintained thick, shiny, dark-colored hair. A common technique for maintaining lustrous hair involves applying coconut oil to preserve and restore a proper moisture balance. Coconut oil prevents hair breakage due to dryness, so it is applied regularly. Women in **India** also avoid shampoo and instead cleanse their hair with a naturally astringent powder made from a seed pod from a fruit called *shikakai* (*Acacia concinna*). Many also believe that regular oil and *shikakai* treatments promote hair growth and delay the onset of gray hairs due to **aging.**

During the mid-1990s in **Japan**, a fad for brown hair (*chapatsu*) inspired both men and women to seek salon services to transform dark black hair to shades of mahogany or chocolate tones (Miller 2016). Dying in streaks of hair in a contrasting shade of gray and pink to accent the darker overall color of the hair was also a popular coloring technique in the early years of the millennium.

Though brunette is usually used to reference the hair color of women, the idiom of "tall, dark, and handsome" also describes ideal physical features for the "traditional" man desirable in Western culture. Where leading ladies of the classic Hollywood era were often blonde, leading men were typically dark-haired. The phrase "tall, dark, and handsome" appears to have first been used in print by novelist M. F. Dickson in 1815 in *Scenes on the Shores of the Atlantic*, though the expression and aesthetic appreciation of this type predates this language considerably (ELU 2011). Possibly, the idea of attractive dark-haired men can be traced to the Iberian occupation by the Moors, as seems to be indicated in Shakespeare's *Othello*.

In the catalog of classic American films, the brunette is often cast as the mild sidekick to the exciting blonde. One stereotype about brunettes, at least in the classic Hollywood era, was that brown hair revealed timidity and meekness. Brunettes were sometimes cast as mothers or matrons, or the "nice girl," who stood behind her more glamorous, dramatic blonde friend. Brunettes are also sometimes stereotyped as competent, intelligent, or reliable.

Another stereotype associated with brunettes is that of the dark-haired "vamp." Theda Bara, a film star during the flapper era, was famous for her sleek black bob, framed with thick bangs that fell seductively to her eyebrows. Bara also adopted dark kohl eyeliner and long fingernails to complement her mysterious, sensuous "femme fatale" look. Fashion icon and pinup model Bettie Page was another famous brunette who popularized a pageboy style with a thick fringe and combined it enticingly, often paired with swimwear worn with heels.

Brunette Elizabeth Taylor portrayed a series of seductive and sexually aggressive women during her film career. The iconic

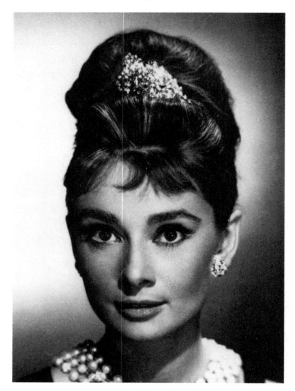

Actress Audrey Hepburn poses as Holly Golightly in the 1961 movie *Breakfast at Tiffany's*. (AP Photo)

brunette wig worn by superstar Taylor during the 1963 filming of *Cleopatra*, a stylized long bob with heavy bangs and braids topped off with heavy golden beads, sold for $16,000 at an auction in 2011 (Owoseje 2011). Nearly 50 different styles of wig made from brown human hair and 26,000 separate costumes were ordered by 20th Century Fox for *Cleopatra*, at the time the most expensive movie ever made.

Audrey Hepburn was another successful film brunette who inspired fashion and style for her era. Hepburn appealed to many women fans and imitators for her elegant simplicity. Her modesty also promoted a "girl next door" appeal that was attractive to both male and female fans. Her iconic hairstyles ranged from a simple ponytail, sometimes worn with bangs, to different versions of a chin-length bob, to a shoulder-length pageboy, sometimes coiled and piled in the bouffant style of the 1960s. As an older woman, Hepburn often wore her hair pulled back in a simple bun.

See also: Hair; India; Japan.

Further Reading

Boone, Sylvia Arden. 1986. *Radiance from the Waters: Ideals of Feminine Beauty in Mende Art*. New Haven, CT: Yale University Press.

English Language and Usage (ELU). 2011. *Stack Exchange*. March 22. Accessed August 15, 2016. http://english.stackexchange.com/questions/17332/whats-the-origin-of-the-stock-phrase-tall-dark-and-handsome.

Manning, Jodi. 2011. "The Sociology of Hair: Hair Symbolism among College Students." *Social Sciences Journal* 10, no. 1: article 11.

McCracken, Grant. 1995. *Big Hair: A Journey into the Transformation of Self*. Woodstock, NY: Overlook Press.

Miller, Laura. 2016. *Beauty Up: Exploring Contemporary Japanese Body Aesthetics*. Berkeley, CA: University of California Press.

Owoseje, Toyin. 2011. "Liz Taylor's Cleopatra Wig Sold at Auction for £10,300." December 13. *International Business Times*. Accessed August 15, 2016. http://www.ibtimes.co.uk/liz-taylor-s-cleopatra-wig-sold-auction-266465.

Sherrow, Victoria. 2006. *Encyclopedia of Hair: A Cultural History*. Westport, CT: Greenwood Press.

BUNDA

"Bunda" or "bumbum" are Brazilian terms for a woman's buttocks, a key part of the general Brazilian ideal of beauty. Often credited to the unique racial makeup of the Brazilian populace, an **hourglass** waist and large, round bottom, paired with small **breasts**, is often cited as the traditional Brazilian model of attractiveness in physical appearance for women (Edmonds 2010). The buttocks are so important an element of physical beauty in **Brazil** that a national pageant exists to name a "Miss Bumbum."

Part of this aesthetic ideal goes beyond the buttocks themselves. The traditional Brazilian preference is for women to have large round buttocks, but also curvy, rounded hips and thighs of a type that are significantly different from the stick-thin beauty ideal promoted by international supermodels such as Chrissy Teigen or Brazilian-born Gisele Bündchen.

Many cite the influence of African and afro-Brazilian culture in the creation of the racially mixed beauty ideal that includes the large *bunda*. Indeed, the preference of a racially mixed form of beauty is a key source of identity to many Brazilians. In 2007, the plastic surgeon Dr. Raul González claimed that "it is indisputable that the feminine bumbum is a national preference reflecting the diversity of ethnicities that compose the Brazilian population. There was a mixture of the exuberant forms of the bumbum of the black race with the slender body of the Aryan" (González 2007).

While 21st-century trends are seeing an increase in the ideal size of breasts in Brazil, the importance of the buttocks remains central to ideas of beauty. The actress and dancer, Carla Pérez, known popularly as the "Bunda Nacional" [National Bottom] in Brazil, credits her success to a physique that embodies the national ideal of beauty, from her bottom to the recent breast implants she received (Edmonds 2010).

In his research on Brazil, the anthropologist Alexander Edmonds calls the *bunda* the "national passion" of Brazilians and key to both male and female success. In interviews, he finds that both men and women find that "the attraction is the *bunda.*" (Edmonds 2010, 136). Many Brazilians see a clear link between attaining an attractively round bottom and both personal and professional success.

The pursuit for men and women of a shapely posterior leads to a variety of beauty work, from exercise, to injections, to plastic surgery. Many Brazilians take to the gyms to not only lose weight, but to engage in body sculpting to "thicken" and define their buttocks and thighs (Edmonds 2010, 136). Brazil is also the world leader in buttocks implant surgeries, having performed nearly 51,000 procedures in 2014 alone (ISAPS 2015).

Exercise and licensed implant surgery, however, are not the only avenues that men and women pursue in their quest for the perfect bottom. Illegal and unlicensed injections of silicone, cooking oil, and other substances are also unfortunately common, often resulting in serious complications. In 2015, the runner-up of the 2012 Miss BumBum pageant, television personality Andressa Urach, nearly died after suffering complications from injections of hydrogel, a substance not approved for that use (Haggerty 2015).

See also: Brazil; Buttocks Lifts and Implants; Butts and Booty; Injections; Plastic Surgery.

Further Reading

Edmonds, Alexander. 2010. *Pretty Modern: Beauty, Sex and Plastic Surgery in Brazil.* Durham, NC, Duke University Press.
González, Raúl. 2007. *Buttocks Reshaping.* Rio de Janeiro: Indexa.
Haggerty, Deidre. 2015. "Brazil's Miss BumBum Runner-Up Almost Dies after Bad Butt Enhancing Injections." Accessed November 19, 2015. http://www.examiner.com/article/brazil-s-miss-bumbum-runner-up-almost-dies-after-bad-butt-enhancing-injections.
ISAPS. 2015. "ISAPS International Survey on Aesthetic/Cosmetic Procedures Performed in 2014." Accessed November 20, 2015. http://www.isaps.org/Media/Default/globalstatistics/2015%20ISAPS%20Results.Pdf.

BURLESQUE

A type of fashion and entertainment that originally dates from the French and German cabarets of the 1920s, burlesque has made a resurgence as a popular style in the 21st century. Burlesque fashion, which is most often worn by women, is characterized by the use of lingerie and fetish apparel and by the playful display of female nudity. **Corsets**, garter belts, fishnet stockings, stiletto **heels**, and feathers are hallmarks of burlesque fashion. The performance and clothing associated with burlesque may be summarized as a "tease"—revealing enough to be provocative while not baring all (Packard and Minx 2015).

Historically, the fashion for striptease performances and styles that bared more female flesh grew from the erotic dances of Hindu culture in **India**, North African belly dancers, and snake dancers in **Brazil** (Ross 2009). These styles and ideas then influenced the development of erotic dancing in Europe and North America, and by the late 1800s, burlesque dancers were performing in bars and public venues such as the Chicago World's Fair and the famous Moulin Rouge in Paris (Turecamo 2015).

By the early 20th century, the burlesque style had gained great popularity. Bare-breasted and skimpily clad chorus line dancers, as well as individual performers, were hugely popular in vaudeville shows such as the Folies Bergère in France and the Ziegfeld Follies in New York City (Ross 2008). From the late 1800s through the 20th century, burlesque shows were designed to be playful, and at times comic, spaces where performers used exaggerated costumes, gestures, and jokes to make fun of society's rules, prudishness, and hypocrisy. The performance of burlesque was designed to be over the top and transgressive in the way it questioned social norms of sexuality, dress, and control of female nudity (Nally 2009).

One of the most common cultural references for burlesque is the Broadway show *Gypsy*, based on the 1957 memoir of the famous true-life artist Gypsy Rose Lee. This show, and the later film, showcased the post-WWII version of burlesque performance, in which the increased incomes and economic strength of U.S. and Canadian citizens helped fuel the market for striptease shows (Ross 2008). This period, sometimes called the "nightclub era," saw the performances move away from large theaters and into more intimate bar settings, combining the smaller space with ever more complex and elaborate performances. These performances were often "narrative" striptease, where the story being told was central to the performance and an element of the playfulness and comedy (Urish 2014).

While burlesque thrived for the decade of the post-war period, it was overtaken by the creation of the pornography industry in the

Moulin Rouge

The Moulin Rouge is a fabulously gaudy, risqué, and provocative French nightclub that has offered adult entertainment since the late 1800s. The club was founded in 1889 as both a dance and music hall and also as a brothel, with the high-end prostitutes offering dances as a display for their services. The can-can dance, in which women lift their skirts to showcase their legs, was invented for this purpose and was made famous by the paintings and prints of the French artist Toulouse Latrec. Since the 20th century, the Moulin Rouge has become synonymous with flamboyant costumes, decoration, and performance and has been the inspiration for more than 10 films, including *Moulin Rouge!* in 2001. In 2016 the club still operates as a dance hall and popular tourist attraction.

1960s with the launch of *Playboy* magazine and the creation of an erotic film industry. The style faded then until the end of the 20th century (Packard and Minx 2015).

Burlesque as a clothing style is often associated with the idea of "tasteful" nudity and celebration of playful female sexuality (Ross 2008). Clothing and fashion associated with the trend also often refer back to the model of 1930s French "can-can" style, featuring lacy corsets, tiered, ruffled skirts held aloft or cut higher in the front, and elaborate feathered or flowered headpieces (Packard and Minx 2015).

Burlesque began a revival and resurgence in popularity in the late 20th century when troupes of burlesque performers began touring the **United States**, Canada, and **Great Britain**. These groups performed a stylish, high-concept form of performance with live orchestras accompanying the choreographed dancing and strip-tease displays. Beyond the music, however, the costumes and clothing continued to be an essential element of the display of female nudity. The use of exotic lingerie-like pasties and g-strings combined with feathers and sequins in these shows teased the viewer without baring all (Ross 2008).

The 20th- and 21st-century versions of burlesque (sometimes referred to as "neo-burlesque") are also notable in the way that the style is considered inclusive of a wide range of ages and body types. At first glance, it is easy to note the prevalence of curvy, voluptuous performers among the most famous burlesque dancers, a body style that stands in strict contrast to the very thin models preferred in the same time period by high-fashion magazines and global designers. The modern inclusiveness goes beyond simple preference for curvier dancers, however. Burlesque troupes of women aged 50 to 80 perform popular shows, and in Canada, wheelchair burlesque has opened up the genre for those with some physical disability (Burgmann 2016).

In the 21st century, burlesque as a style and fashion choice has been making an increasingly big comeback. In the United States, a high-profile Hollywood film starring Cher and Christina Aguilera, called *Burlesque*, was released. In addition, in nations such as Great Britain young designers are fashioning whole lines of clothing

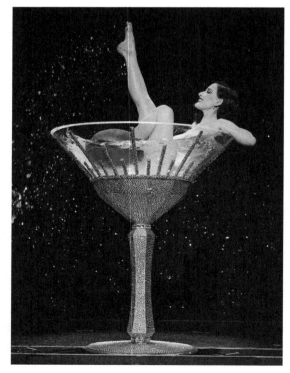

Dita Von Teese appears on stage in her signature martini glass at "Burlesque: Strip Strip Hooray!" in Los Angeles, June 21, 2013. (Todd Williamson/Invision/AP Photo)

based on the burlesque aesthetic, and the annual "Dirty Red Ball," a masquerade that encouraged participants to dress in burlesque attire, drew a high-profile crowd of participants in London (Associated Press 2008).

In the world of burlesque performance and style, Dita Von Teese is perhaps the best known and most famous contemporary celebrity. Von Teese, known sometimes as the "Burlesque Superheroine," is credited for helping to repopularize burlesque performance and fashion. She is particularly famous for her performances of old-fashioned, narrative striptease dances, which typically culminate in immersing herself in an oversized champagne or martini glass (Associated Press 2008).

In 2016, there were many U.S. and international competitions designed to showcase neo-burlesque performers, from burlesque festivals in Las Vegas, Austin, and Denver, to competitions such as "Miss Viva Las Vegas" or "Miss Exotic World." In 2011, the Burlesque Hall of Fame, celebrating the tradition and showcasing many costumes, opened in New Orleans, Louisiana (Burlesque Hall of Fame 2016).

See also: Corsets, Shapewear, and Waist Trainers; Fetish; High Heels; India; United Kingdom.

Further Reading

Associated Press (Producer). 2008. "Burlesque Increasingly Fashionable in the UK" [Streaming video]. Retrieved from Associated Press Video Collection database July 11, 2016.

Burgmann, Tamryn. 2016. "Wheelchair Burlesque Strips Down Stigma." May 12. *Toronto Star (Canada)* Accessed October 14, 2016. http://www.theglobeandmail.com/news /british-columbia/wheelchair-burlesque-aims-to-   strip-down-stigma-sex-up-disability/ article29987021/.

Burlesque Hall of Fame. 2016. "About." Accessed July 11, 2016. http://www.burlesquehall .com/category/exhibitions.

Nally, Claire. 2009. "Grrrly Hurly Burly: Neo-Burlesque and the Performance of Gender." *Textual Practice* 23, no. 4: 621–43.

Packard, Morgan and Trixie Minx. 2015. "Burlesque." *New Orleans Magazine* 49, no. 12: 56.

Ross, Becki. 2009. *Burlesque West: Showgirls, Sex and Sin in Postwar Vancouver*. Toronto: University of Toronto Press, Scholarly Publishing Division.

Turecamo, David. 2015. "The History of the Can-Can." CBS News. Accessed July 11, 2015. http://www.cbsnews.com/news/the-history-of-the-cancan.

Urish, Ben. 2014. "Narrative Striptease in the Nightclub Era." *Journal of American Culture* 27, no. 2: 157–65.

BURQA

In 2015, presidential candidate Donald Trump asserted that Islamic women prefer to wear the burqa so that they do not have to trouble themselves with wearing makeup (Schleifer 2015). Trump's statement reveals profound misunderstandings in the Western world about women, beauty standards, veiling, and Islam. As with all cultural practices, veiling and the use of the burqa is a complex, historically grounded practice that is not the same in all cultures, nations, or time periods.

Because of this, it is crucial to consider the lived experiences of women and to resist the urge to make big generalizations about their identity based only on a visible garment.

Across India, the Middle East, and North Africa, traditional cultures have been engaging in strict behavioral taboos that anthropologists classify as "honor-shame" taboos well before the onset of Islam. Within these traditions, the behavior of individuals was expected to match with rigid gendered guidelines that reflected upon the reputation of the entire family lineage. Not surprisingly, many of the standards for honor and shame revolved around standards for proper gendered and sexual behavior. Any deviations from these norms, especially concerning the virginity or sexual purity of young women (or even a rumor or suggestion that proper behavior had not been observed), could result in shame and dishonor falling upon the entire family (Shirazi 2001).

These allegations could demand dire consequences from the family in order to "save" face in the community, including "honor killings," where the accused young woman was put to death. Many honor-shame cultures require the observation of *purdah*, the seclusion of women, in order to maintain the sexual purity of unmarried women and to avoid the possibility that the family's honor could be called into question by the inappropriate behavior of a woman. (The word "burqa" is an Arabized version of the Persian word "parda," which means curtain or veil.) Veiling is a part of this tradition: by shielding the woman from the gaze of unrelated men, women are both symbolically and literally protected from any potentially sexual, lewd, or untoward behaviors. Veiling was designed not only to protect the woman, but perhaps more importantly, veiling ensured the wealth, status, and honor of the family name (Goldman 2016).

> "I remember when the wave of Jennifer Lopez, Salma Hayek and these beautiful Hispanic women came into light, and I looked up to them and I loved them, but I was like, 'Where are Middle Eastern women?'"
>
> —KIM KARDASHIAN

Within Islam, according to Qu'ranic scripture, women are expected to dress modestly in public. Veiling is a part of this expectation, though the range of veiling options expected of women varies according to the culture. *Hijab* is a form of veiling that covers the hair of the woman, usually with a headscarf. Niqāb is a form of veiling that covers the entire face but leaves openings for the eyes to see without obstruction. Burqas are veils that cover both the face and the body worn by Muslim women and represent the most extreme form of veiling in the contemporary world, typically associated in the West with oppressive Islamist regimes that favor militarism. A panel of netting at eye level allows women to see out. The burqa of Afghanistan, light blue in color, is locally called a *chadri* and was rarely worn in public prior to the rise of the Taliban, when it became mandated in public (Goldman 2016).

However, women are not obliged to wear the burqa within their own homes or in the presence of close family members. In her 2007 book about post-war Kabul,

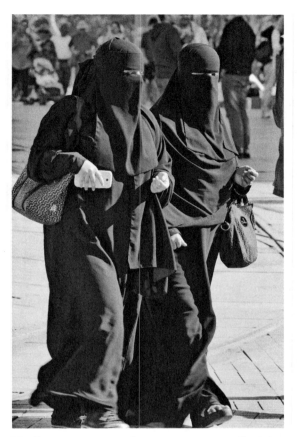

Muslim women wear burqas to preserve feminine modesty while appearing in public, Istanbul, Turkey. (Meunierd/Dreamstime.com)

Deborah Rodriguez highlights how valuable beauty practices remain to women who are living lives of extreme deprivation. She argues that for these women who have enrolled in her unusual "beauty school," maintaining control of their looks is one of the only options available to them in a cataclysmic world. Women who come to her salon to learn to be beauticians spend the day perfecting beauty practices on themselves and each other and shroud themselves in burqas to leave the female-only space and head back to their homes in Kabul. The only people who see them and the results of their exertions are other members of the beauty school and their husbands (Rodriguez 2007).

Today, extreme forms of veiling through the use of the burqa have become an increasingly politicized issue. The republic of France has long been concerned with secularity and discouraging the display of conspicuous religious symbols in civic space. In 2010, France banned face coverings in public spaces, including masks, helmets, balaclava, niqāb, and the burqa. The French National Assembly supported this decision by arguing that these types of face coverings pose a significant security risk because they do not allow for clear identification of a person and also represents a social hindrance within the society, as it does not allow expression in communication and civic life. Exceptions to the ban allow women to wear the burqa while traveling in a private car or while worshiping in a religious place (BBC 2014).

Opponents of the legislation argue that the ban encroaches on individual and religious freedoms. Debates about the burqa continue in other Western countries too. In 2011, a poll in the United Kingdom revealed that 66 percent of British people favored legislation to ban the burqa in public places. In 2015, the Netherlands passed a law banning burqas in some public places, including public transportation, educational institutions, public health facilities, and government buildings. Additionally, Dutch police reserve the right to request that wearers remove the burqa for identification purposes at any time (BBC 2014).

See also: The "Other."

Further Reading

BBC. 2014. "The Veil Across Europe." Accessed October 14, 2016. http://www.bbc.com /news/world-europe- 13038095.

Goldman, Russell. 2016. What's That You're Wearing? A Guide to Muslim Veils. May 3. *New York Times,* Accessed May 5, 2016. http://www.nytimes.com/2016/05/04/world /what-in-the-world/burqa-hijab-abayachador.html?smid=fbnytimes&smtyp=cursmvar =witw1&_r=1.

Kaukab, Samar. 2016. A Review of New York Times "What's That You're Wearing? A Guide to Muslim Veils. AltMuslimah. May 4. Accessed May 5, 2016. http://www.altmuslimah .com/2016/05/review-nyts-whats-youre-wearing-guide-muslim-veils/.

Mcafee, Tierney. 2015. "Donald Trump's Take on Women Wearing Burkas. 'It's Easy— You Don't Have to Wear Makeup.'" October 28, 2015. *People Magazine* [Web site]. Accessed May 5, 2016. http://www.people.com/article/donald-trump-women-burkas -makeup.

Rodriguez, Deborah. 2007. *Kabul Beauty School: An American Woman Goes Behind the Veil.* New York: Random House.

Schleifer, Theodore. 2015. "Donald Trump's Take on Burka's: Islamic Women Might Prefer Them." *CNN* [Web site]. October 26. Accessed May 5, 2016. http://www.cnn.com/2015 /10/26/politics/donald-trump-burkas-new-hampshire.

Shirazi, Faegheh. 2001. *The Veil Unveiled: The Hijab in Modern Culture.* Gainesville, FL: University of Florida Press.

BUTTOCKS LIFTS AND IMPLANTS

Most popular in nations where the beauty ideal for women includes a round bottom, buttocks implants are a surgical procedure designed to help women achieve that ideal. The implants, also known as gluteal implants, are designed to "improve the size and appearance of the buttocks by placing silicone implants under, in between or above the gluteal muscle producing a cosmetic enhancement" (IASPS 2015).

The nation where the majority of these procedures is performed is **Brazil**, a country with a specific beauty ideal attached to the bottom, or *bunda*. In Brazil, the appearance of a woman's buttocks is so central to the ideal of beauty that a specific national beauty pageant is held every year to select a national "Miss BumBum." In 2014, more than 50,000 buttocks implant procedures were performed in Brazil, compared to only 19,000 in the United States.

Another type of procedure, known as a "butt lift," often involves analogous fat transfer, or lipofilling, where fat from a person's own body is removed and injected into another area of a that person's body. In the case of a butt lift, the necessary fat is suctioned out via **liposuction** and reinjected into the buttocks (Jacobson 2015).

The popularity of the procedure in the United States is growing, however, in part due to the shift in body ideals presented by celebrity beauty icons. **Butt** lifts still outpace butt implants among U.S. patients, who are mostly women. In the United Kingdom, however, surgeons report that more men are seeking buttocks implants in the 21st century (Samson 2012).

A standard buttocks implant procedure in a licensed surgeon's office takes between one and two hours and must be performed under general anesthesia. The surgery can be done as an outpatient procedure, but often requires a hospital stay. After the surgery, the patient must not sit for at least 72 hours and should only stand or lie on the back to avoid both pain and displacement of the implants. Patients must also wear tight clothing on the buttocks and use special devices to sit for the first two weeks. The risks associated with approved butt implants can be serious, including the formation of painful scar tissue, rupture of the implant, or life-threatening infection (ISAPS 2015).

While the placement of silicone implants in the buttocks is the medically improved way to increase the size and shape of the buttocks for women, an unfortunate fact is that some transgendered persons seeking to transition to female undergo unsafe procedures to achieve this effect. Worldwide, unlicensed practitioners often inject a range of substances into individuals seeking to create the same effect as silicone implants. Silicone, glue, and other substances have been known to be injected into those who, for whatever reason, do not have access to the licensed implant procedure.

A review of police and media records in many nations shows that these dangerous procedures can happen at beauty salons, illegal storefront clinics, and events known as "butt-pumping parties," where participants line up to have the practitioner inject them (Samson 2012). The side effects and medical dangers of these injections can be severe, from infections and cancer to even death.

The danger and cost of the unapproved substances became more public in Brazil in 2015, when a former "Miss Bumbum" runner-up in Brazil nearly died of infection and septic shock after receiving injections of hydrogel, a chemical substance not officially approved in Brazil or the United States (AP 2015).

See also: Brazil; Bunda; Butts and Booty; Injections; Plastic Surgery.

Further Reading

Associated Press (AP). 2015. "Brazil Miss Bum Bum Contestant's Botched Plastic Surgery Sheds Light on Cosmetic Procedure Dangers." Accessed November 19, 2015. http://www.nydailynews.com/news/world/brazil-bum-bum-botched-plastic-surgery-shows-dangers-article-1.2095071.

ISAPS. 2015. "Buttocks Implants." Accessed November 17, 2015. http://www.isaps.org/procedures/buttocks-implants.

Jacobson, Sherry. 2015. "Buttock Procedures Can't Be Taken Lightly, Doctors Say." *Dallas Morning News, The (TX)*. March 20.

Miss BumBum. 2015. "*Com destaque para miss Bumbum Evangélica, imprensa internacional noticia chegada de fim da competição e a marca de 2 milhões de votos.*" Accessed November 10, 2015. http://missbumbumbrasil.com.br/com-destaque-para-miss-bumbum-evangelica-imprensa-internacional-noticia-chegada-de-fim-da-competicao-e-a-marca-de-2-milhoes-de-votos/.

Samson, Peter. 2012. "'Booty Butcher' Arrested at Butt-Pump Party." March 2. Accessed October 14, 2016. https://www.thesun.co.uk/archives/news/416454/booty-butcher-arrested-at-butt-pump-party/.

BUTTS AND BOOTY

In a study of eighteen different cultures, evolutionary psychologist Devendra Singh tested men's preference for body shape in women. His findings revealed an overwhelming preference for a narrow waist and a large, round bottom with wide hips

(Singh 1993). Evolutionary psychologists argue that a pervasive preference for a wide and round rear end can be explained by the male drive to procreate and his desire to select a mate who will bear many children. Narrow waists with full hips and bottoms signal high fertility, high estrogen, and low testosterone, all strong indicators of a woman's ability to bear children (Etcoff 2000).

Perhaps because of the deep connections between rounded hips and buttocks and sexual attraction, the butt has been a sexually attractive element of consideration and appreciation in painting, photography, and modeling for centuries. As an element of the appearance of a woman that signals both femininity and eroticism, the backside is a key aspect of physical beauty.

Ancient Greek and Roman statues from as early as the BCE second century show how artists have showcased women's butts in sculpture and painting, a trend that continues through the present day. The significant attention to the single body part, placed front and center in art, draped decoratively, and in modern times, described in song, is part of a widespread fetishism of the female backside (Dopp 2011). Twenty-first-century songs such as Sir Mix-a-Lot's "Baby Got Back," in which the rapper waxes poetic about the beauty of women's rear ends are just one example of the focus on the sexual attractiveness of the body part (Sir Mix-A-Lot 1992).

This ongoing phenomenon of the identification and self-identification of women, and especially women of color, by singular body parts can be problematic and reductive. The most famous example of this is Saartjie "Sarah" Baartman, a Khoikhoi woman born in 1790 in the Dutch colony of what is now South Africa, who came to be known as the "Hottentot Venus." Accompanied by the entrepreneurial showman Hendrik Cesars, Baartman was exhibited publicly across Europe between 1811 and 1815 in the equivalent of a "freak show" to the delight and disgust of audiences. Baartman's display linked the notion of the wild or savage female with dangerous, uncontrollable sexuality, evidenced by her generous buttocks, which had become a clear symbol of female sexuality by the middle part of the century (Fausto-Sterling 1995, 31). She died, possibly of smallpox, in 1815 at the age of 25.

Baartman's genitals (characterized by stretching) and generous backside (sometimes referred to as "steatopygia," from the root words for fat and buttocks) were so fascinating to scientists that she was dissected by a distinguished "father" of modern biology, Georges Cuvier (Fausto-Sterling 1995). Baartman's genitalia were preserved for further study after her death and continued to be on display until the mid-1970s. The emerging field of physiological science of the Victorian era equated notions of the "noble savage," or those outside of the conventions of the "civilized" world, to be closer to nature and created considerable excitement about the possibility of the Hottentot as the "missing link" theorized by Aristotle's Great Chain of Being (Hobson 2005, 29). The tragedy of Sarah Baartman's sad life and early demise is that she was evaluated, judged, identified, and racialized according to racist curiosity about her body parts, and she clearly had no choice in the matter (Henderson 2014). Women in the 21st century, however, although finding themselves also evaluated by their individual physical features, can exercise some agency to leverage that focus in order to achieve some practical and strategic goals.

One example discussed by many is that of the 21st-century pop artists Nicki Minaj and Jennifer López, two women celebrated for their behinds. Minaj has a clothing line specifically designed to be curve hugging and "fit all body types," and is clear in how she recognizes the power of her butt in songs such as "Anaconda," which samples Sir Mix-A-Lot's earlier song (Minaj 2014). Other celebrities, including Kim Kardashian and Jennifer Lopez, are also associated with large butts. Lopez, the highest-paid Latina actress ever, maintains that her large rear end "is a sign of identity and pride . . . a 'kiss my ass' as a form of revenge against a hostile cultural gaze, and 'I'm going to kick your ass'" by making money in the same system that is trying to keep her down (Negrón-Muntaner 1997).

In the contemporary United States, tension between racialized **fetishism**, exploitation, and self-identification is strong. Attention on the "butt" is often a substitution for race, though mainstream discussions may avoid such blunt terms (Barrera 2000, 412). For women who are seeking success within the structure that seeks to identify them only by a certain part of their anatomy, it can be challenging to rebrand or skewer racist images and the system's power to force those images on female artists.

See also: BBW; Brazil; Bunda; Buttocks Lifts and Implants; Fetish; Hourglass Shape; Injections; Pageants—International, National, and Local Contests; Plastic Surgery; Supermodels.

Further Reading

Barrera, Magdalena. 2000. "Hottentot 2000: Jennifer Lopez and Her Butt." In: *Sexualities in History*, edited by Kim M. Phillips and Barry Reay. New York: Routledge, 407–17.

Dopp, Hans-Jurgen. 2011. *In Praise of the Backside*. New York: Parkstone International.

Etcoff, Nancy. 2000. *Survival of the Prettiest: The Science of Beauty*. New York: Anchor.

Fausto-Sterling, Anne. 1995. "Gender Race, and Nation: The Comparative Anatomy of 'Hottentot' Women in Europe, 1815–1817." In: *Deviant Bodies*, edited by Jacqueline Urla and Jennifer Terry. Bloomington, IN: Indiana University Press, 19–48.

Henderson, Carol E. 2014. "AKA: Sarah Baartman, The Hottentot Venus, and Black Women's Identity." *Women's Studies* 43, no. 7: 946–59.

Hobson, Janelle. 2005. *Venus in the Dark: Blackness and Beauty in Popular Culture*. New York: Routledge.

Minaj, Nicki. 2014. "Anaconda." Song. Young Money/Cash Money Records. Accessed August 22, 2016. https://www.youtube.com/watch?v=LDZX4ooRsWs.

Negrón-Muntaner, Frances. 1997. "Jennifer's Butt." *Aerlán* 22: 189.

Press, Julie E. 2004. "Cute Butts and Housework: A Gynocentric Theory of Assortative Mating." *Journal of Marriage and Family* 66, no. 4: 1029–33.

Singh, Davendra. 1993. "Adaptive Significance of Female Physical Attractiveness: Role of a Waist-to-Hip Ratio." *Journal of Personality and Social Psychology* 65: 293–307.

Sir Mix-A-Lot. 1992. "Baby Got Back." Song. Def American. Accessed August 22, 2016. https://www.youtube.com/watch?v=kY84MRnxVzo.

C

THE CARIBBEAN

Most nations of the Caribbean entered the 20th century in a state of tension between centuries-old colonial ideas of European superiority and nascent ideas of the value of native and African culture. Whether the former colonies of Britain, Spain, France, Holland, or the territories affected by U.S. influence, these dynamic, changing ideas of heritage and worth affect images and ideals of beauty across the islands of the region.

Nations such as Jamaica, Trinidad, Cuba, the Dominican Republic, and Barbados were, until the mid-to-late 1800s, colonies of European nations that held Afro-descended people as slaves and controlled the power, wealth, and governmental structure of the islands. The governmental and social structure of the Caribbean islands was, by and large, plantocratic—large plantations of sugar, bananas, or other crops owned by a small number of elite, Euro-descended, white families who controlled large numbers of African and Afro-descended slaves. Even after the abolition of slavery, the population of Afro-descended peoples far outnumbered the amount of white landowners, though those landowning families continued to run and control the island nations (Klein 1986).

This control of the islands and the institutions that were put in place in the plantocracy were important elements in the early creation of the idea of national identity. The elite landowners sought to portray the aspirational identity as white and rich, dismissing or diminishing the contributions and lives of the former slaves. This preference is evident in the values placed on elements of appearance. Centuries of hierarchical privilege for European whiteness naturally found its way into preferences for elements of a "white" appearance (Barnes 2006).

Early 20th-century beauty pageants across the Caribbean were specific vehicles for reinforcing the social norms of beauty that privileged a European appearance of light skin, soft and flowing hair, and light-colored eyes. Indeed, in nations such as Jamaica, contests existed to give prizes to women with the "best eyes"—prizes that were never awarded to women with brown or black eyes (Barnes 2006). The routine selection of blonde-haired, blue-eyed women as Miss Jamaica or Miss Barbados helped solidify the European ideal of beauty in the Caribbean through the 20th century.

In the 1960s, enthusiasm over independence and nationalism across Jamaica raised the question, especially in a postcolonial context, "How do young people perceive their bodies and physical beauty in relation to their skin color?" In 1955, ten separate beauty contests were held under the title "Ten Types—One People" in Jamaica. Each winner represented an ideal for each specific skin tone, including

Miss Apple Blossom, Miss Allspice, and Miss Ebony. In a 1960s study of Kingston high school–aged students, researchers found that across ethnic groups, there was a remarkable standardization of beauty. Members of each group preferred physical features that included a straight nose, "fair" or "clear" (but not "white") skin, and straight hair (Miller 1969).

Despite widely publicized notions that female fatness has historically been a "potent generator of male heterosexual desire" in geographic areas where women's **weight** could be read as an indicator of economic well-being, some ethnographic evidence shows that this preference is beginning to change (Shaw 2012, 140). At least in the context of 21st-century dance-hall music, new male narratives of desire suggest that "fatness is a degenerative condition that diminishes a woman's sexual appeal" (Shaw 2012, 145).

Possibly due to the location of the **male gaze** outside the Caribbean in an era of global media, dance-hall lyrics aggressively demand remedy to the toxicity of fat and a rising imperative for toned slenderness. Accordingly, **liposuction** has quickly become the most requested **plastic surgery** procedure in Jamaica (Shaw 2012). The current demand for cosmetic surgery in Jamaica extends far beyond the country's capacity to deliver these services.

See also: "Black Is Beautiful Movement," or Black Power; Liposuction; Plastic Surgery; Skin Whitening; Weight.

Further Reading

Barnes, Natasha. 2006. *Cultural Conundrums: Gender, Race, Nation, and the Making of Caribbean Cultural Politics*. Ann Arbor, MI: University of Michigan Press.

Klein, Herbert S. 1986. *African Slavery in Latin America and the Caribbean*. New York: Oxford University Press.

Miller, Errol. 1969. "Body Image, Physical Beauty, and Colour among Jamaican Adolescents." *Social and Economic Studies* 18, no. 2: 72–89.

Rowe, Rochelle. 2009. "Glorifying the Jamaican Girl: The Ten Types—One People Beauty Contest, Racialized Femininities, and Jamaican Nationalism." *Radical History Review* 103: 36–58.

Shaw, Andrea. 2012. "Tuck in Yuh Belly": Imperatives of Female Slenderness in Jamaican Dancehall Music." *Fat Studies* 1: 140–152.

CHEMICAL PEELS AND FILLERS

Both chemical peels and fillers are treatments designed to enhance the appearance of facial skin. After botulism toxin (or **Botox**), hyaluronic acid and chemical peels are the most common nonsurgical cosmetic procedures performed around the world. Whereas chemical peels remove layers of skin, decreasing lines and **wrinkles**, fillers increase the size, firmness, and fullness of skin.

Fillers are injectable substances that are used to improve the appearance of skin by making it look more hydrated and plumper. According to the International Society of Aesthetic and Plastic Surgery (ISAPS), fillers are used to replace volume under the skin to fill wrinkles or enhance facial features (ISAPS 2016b). The most common filler agent used worldwide is hyaluronic acid. Hyaluronic acid works by binding moisture to skin cells, making them appear plumper. Hyaluronic acid can be injected into the skin, and often the lips, but can also be used in a cream or lotion that is applied topically to the skin. Hyaluronic acid is often combined with other materials naturally occurring in the body, making it a lower-risk procedure, but meaning that the results are not permanent (Lipham and Melicher 2015).

Hyaluronic acid **injections** are low-risk outpatient procedures that take less than an hour. After botulism toxin, hyaluronic acid injection is the second most common nonsurgical medical cosmetic procedure performed worldwide, with more than 2 million treatments given in 2015. The United States, Brazil, Japan, and South Korea all performed more than 150,000 hyaluronic acid injections in 2015 (ISAPS 2016c).

Chemical peels are a nonsurgical medical procedure designed to improve the appearance and texture of the skin, usually on the face of the patient. According to the ISAPS, chemical peels use a chemical solution to peel away the top layers of the skin in order to improve the appearance of wrinkled, blemished, unevenly pigmented, or sun-damaged faces (ISAPS 2016a).

Chemical peels are most often an outpatient procedure that takes approximately an hour to two hours. The two most common forms of peel are the TCA and phenol peel. In the TCA peel, practitioners use a solution of trichloroacetic acid (TCA), mixed with a lotion or mud, which is applied to the face and produces a sloughing reaction, causing layers of skin to peel off. This procedure may be done by an aesthetician or beautician, but typically those practitioners will only use a 20 percent TCA solution. A physician will put the patient under anesthesia and apply up to a 35 percent TCA solution. The stronger level of acid is more painful and takes longer to heal, but removes more fine lines and brown spots (Held 2014).

Phenol peels use a form of carbolic acid to achieve the same results as the TCA peels, though in a stronger and more penetrating way. Because of this some physicians recommend phenol because deeper and more long-lasting effects can be achieved. A phenol peel can reduce the appearance of **acne** scars or deeper wrinkles (Petrou 2006). Indeed, because the phenol may peel off much more of the skin, some doctors who perform phenol peels insist that patients must be ready for the unattractive appearance of their face for up to a month after the procedure. Post–phenol peel faces are bright red and may have a blistered appearance until the skin is healed, which may take several weeks (Petrou 2006). Full-face phenol peels may even require hospital admission for a short time (ISAPS 2016a).

Both types of chemical peel work best on fair, thin skin with only superficial wrinkles. Both procedures carry similar side effects or dangers, as well. The risks for both kinds of chemical peel include infection, scarring, flare-up of skin allergies, and cold sores. In addition, a full phenol peel carries the risk of producing permanent abnormal color changes, a permanent loss of color in the face, or the loss of the ability to tan (ISAPS 2016a).

Despite the risks, chemical peels are relatively common worldwide. In 2015, the ISAPS reported that almost half a million chemical peels were performed throughout the world, making the procedure the third most common nonsurgical treatment after botulism toxin and hyaluronic acid. The **United States** and Japan were the nations with the most recorded chemical peel procedures (ISAPS 2016c).

See also: Acne; Botox; Injections; Plastic Surgery; United States.

Further Reading

Held, Shari. 2014. "Preferred Procedures." *Indianapolis Monthly* 37, no. 9: 89.

ISAPS. 2016a. "Chemical Peels." Accessed June 13, 2016. http://www.isaps.org/procedures
/chemical-peels.

ISAPS. 2016b. "Fillers" Accessed June 13, 2016. http://www.isaps.org/procedures/dermal
-fillers.

ISAPS. 2016c. "Global Statistics." Accessed June 13, 2016. http://www.isaps.org/Media
/Default/global-statistics/2015%20ISAPS%20Results.pdf.

Lipham, William J., and Jill S. Melicher. 2015. *Cosmetic and Clinical Applications of Botox
and Dermal Fillers: Third Edition*. Thorofare, NJ: SLACK Incorporated.

Petrou, Ilya. 2006. "Chemical Lift with a Phenol Peel." *Dermatology Times* 27, no. 11 (November): 84.

CHINA

Chinese history spans thousands of years and offers many examples of beauty work and beauty ideals. From the imperial dynasties of thousands of years ago to the present day, beauty and appearance form an important part of Chinese culture.

Chinese folklore recounts tales of Four Beauties of ancient China renowned for their beauty. These women lived hundreds of years apart, and each of their heart-breaking stories has been embellished and retold for generations. Xi Shi (also Hsi Shih, whose name is synonymous with "beauty" in China) lived in the fifth century BCE and was believed to be so beautiful that when she looked at a reflection of herself in the water, the fish forgot how to swim and sank to the bottom of the pool. Xi Shi was part of a tribute from a defeated king to a warlord. Her beauty and kindness inspired the warlord to abandon his plans of military domination. Instead he constructed Guanwa Palace (The Palace of Beautiful Women). Later, his army was defeated, and the warlord committed suicide. Legend says that the beautiful Xi Shi, who once charmed fish, later drowned in the Huansha River.

The second of the Four Beauties, Wang Zhaojun, lived during the Han Dynasty in the first century BCE. Born when her father was very old, she enjoyed a childhood of indulgence as "a pearl in his palm." As an adventurous young woman, Wang Zhao-jun entered the harem of Emperor Yuan, where she quickly volunteered to leave the Han Empire to serve as a tribute to the Xiongnu government, located far to the north in the grasslands. On her journey north by horseback, it is said that she was so beautiful that geese who glimpsed her loveliness forgot how to fly and fell from the sky. She had several children with the leader of the Xiongnu, who was charmed by her beauty.

Later in Chinese history, similar stories surround a woman named Diaochan, a woman who was so beautiful that it was said the moon turned away in embarrassment at her loveliness. In Chinese culture Diaochan is a composite of several fictional characters and also a cautionary tale about the potential dangers of being too beautiful. Her tragic story is memorialized in a famous classic Chinese novel (*Romance of the Three Kingdoms* by Luo Guanzhong) written sometime between 1330 and 1400. As a young woman, Diaochan found herself betrothed to the much older, tyrannical warlord Dong Zhuo. Aware of her beauty and allure, Diaochan persuaded her handsome young lover, Lü Bu, to resist Dong Zhuo, his foster father. The ensuing sexual jealousy created betrayals, suicide, and murder. The story of this heartless, beautiful woman has been told over and over in songs, poems, operas, and most recently, a popular Chinese television series.

The most recent of the legendary Chinese Four Beauties, Yang Guifei (also Yang Kuei-fei), lived from 719 to 756 and was the celebrated consort of Emperor Xuanzong during the Tang Dynasty. Her face was compared to the beauty of flowers, and her body was celebrated for being full-figured and fleshy with large breasts and rounded curves, considered attractive feminine qualities of the era. Originally arranged as a consort for his son, the emperor found Yang Guifei so enchanting that he took her as his own lover. As a tribute to her singular beauty, the emperor forbade all other women in the kingdom to wear pink jade (Harris 2004).

Yang Guifei spent lavishly and enjoyed the finer things in life, including beautiful clothing and jewels. She succumbed to an attraction to a young general of Turkish origin called An Lushan, whom she initially adopted as her legal son but allegedly took as a lover. Through a series of misunderstandings and miscommunications during a military defeat to the traitorous An Lushan and a mutiny of the Imperial Guard, the soldiers of the army forced the emperor to have his beloved concubine strangled because of her family's role in the uprising. Seized by remorse, the emperor spent the rest of his life and much of his fortune trying to contact Yang Guifei in the afterlife. In legends, a Taoist priest was said to able to contact her and brought back half of a golden hair comb to the bereaved Xuanzong. The palace of Emperor Xuanzong at Huaqing Hot Springs is now a tourist attraction, where visitors can glimpse Yang Guifei's private bath, originally rimmed in pink jade, and an outline of her right hand etched in stone.

In ancient times, both men and women took great care with their skin and personal odors, cultivating elaborate bathing routines. Women routinely removed all of their body hair and remade their complexions as to be as light as possible with rice powder, colored their cheeks with red powder (sometimes made of cinnabar), and sported sharply arched eyebrows, painted on with blackened grease (Louie 2002).

Hair was also a consideration for beauty practices. Men shaved most of their head, leaving a long ponytail that was occasionally bound up into an elaborate top knot. Women preferred to grow their **hair** as long as possible and to dress it into elaborate styles. Occasionally, women of means also made use of wigs to enhance their coiffure. Most of the hairstyles were set with oils or wax and affixed using combs, hair sticks, and other hair ornaments. Some of this hair **jewelry** was heavily decorated. The Chinese Fakien the custom of triangular hairpins was banned during the 1920s. These massively long hair sticks were originally used to keep the hair tidily in place; however, in times of crisis, these hair pins could also be used as lethal darts. Wealthy women at court during the T'ang Dynasty adorned their hair with ornaments known as *buyao*. Some ancient love stories discuss how hair pins were cherished gifts given by lovers: when they were parted, they sometimes split the pin, to be restored upon the reunification of the lovers (Cultural China 2015).

During the Shang Dynasty, feminine beauty became closely linked with extremely small feet. From childhood, women trained their feet to grow so that the bottom of the heel joined the bottom of the toes. Frequently, the instep was intentionally broken and tightly bound to conform to this aesthetically pleasing standard of **body modification.** Feet were coaxed into tiny, pointed slippers that were celebrated for their degree of daintiness and did not allow the woman to place her weight on the sole of her foot. Although the small feet were undoubtedly considered to be an attractive form of **fetish** in many ways, the practical implication of the practice was to keep women immobile and dependent. The practice of footbinding lasted for hundreds of years until it was finally outlawed in 1928 (Levi 1966).

In 1949, with the formation of the current People's Republic of China and the end of the Chinese Revolution, traditional attitudes about family, gender, and beauty transformed almost overnight. Communist leaders preferred simplicity in dress and personal grooming, and they regarded the excesses of materialistic beauty culture as incompatible with their communalistic values. The party celebrated plain and natural-looking people. However, with the rise of the Asian market in recent years, China registers a large and growing market in the consumption of Western **cosmetics** and grooming products, many of which are imported.

One area in which the demand for global products is evident in China is in the 21st-century rise in the prevalence of cosmetic surgery. Whereas in pre-1980s China, **plastic surgery** was looked down on as a sign of bourgeoisie decadence, in the late 20th and early 21st centuries, consumption of both cosmetics and cosmetic surgery are seen as indicators and celebrations of consumer freedom and individuality (Jha 2016). In December 2004, China celebrated the first "Miss Artificial Beauty Pageant" in Beijing, a competition only open to women who had undergone plastic surgery.

The pageant is just one indication of a growing interest in and acceptance of the use of cosmetics and cosmetic procedures. Chinese celebrities, like those in Korea, are open about their favorite products and the surgeries that they have undergone, and the Chinese state tacitly approves of the increase in beauty work by labeling it a sign of the improved economic status of its citizens (Hua 2013).

See also: Body Modification; Fetish; Footbinding; Hair; Makeup and Cosmetics; Plastic Surgery.

Further Reading

Cultural China. "Historical Hair Ornaments and Their Social Connotations." Accessed November 17, 2015. http://traditions.cultural-china.com/en/15Traditions7948.html.

Harris, Rachel. 2004. *Singing the Village: Music, Memory, and Ritual Among the Sibe of Xinjiang.* London: Oxford University Press.

Hua, Wen. 2013. *Cosmetic Surgery in China.* Hong Kong: Hong Kong University Press.

Jha, Meeta Rani. 2016. *The Global Beauty Industry: Colorism, Racism and the National Body.* New York: Routledge.

Levi, Howard S. 1966. *Chinese Footbinding.* New York: Walton Rawls.

Louie, Kam. 2002. *Theorizing Chinese Masculinity: Society and Gender in China.* Cambridge, MA: Cambridge University Press.

CLASS

What is considered "beautiful" in a given culture at any particular time conforms to how that culture interprets "taste." French social theorist Pierre Bourdieu (1987) described how taste for clothing, furniture, leisure activities, and personal grooming is shaped by social class and used as the basis for social judgment.

One compelling example of the ways that class informs popular tastes and determinations of physical beauty comes from examining the growth of the **barber** and hairdressing trades in 20th-century France. Census data confirm that even prior to the 20th century, a healthy number of people worked in the "tonsorial professions." Barbers were overwhelmingly male, working long hours to earn a meager wage. Over time, hairdressers professionalized and established fancy salons to exploit the growing popularity of *coiffure pour dames*, employing women as beauticians. Whereas the "feminization" of most trades signals impoverishment, in hairdressing, the influx of women accompanied both growth and prosperity (Zdatny 1993, 56).

Women's coiffure became a growth industry offering high wages and expensive services. This expanding market created a new class of "middle-class woman" with the resources to get her hair "done" professionally. New hairstyles, like the so-called "Marcel wave" invented by Marcel Grateau in a salon in Montmartre, became the hallmark of class achievement. New technologies followed (Zdatny 1993, 58), and women began wearing shorter haircuts, which required more frequent maintenance in a professional setting. The luxury beauty parlor was born, and 20th-century developments pointed to the evolution of patterns of consumption that encouraged individuals to consume and **perform** their class aspirations.

See also: Barbershop; Hair; Performance/Performativity.

Further Reading

Bourdieu, Pierre. 1987. *Distinction: A Social Critique of the Judgment of Taste*, translated by Richard Nice. Boston: Harvard University Press.

Corson, Richard. 1965. *Fashions in Hair: The First Five Thousand Years*. London: Peter Owens Publishing.

Zdatny, Steven. 1993. "Fashion and Class Struggle: The Case of *Coiffure*." *Social History* 18, no. 1: 53–72.

CORN ROWS ("CANE ROWS")

Corn rows refer to the hairstyle achieved when hair is braided or plaited into narrow strips that lie flat against the scalp, creating a wide range of geometric patterns. Though the braids may take several hours to create, they are easily maintained for up to several weeks. Though any texture of hair may be arranged into corn row styles, the practice is most closely associated with hair types common to African descent.It is technically possible to braid one's own hair into corn rows; however, achieving the distinctive, "sharp" look of corn rows typically takes another person to complete. The braids are formed by first dividing and gathering the hair into thin sections: the more sections that are made, obviously, the thinner the braid and the longer it will take to achieve the overall hairstyle. Microbraids, especially those that incorporate artificial hair and add length to the hairstyle, can take ten hours or more to complete. As the stylist begins braiding, other sections of hair are added to the original braid in order to keep the hair flat to the scalp. The stylist must maintain a fair degree of tension in order to secure the braids, thus causing some discomfort for some corn row wearers. As with other techniques that pull sections of hair from the scalp, including ponytails and braids, cornrows are associated with traction alopecia, which may cause temporary baldness if they are too tight or are not released from their shape after a certain length of time.

In West Africa, elaborate braids and plaits were historically an important part of a woman's hairstyle (*ngu-fèlè*). Evidence of such braids endures on in wooden

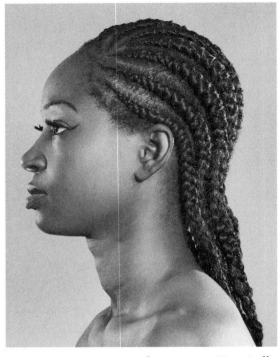

A Cameroonian woman with corn rows. Historically, elaborate braids were an important part of a West African woman's hairstyle, and could act as an indicator of age and ethnicity. (Matthias Ziegler/Dreamstime.com)

masks from the region. An involved coiffure could take many days to complete, and the pattern created can confer information about the wearer's age and ethnicity. Elaborate plaited hairstyles are also emulated in the carved wooden masks that are central to important ceremonies (Boone 1986). To the Mende aesthetic eye of West African cultures, the artistry of corn rows should display axial symmetry around the face in order to illustrate harmony and balance that is considered to be beautiful.

Hair has long been used as a proxy of "otherness" of people of African descent. Racist cartoons of diasporic Africans that appeared in the popular media during the 19th and early 20th century depicted black subjects with wild, unkempt hair as a symbol of supposed degenerate savagery (Dash 2006, 28). Discrimination for such hairstyles as dreadlocks, corn rows, and braids has been common for many years. Some legal evidence exists that certain hairstyles create a punitive sexist and racist reality for black women in court litigations in the United States (Caldwell 1991). In 2011, a court in the United Kingdom ruled that male students had the right to wear corn rows as an accommodation to ethnic and cultural practices, despite concerns on the part of school administrators that such hairstyles might indicate membership in gangs or other illegal groups.

African women, especially those of the diaspora who find themselves living in mainstream white contexts, often struggle with complicated feelings about the nature of their hair. "Competing mythologies around something as deceptively insignificant as hair still haunt and complicate African Americans' self-identities and their ideals of beauty, thus revealing broad and complex social, historical, and political realities" (Lester 2000, 203). References to "good" hair as a deeply intimate index of anxiety about beauty, belonging, and self-worth can be found in novels (Adichie 2014), documentaries (Rock 2009), and pop songs (Swann 2016).

Since the 1970s, a number of children's books have relied on autobiography and fiction to create Afrocentric celebration of black hair types and to treat seriously the complicated political, personal, and social implications of growing up in a culture that may not value certain types of hair as "beautiful." These books, from Camille Yarbrough's thoughtful *Cornrows* (1979) to bell hooks' joyful *Happy to Be Nappy* (1999), to the sweet, coming-of-age tale *Bintou's Braids* by Sylviane Diouf 2001, aim to recast the experience of black hair as a celebration of identity.

Today, there has been a notable return to the "traditional" styles of African hairdressing in some urban centers (Dash 2006). Prominent male basketball stars and Ultimate Fighting Championship (UFC) celebrities also began wearing corn rows as a practical hairstyle for high-profile, close-contact sporting events. However, critics note that there is also a degree of cultural appropriation of the hairstyle, as well as related styles like "baby hair," "Senegalese twists," and "Bantu knots" (Finley 2015). Cultural appropriation arises when members of a dominant group "borrow" or adopt some element from a minority group for their own purposes, often because the minority group represents an "**exotic**" identity whose experiences may be flattened out, manipulated, and "owned" by the member of the dominant group, typically through consumption. In this way, corn rows were controversially worn by white model/actor Bo Derek in the 1970s blockbuster sexual-fantasy movie *10* and also modeled by white, internationally known soccer star David Beckham in the 1980s. Popular magazines and style Web sites geared toward white female consumers began calling the traditional corn row style "boxer braids," or "double French braids," when the style appeared on reality TV celebrity Kim Kardashian in 2016 (Brown 2016).

See also: "Black Is Beautiful Movement," or Black Power; Dreadlocks; Exoticize; Hair; The "Other."

Further Reading

Adichie, Chimamanda Ngozi. 2014. *Americanah*. New York: Anchor Books.

Boone, Sylvia Arden. 1986. *Radiance from the Waters: Ideals of Feminine Beauty in Mende Art*. New Haven, CT: Yale University Press.

Brown, Kara. 2016. "White People Are Rebranding Cornrows as 'Boxer Braids.'" *Jezebel*. March 15. Accessed July 22, 2016. http://jezebel.com/white-people-are-rebranding -cornrows-as-boxer-braids-1765012240.

Caldwell, Paulette W. 1991. "A Hair Piece: Perspectives on the Intersection of Race and Gender." *Duke Law Journal* 40, no. 2: 325–65.

Dash, Paul. 2006. "Black Hair Culture, Politics, and Change." *International Journal of Inclusive Education* 10, no. 1: 27–37.

Diouf, Sylviane. 2001. *Bintou's Braids*. San Francisco: Chronicle Books.

Finley, Taryn. 2015. "8 Times Black Hairstyles Have Been Culturally Appropriated," *Huffington Post*. July 17. Accessed July 22, 2016. http://www.huffingtonpost.com/entry/9-times-white -people-have-appropriated-black-hairstyles-since-2014_us_55a81211e4b0896514d0c3ca.

The Guardian. 2011. "School's Refusal to Let Boy Wear Corn Row Braids Is Ruled Racial Discrimination." June 17. Accessed July 22, 2016. https://www.theguardian.com/uk/2011 /jun/17/school-ban-cornrow-braids-discrimination.

hooks, bell. 1999. *Happy to Be Nappy*. New York: Jump at the Sun Press.

Lawson, Helene. 1999. "Working on Hair." *Qualitative Sociology* 22, no. 3: 235–57.

Lester, Neal A. 2000. "Nappy Edges and Goldy Locks: African-American Daughters and the Politics of Hair." *The Lion and the Unicorn* 24: 201–24.

Picardi, Phillip. 2014. "The Thin Line between Fashionable and Offensive." *Refinery 29*. October 8. Accessed April 5, 2016. http://www.refinery29.com/cornrows-cultural -appropriation.

Rensselaer Polytechnic Institute. 2016. "History of Cornrow Braiding." *Culturally Situated Design Tools*. Accessed April 5, 2016. http://www.csdt.rpi.edu/african/CORNROW _CURVES/culture/african.origins.htm.

Rock, Chris. 2009. *Good Hair* [videorecording]. Directed by Jeff Stilson. HBO Films.

Sherrow, Victoria. 2006. *The Encyclopedia of Hair: A Cultural History*. Santa Barbara, CA: Greenwood Press.

Swann, Jennifer. 2016. "The Complete History of 'Becky with the Good Hair,' From the 1700s to Lemonade. *Fusion* [Web site], May 4. Accessed May 6, 2016. http://fusion.net /story/298448/history-becky-with-the-good-hair-beyonce-lemonade.

Wright, Dakara Rucker, Raechele Gathers, Alissa Kapke, Dayna Johnson, and Christine L. M. Joseph. 2011. "Hair Care Practices and Their Association with Scalp and Hair Disorders in African American Girls." *Journal of the American Academy of Dermatology* 64, no. 2: 253–62.

Yarbrough, Camille. 1979. *Cornrows*. New York: Puffin Books.

CORSETS, SHAPEWEAR, AND WAIST TRAINERS

Nineteenth-century corsets and 21-century shapewear are both designed to control and enhance the shape of a woman's torso, from the hips (or below) to the breasts (or above). Although the corset fell out of favor in the early 20th century in fashion, in the 21st century, a resurgence in the popularity of garments designed to fulfill a similar role speaks to the staying power of the idea of undergarments that restrict and plump out certain parts of a woman's anatomy.

Corsets, a close-fitting undergarment that is stiffened with whalebone or similar material and is often capable of being tightened by lacing, are designed to enclose the torso of the wearer, at times enhancing the appearance of the breasts while shaping and supporting the body. Corsets have traditionally been worn by women, and the effect has been that the body is actually molded, over time, into the shape of the corset.

The earliest precursor to the corset was a garment called the cote, which was a tightly laced bodice worn by women in medieval times on the outside of their dress. This garment, worn from the 5th to the 15th centuries in Europe, was made of stiff material but lacked stays, or pieces of metal, to keep them rigid. The advent of corsets in the 16th century incorporated pieces of whalebone, wood, and steel to keep the corset stiff while flattening both the stomach and the **breasts** (Mahe 2013).

After the 16th century, corsets were redesigned to flatten the belly and slim the waist but push up and enhance the breasts, creating an **hourglass** figure. This type of corset was made even more popular by Queen Victoria of England, who ruled from 1837 to 1901 (Ricketts 2014). Fashionable through the late 19th century, this style of garment undoubtedly had health repercussions for those who wore it, especially at the height of the corset's popularity, when women began to put restrictive belts on female infants and young girls wore corsets starting at the age of seven (Caelleigh 1998).

Napoleon Bonaparte decried the wearing of corsets as damaging to a woman's reproductive capacity. The tightly laced, restrictive shape altered women's bodies, compressing their rib cages and putting pressure on internal organs. Health problems related to regular corset wearing included infertility, endometriosis, breathing problems, and digestive trouble (Mahe 2013).

In the 20th century, corset-type garments continued to be manufactured and worn in different fabrics and styles, often called "girdles" or "foundations." By the 1930s, most corsets manufactured included an attached bra, and many also had garters attached for the use of stockings (Mahe 2013). These new undergarments made use of elastic materials in combination with the rigid stays of older versions of the corset garment, with zippers replacing the old laced style.

As technology for creating high-performance fabric progressed, so, too, did the materials used in girdles and corsets. By the 1950s, new synthetic fabrics such as polyester and elastics were commonly used, and whalebone was no longer a stiffening agent. When the garter belt, and then later pantyhose, were introduced in the 1950s and 1960s, allowing women to wear stockings without a girdle, the corset undergarment became even less common (Mahe 2013).

In the 21st century, 19th-century-style corsets can still be found in lingerie stores that seek to sell "sexy" undergarments, demonstrating how the corset has changed from daily clothing worn by women to a fashion statement that is considered sexually provocative, edgy, or part of a costume and visible to others. **Burlesque** dancers often wear corsets, as do those participating in steampunk fashion.

The British designer Alexander McQueen became famous with his rebellious designs that often featured corsets. When the designer's label was called upon to design the wedding gown for Kate Middleton, who married Prince William of England, the resultant gown had McQueen's signature corset as part of the bodice.

In 2012, young entrepreneur Sara Blakey founded a new, massively successful "shapewear" company. Blakey's brand, known

---

Steampunk Fashion

Steampunk is a 21st-century style based on a vision of the future in which Victorian ideas of science and culture, including steam power and fashion, characterize daily life. Steampunk can be understood as what the science fiction authors H. G. Wells, Jules Verne, or Mary Shelly believed the future would look like. In the 21st century, steampunk fashion has developed from movies and illustrations that portray a future that combines advanced steam and clockwork technology with Victorian aesthetics. Famous fictional works that provide inspiration include the films *Sky Captain and the World of Tomorrow* and *The League of Extraordinary Gentlemen*. Steampunk fashion often combines modern styles and pieces of steam or clockwork technology with Victorian elements such as corsets, petticoats, bustles, waistcoats, top hats, and spats.

as "Spanx," offers body-shaping undergarments that slim waists and bellies while enhancing breasts in much the same way as the girdle. Spanx exploded with success and was available in 50 countries worldwide by 2016. Blakey was declared the first female self-made billionaire by *Forbes* magazine and named one of *Time* Magazine's 100 most influential people in the world (Blakey 2016).

Another indicator of this continuing preference for the "Coke-bottle" figure is the 21st-century advent of "waist trainers," devices that remind many of the 19th-century practice of molding young women's waists into tiny sizes. The garments, made of high-tech stretchable fabrics, are worn by many women, including notable celebrities such as Kim Kardashian and Jessica Alba, to lose weight and regain the hourglass figure after childbirth (Armstrong

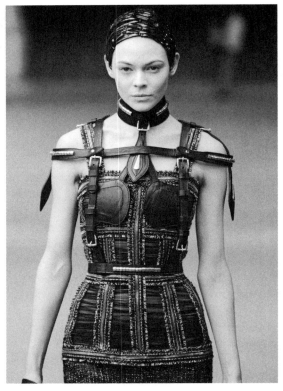

British fashion designer Alexander McQueen is known for his bold designs, as in this corset-inspired dress, Paris, March 2011. (Pavel Bendau/Dreamstime.com)

2014). Fans of the garment say that it helps in weight loss through perspiration and reducing appetite, but experts warn that the health risks of waist training, called "tight-lacing" in extreme circumstances, remains the same as the risks for corsets in previous centuries.

See also: Breasts; Burlesque; Weight.

Further Reading

Armstrong, Jenice. 2014. "It's a Cinch: Waist Trainers Mark Return of the Corset, for Better or Worse." *Philadelphia Daily News, The (PA)*, September 11.

Blakey, Sarah. 2016. "Spanx by Sara Blakey." Accessed June 15, 2016. http://www.spanx .com/about-us.

Caelleigh, Addeane S. 1998. "Too Close for Comfort: 500 Years of Corsets." *Academic Medicine* 73, no. 12: 1228.

Mahe, Yvette. 2013. "History of Women's Corsets." Accessed June 15, 2016. http://www .fashionintime.org/history-of-womens-corsets-part-1.

Ricketts, Laura. 2014. "Vicky's Knickers, or Queen Victoria's Secret." *Piecework* 22, no. 6: 25–31.

Turner, Mimi. 2011. "Kate Middleton's Wedding Dress by Sarah Burton for Alexander McQueen." Accessed June 15, 2016. http://www.hollywoodreporter.com/news/kate-midd letons-wedding-dress-by-183649.

D

DANCE-HALL BEAUTY: SKIN OUT AND BLING

A Jamaican tradition in which women enact performances of beauty and sexuality, the "skin out" is a display of fashion and appeal unique to Jamaican culture. In popular dance clubs, men, often called *dons* or *shottas*, seek to present an aspirational level of wealth and power seen as hypermasculine. The dance hall is a place where the poorer of Jamaica's citizens parade their best clothing and jewelry in a show of conspicuous consumption and erotic energy designed to impress others and gain success (Hope 2010). The "skin out" is an informal beauty pageant and opportunity for women to display the unique, local standard of beauty that is prized by the less advantaged socioeconomic classes of Jamaican society.

Dance-hall culture and music developed from the reggae dance clubs where young DJs, known as "rude boys," would talk or sing over a popular reggae rhythm, often freestyling, commenting on the members of the crowd and making up lyrics in the moment (Nichols and Robbins 2015). Dance-hall music is notable for a combination of intensely masculine and macho lyrics that sexualize and objectify women. The environment also creates opportunities for social advancement of both men and women who conform to gendered standards of behavior and appearance.

Going to the hall, or club, is a social event and fashion show and is as much about seeing and being seen as it is about the music. The event is a form of public **performance**, where community members show off new clothing, seek sexual partners and mates, and showcase their wealth and success (Nichols and Robbins 2015). For men, this often is about driving in on a fancy, tricked-out motorcycle or wearing expensive designer clothing, and for women this is on display in the tradition of the "skin out."

In contrast to some sectors of Jamaican society, and in particular the middle and upper **classes**, dance-hall culture privileges a style of beauty for women known as *mampy* or *mampy-sized* (Hope 2006a). The ideal body standard for women in this context is large, full bodied, round, and with large **breasts**. Within dance-hall culture, extra weight and body fat are associated with prosperity and wealth, the ability to not just eat but eat well, and the lack of need to work so much that muscles become too pronounced. Beauty norms for women include big breasts, hips, and "bumpers"—backsides or **butts**. The social ideal is to be "*trang*," a word meaning "strong" and used as a compliment for women with round hips and backsides. To achieve this state, some women in Jamaica regularly take "fowl pills," hormone supplements used in the chicken industry to increase breast size in poultry (Hope 2006a).

As a standard norm of beauty, skin color is also symbolically important. As a marker of class and status, preferences for skin color are a matter of great tension and a source for debate on bleaching, color, and identity in Jamaican culture. Historically, the social preference across the **Caribbean** was for lighter skin; to be a "browning" (with lighter, brown skin and not darker black skin) is widely recognized as a symbol of higher social class and status. For men, there is prestige and added respect for having a wife or lover who is a browning. Many Jamaicans are critical of the higher status of lighter skin as a measure of social importance, arguing that seeking lighter skin is a way of rejecting African heritage and submitting to colonial, European preferences (Hope 2006a).

The dance-hall competition to identify the most *mampy, trang,* and beautifully sexual woman at the club is called the "skin out." The skin out is a contest where provocatively and erotically dressed women dance and display their bodies for the evaluation and judging of the male audience. In keeping with the standard of being *mampy,* skin out competitors are also judged on their *phatness,* a term that refers to the erotic appeal of their hips, backsides, breasts, and labia (the acronym PHAT sometimes stands for P*ssy, Hips, A**, and Tits). **Elongated labia**, as in many parts of Africa, are considered especially appealing, as they promise heightened sexual pleasure for both partners. The size of a woman's labia is so important to winning the skin out, that contestants have been known to enhance their vaginas with sanitary pads to enhance their *phatness* as part of their costumes (Hope 2006a). Women's clothing is especially important as part of the evaluation of her beauty, with more revealing, skimpier, and more sexually suggestive clothing being preferred, as well as clothing that communicates success. Women will spend a great deal on designer clothing or go to great lengths to have reproductions of designer clothes made (Hope 2006a).

Women who win the "skin out" contests are rewarded not only with the admiration of their peers, but also often with trophies, cash, and trips abroad. Winning can also turn into paid employment, as the victor is often paid to appear in music videos, on posters, or in other advertisements. Winners may even be paid to simply attend parties, dances, and events to lend their fame and erotic appeal to the venue (Hope 2006a). A dance-hall queen achieves a great deal of status and fame within the community, directly related to her personal and professional success (Stanley-Niaah 2009). These real rewards for performing and achieving the social ideal are part of the intellectual debate on whether the practice is an example of exploitation of women through objectifying their sexuality, or an example of how women take control of their own bodies to navigate existing social norms to seek and achieve power through the politics and "erotics of the carnal" body (Bakare-Yusuf 2005).

See also: Breasts; Butts and Booty; The Caribbean; Elongated Labia; Jewelry; Skin Tone; Skin Whitening.

Further Reading

Bakare-Yusuf, Bibi. 2005. "'I Love Myself When I Am Dancing and Carrying On': Refiguring the Agency of Black Women's Creative Expression in Jamaican Dancehall Culture." *International Journal of Media & Cultural Politics* 1, no. 3: 263–76.

Hope, Donna. 2006a. "Dons and Shottas: Performing Violent Masculinity in Dancehall Culture." *Social & Economic Studies* 55, no. ½: 115–31.

Hope, Donna. 2006b. *Inna Di Dancehall: Popular Culture and the Politics of Identity in Jamaica.* Mona, Jamaica: University of the West Indies Press.

Hope, Donna. 2010. *Man Vibes: Masculinities in the Jamaican Dancehall.* Kingston, Jamaica: Ian Randle Publishers.

Nichols, Elizabeth Gackstetter, and Timothy R. Robbins. 2015. *Pop Culture in Latin America and the Caribbean.* Santa Barbara, CA: ABC-CLIO.

Stanley-Niaah, Sonjah. 2009. "Negotiating a Common Transnational Space." *Cultural Studies* 23, no. 5/6: 756–74.

DÉCOLLETAGE

Décolletage refers to the exposed part of a woman's torso, neck, and shoulders, usually intentionally, and enhanced by clothing designed to highlight femininity. The term references a broader area of exposed skin than the related term "cleavage," which refers only to the exposed area of a woman's **breasts**. In addition to the front, décolletage may refer to the deliberate exposure of a woman's back. Certain other garments are often specifically designed to highlight the breasts of a woman's body through specially designed evening gowns, lingerie, and swimwear. The degree to which décolletage is encouraged in women's fashion relates directly to specific standards of modesty and cultural notions about exposure of the breasts.

Indian women have long worn backless styles of garments, including *choli, sari,* and *ghagra.* The back can be partially exposed with a low cut or fully exposed by the use of thin strings, which may cascade down the back (Keshavrao 2005). In Europe of the early Middle Ages, men and women wore similar, long, loose-fitting unisex robes. Fashion began to change in the mid-14th century, when men adopted shorter jackets and leg-skimming breeches and women's long garments became more tailored to the body with a plunging neckline (Savacool 2009). Newly gender-specific fashions spread across western and northern Europe with remarkable speed and marked the beginning of fashion's influential role on ideal body shape. Individuals became invested in the ways that social value was placed on being "fashionable" as an index of who a person is, what **class** he or she belonged to, and what kind of resources he or she has at his or her disposal.

Agnes Sorel, a mistress of French king Louis VII, first popularized the low, square-cut décolletage gown, which fully exposed her breasts to the French court in the 1450s. Women of means during the centuries that followed squeezed into luxurious fabrics to highlight tiny waistlines and exposed cleavage pushed up by stiff, tight bodices. In the 1730s, the *robe volante* ("flying dress") was introduced. Though it still featured a plunging V-neck to show off a daring décolletage, otherwise the dress, which did not include tight bindings or corsets, was considered as comfortable as the yoga pants of today (Stamberg 2016).

Fashionable styles featuring much or all of a woman's bared breasts and exposed necks remained popular through the 18th century, when the French Revolution changed standards of modesty across Europe. During the Victorian period, for example, norms of modesty and respectability discouraged women from showing

any décolletage in public, and the fashions of the era featured high, buttoned necklines. Décolletage did not return to fashion until after World War I, when rounded
necklines reappeared, especially in women's formal and evening wear. Backless
dresses were also popular in the 1920s and 1930s, when the halter neck style became
a way to show off tanned skin without tan lines.

The skin exposed by décolletage is very delicate and does not produce oil as
readily as the face. As such, the neck, shoulders, and tops of the breasts are readily
susceptible to **wrinkles**, "crepey" skin, and other signs of **aging**. Many skin care
experts suggest a specialized regimen to care for this sensitive skin, emphasizing the
motto "your face starts at your nipples" (Savacool 2009) To enhance **youthful**-looking
skin, most regimens recommend careful cleansing, exfoliating, moisturizing, protecting with sunscreen, and highlighting or bronzing.

See also: Breasts; Class; India; Wrinkles; Youth.

Further Reading

Keshavrao, Dhanwanti. 2005. "Dressed for Dandiya." *The Tribune* [India]. October 8.
    Accessed October 24, 2016. http://www.tribuneindia.com/2005/20051008/saturday
    /main4.htm.
Savacool, Julia. 2009. *The World Has Curves: The Global Quest for the Perfect Body.* New York:
    Rodale.
Stamberg, Susan. 2013. "Vive le Confort: For Corseted Courtiers, This Dress Was a French
    Revolution." NPR Morning Edition. August 9. Accessed October 24, 2016. http://www
    .npr.org/2016/08/09/489179987/vive-le-confort-for-corseted-courtiers-this-dress-was
    -a-french-revolution.

DENTAL HYGIENE AND COSMETIC DENTISTRY

Attractive teeth symbolize both health and wealth. Sociologists note that in the
industrialized world, the preoccupation with self-image is particularly evident in the
"prevailing fixation with straight, white teeth" (Khalid and Quiñonez 2015).

The oldest evidence of a dental filling was found at an archaeological site in Slove-
nia (Choi 2012). The 6,500-year-old filling was made with beeswax, not for beauty
enhancement, but to probably to ameliorate the pain and swelling associated with a
dental cavity. Much later, the French surgeon Pierre Fauchard became the Father of
Modern Dentistry in 1723, the first to describe a comprehensive system of caring for
and treating damage to teeth (Holloway 2014).

During the 18th century in Europe, artificial teeth designed to disguise tooth loss
by "plumping" up the cheeks were made of cork (Downing 2012, 29). These were
frequently worn by older people who lost their molars to tooth decay. Missing front
teeth were replaced by a row of artificial teeth carved from hippo ivory imported
from Africa. The color was closer to the natural shade of human teeth than other
types of ivory.

In the 21st century, dental hygiene promotes the care of teeth for health reasons
but also to promote a beautiful smile. Brushing regularly with fluoride toothpaste,
flossing, and getting fillings in teeth with cavities have become normative hygiene
standards. The practice of dental hygiene also prevents and cures gum and tooth

disease such as gingivitis and periodontitis, which are conditions that can cause swollen or bleeding gums, and addresses cavities and tooth decay, which can lead to teeth rotting or falling out (Wolf and Hassell 2006).

Cosmetic dentistry is a combination of practices and products specifically designed to improve the appearance of the teeth. The most popular cosmetic dentistry procedures straighten misaligned teeth, fill gaps and cracks, and whiten the color of the teeth (Cosmetic Dentistry 2004). Teeth whitening has grown extensively in popularity in the 21st century, with in-office whitening making up a $371 million industry in the United States in 2006 alone (Khalid and Quiñonez 2006).

One way dentists can provide whiter teeth while fixing gaps and cracks or chips is with crowns, bonding, and veneers. Each of these is a type of covering for a broken, damaged, or misaligned tooth. A crown is a type of cap that is fitted over the tooth. Bonding is a technique in which a dentist applies a puttylike material over the tooth to fix cracks or chips. Veneers, the most elaborate and expensive option, are custom-made shells of porcelain or resin that fit over teeth much like a false fingernail. Veneers are used not only in the case of broken teeth, but also to mask permanently stained or discolored teeth (Cosmetic Dentistry 2004).

In the 21st century, the appearance of broken, discolored, or missing teeth is often understood as a commentary on social class and status. Straight, white teeth across North America, for example, is a symbol that reinforces **class** differences and is an example of how society exercises a **disciplinary power** on individuals through management of their bodies.

In the **United States** and other nations, dental care is provided separately from general health care and often not covered by state-run health programs or insurance providers. For this reason, access to dental care is uneven, with richer people having a better chance at receiving hygienic dental care and being able to afford cosmetic dentistry.

Dental care is also often linked to the wealth of the area in which a person grew up and lives. In the United States and in nations such as **Brazil** and **Mexico**, dentists and dental practices are concentrated in the most economically developed regions of those nations. Poorer and more rural citizens have less chance to receive care, and so poor dental hygiene or a poor appearance of teeth can become linked to the idea of poverty and lack of education (Saliba, et al. 2009).

Tooth Bleaching

In the 21st century, one of the most widely practiced types of cosmetic dentistry is tooth bleaching. Although people have been seeking to make teeth whiter since the 1800s, it is in this century that the techniques have exploded in type and popularity. Over time teeth become stained by drinking tea, coffee, and red wine and can also become stained by smoking and some medications. To remove stains and whiten teeth, individuals can choose remedies performed by a dentist or in their own homes. In dental offices, dentists most commonly use hydrogen peroxide or carbamide peroxide in gels to whiten teeth. These peroxides are also available for home use in weaker formulations. Home remedies also include rinses or adhesive strips that contain peroxides. Dentists may use lasers in combination with bleach to achieve more dramatic results, but results that leave many teeth oversensitive.

It is not surprising, then, that celebrities or athletes who may have grown up in poorer households or areas often seek out dental care and cosmetic dentistry to improve the appearance of their teeth once they become wealthy (Knight 2003).

See also: Brazil; Class; Disciplinary Practices/Disciplinary Power; Mexico; Teeth Blackening; Tooth Chipping; United States.

Further Reading

Choi, Charles Q. 2012. "Beeswax Filling May Be Oldest Hint of Dentistry." Live Science. September 19. Accessed July 13, 2016. http://www.livescience.com/23321-ancient -dentistry-beeswax-filling.html.

"Cosmetic Dentistry." 2004. In: *The New Harvard Guide to Women's Health*, 175–178, edited by Karen J. Carlson, Stephanie A. Eisenstat, and Terra Ziporyn. Cambridge, MA: Harvard University Press.

Downing, Sarah Jane. 2012. *Beauty and Cosmetics 1550–1950*. Oxford, England: Shire Publications.

Holloway, April. 2014. "From Jewel Capped Teeth to Golden Bridges: 9000 Years of Dentistry." *Ancient Origins*. Accessed July 13, 2016. http://www.ancient-origins.net/human -origins-science/jewel-capped-teeth-golden-bridges-9000-years-dentistry-001427?page =0%2C1.

Khalid, Abeer, and Carlos Quiñonez. 2015. "Straight, White Teeth as a Social Prerogative." *Sociology of Health & Illness* 37, no. 5: 782–96.

Knight, Mike. 2003. "Beauty and the Teeth." *Indianapolis Monthly* 26, no. 6: 90.

Saliba, N. A., Moimaz, S. A., Garbin, C.A., and Diniz, D. G. 2009. "Dentistry in Brazil: Its History and Current Trends" *Journal of Dental Education* 73, no. 2 (February 1): 225–31.

Wolf, Herbert F., and Thomas M. Hassell. 2006. *Color Atlas of Dental Hygiene*. Stuttgart, Germany: Thieme.

DEODORANT AND ANTIPERSPIRANTS

The $18 billion contemporary deodorant and antiperspirant industry has a long history (Everts 2012). For much of history, body odor was prevented or curtailed by washing regularly or by covering the odor with **perfumes**. Sea-faring Phoenicians invented soap in BCE 600, and the ancient civilizations of Egypt, Greece, and Rome all prized bathing and routinely cleaned their bodies (Ramirez 1990). During the Middle Ages in Europe, religious fervor about the evils of nudity and popular notions about the increased susceptibility to illness while wet diminished the zeal for regular bathing. Later, out of concern for perspiration staining clothes, some companies did a brisk trade in dress shields, cotton pads placed in the armpit areas to prevent sweat from being visible.

"Mum," the first trademarked deodorant, was a cream paste created in 1888. The product was designed to be rubbed into the armpit, and although it did prevent odor, it also left a sticky, greasy residue on clothing (Fontanez 2008). The first antiperspirant, "Odorono," was designed to be dabbed onto the underarm with a cotton swab and was introduced in 1912. The original formula, high in aluminum chloride, stopped sweat for up to three days, but could also irritate the sensitive skin in the armpit and damage clothing (Everts 2012).

Marking the beginning of a uniquely North American obsession with armpit sweat, an **advertising** agency in New York City created a sales campaign to present body odor as an unwitting form of social suicide that caused others to gossip behind your back (Everts 2012). The campaign boosted sales and also created something of a stir, as "vulgar" issues like body odor were not frequently discussed in polite society. Nevertheless, the campaign was effective and among the first to exploit women's insecurity and potential embarrassment about their bodies as a way to both create a need and to offer a solution that was available for a price, setting a precedent for many later advertising campaigns. By 1927, the company made $1 million a year.

Men were not initially targeted by the campaign, as sweat and body odor in general were accepted as a masculine reality. However, as profits rose in the lucrative deodorant and antiperspirant market, advertisers set their sight on male customers. Top-Flite, the first men's deodorant, debuted in 1935 in the throes of the Great Depression. The advertising campaign focused on a man's fear of being fired in an unstable economy and linked this fear to the possibility of being considered poorly groomed or "stinky" in the office place. Male deodorants linked smelling good with masculinity by establishing a disciplined grooming routine for men who no longer worked as farmers or laborers (Everts 2012). New products with names like Sea-Forth, Shun, Hush, Veto, Slick, and Zip appeared on the market, and advertisers packaged these masculine-smelling deodorants and antiperspirants in interesting bottles, like faux ceramic whisky jugs, to deliberately appeal to manly sensibilities.

Between the 1940s and the 1970s, new techniques were invented for deodorant delivery, including sticks, roll-ons, sprays, and aerosols (Ramirez 1990). The 1940s introduced the first liquid deodorants, delivered by a pump spray in order to prevent the sticky concoction from getting on the fingers. In the 1950s, inspired by ballpoint pen technology, Ban introduced the first roll-on. Roll-ons were clean, quick, and easy to apply, but they did have a tendency to trap armpit hair in the applicator, making them less popular with male customers. Gillette introduced Right Guard in an aerosol can in the early 1960s, and aerosols were popular for a few decades, until environmental concerns about the deleterious effects of chlorofluorocarbons upon the ozone layer were better understood. Solid-stick deodorants became available in the late 1970s, usually with an active ingredient called triclosan, which fights odor-causing bacteria, delivered in a propylene glycol base that is thickened with sodium stearate and topped off with a pleasant scent.

In the 1990s, new solid-stick formulas offered customers specialized formulas like Degree, which accommodates to the body heat needs of the individual wearer, and Revlon's now-defunct product called No Sweat, which used a time-release formula to provide longer anti-odor coverage. These products were designed to be marketed to both men and women.

See also: Advertising; Bathing and Showering; Perfumes and Scented Oils.

Further Reading

Everts, Sarah. 2012. "How Advertisers Convinced Americans They Smelled Bad." *Smithsonian*. August 2. Accessed September 22 2016. http://www.smithsonianmag.com/ist/?next =/history/how-advertisers-convinced-americans-they-smelled-bad-12552404.

Fontanez, Stefanie. 2008. "Body Odor through the Ages: A Brief History of Deodorant." *Mental Floss.* 2008 [Web site]. Accessed September 22, 2016. http://mentalfloss.com /article/18081/body-odor-through-ages-brief-history-deodorant.

Ramirez, Anthony. 1990. All About Deodorants: The Sweet Smell of Success. *New York Times.* August 12. Accessed September 22, 2016. http://www.nytimes.com/1990/08/12/business /all-about-deodorants-the- success-of-sweet-smell.html?pagewanted=all.

DISCIPLINARY PRACTICES/DISCIPLINARY POWER

French philosopher and social theorist Michel Foucault's study of European penal systems and other social institutions allowed him to formulate a theory about how everyday people internalize the ideas of the powerful. Interested in the evolution of power since the Industrial Revolution, Foucault argued that Western cultures exercise control over individuals through "practices of discipline" that have shifted from external controls (including, for example, the threat of violence, incarceration, and death) to internal self-regulation.

Foucault identified "surveillance" as the primary method of discipline in the contemporary era, where the possibility of corporal punishment is traded for the symbolic identification of the transgressor as a "deviant" through public shaming. He argued that because individuals care deeply about what others think of them, most people in any given society will learn to inhibit or curb their own impulses and behaviors in an attempt to be "normal." Foucault characterized the condition of modern society as living with a continual awareness of being watched, assessed, and judged by others.

When it comes to establishing so-called "proper" behaviors, Foucault suggests that most individuals learn to develop "docile" bodies that voluntarily adhere to social norms. When everyone in the society internalizes shared values about how to behave, Foucault said, there "is no need for arms, physical violence, material constraints. Just a gaze. An inspecting gaze, a gaze which each individual under its weight will end by interiorizing to the point that he is his own overseer, each individual thus exercising this surveillance over, and against himself" (Foucault 1977, 151).

When people discipline themselves, they think of their behavior as "good" or "bad" by measuring themselves against the collectively held standards. There are also significant social rewards—including acceptance, admiration, and popularity—that may be conferred upon those who are the most perfectly compliant to the normative standards of the society.

Not surprisingly, many **feminist** theorists are drawn to Foucault's theories as a way to explain the seemingly contradictory way that women participate in their own physical objectification. Sandra Lee Bartky (1988) identified the many ways that disciplinary power works on women's lives differently than those of men. She argued that disciplinary practices produce a feminine body that is recognizable as ideally "female" in three distinct ways: it adheres to a certain size and proportion ("taut, small-breasted, and narrow-hipped"); it follows a certain repertoire of gestures, postures, and movements ("a reluctance to reach, stretch, and extend the body to meet resistances of matter in motion—as in sport or in the performance of physical tasks—and in a typically constricted posture and general style of movement"); and it is most often displayed as an ornamented surface ("skin must be soft, supple, hairless, and smooth; ideally, it should betray no sign of wear, experience, age, or deep thought . . . The crown and pinnacle . . . is, of course, the arrangement of the hair and the application of cosmetics . . . A woman must learn the proper manipulation of a large number of devices . . . and the correct manner of application of a wide variety of products)" (Bartky 1988, 191).

In *Unbearable Weight* (1993), feminist philosopher Susan Bordo used Foucault's idea of disciplinary power to explain why so many Western women internalize feelings of self-loathing, particularly around the issue of their weight, thus driving a multibillion-dollar fitness and weight loss industry. She observed that women try to conform to an unrealistic standard of female beauty by exercising increasing amounts of control over their appearance, which inevitably takes enormous amounts of time and resources to achieve, if at all. Through this lens, the ultimate disciplinary act might be viewed as a mechanism contributing to the rise in eating disorders in Western culture, which are frequently medicalized as disorders that rise from a lack of individual control. Bordo argues that the current disciplinary practices of Western culture train the female body to focus intentionally on "flaws" and to obey cultural demands to reduce their very presence. Anorexia nervosa is literally an attempt to starve the body to create a "size 0."

See also: Eating Disorders; Feminism.

Further Reading

Bartky, Sandra Lee. 1988. "Foucault, Femininity, and the Modernization of Patriarchal Power." In: *Feminism and Foucault: Paths of Resistance*, edited by Lee Quinby and Irene Diamond, 61–86. Boston: Northeastern University Press.

Bordo, Susan. 1993. *Unbearable Weight: Feminism, Western Culture, and the Body*. Berkeley, CA: University of California Press.

Foucault, Michel. 1977. "The Eye of the Beholder." In *Power / Knowledge*, edited by Colin Gordon. New York, Pantheon.

Foucault, Michel. 1995. *Discipline and Punish: The Birth of the Prison*. Translated by Alan Sheridan. New York, Vintage Books.

DOVE CAMPAIGN FOR REAL BEAUTY

The Dove Campaign for Real Beauty emerged in 2004 as an effort by parent company Unilever Corporation to revitalize the fifty-year-old Dove brand. Rather than going with the usual aspirational tactics of most advertisement pitches, Dove chose to promote a more generous standard of "real beauty" by capitalizing on the now-mainstream critiques from **feminist** commentators about the troubling health implications of unrealistic beauty ideals, particularly the high costs of **eating disorders** among young women.

The multimillion-dollar **advertising** campaign was launched in the **United Kingdom** and quickly spread to the **United States**, drawing a great deal of public attention through billboard, television, and magazine advertisements depicting

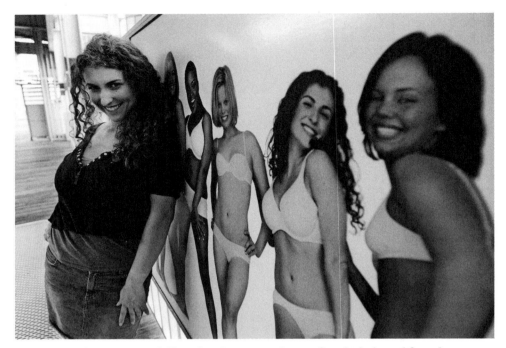

Gina Crisanti leans against a billboard in downtown Chicago, for which she and five other women posed in an ad campaign for Dove Beauty products, July 26, 2005. The ads, featuring "real" women and not models, were designed to prompt a national conversation about unhealthy beauty standards. (AP Photo/Nam Y. Huh)

women who were wrinkled, freckled, pregnant, had stretch marks, or could be considered "fat," at least according to conventional standards of beauty for the media.

The women selected for the advertisements were all in their twenties or thirties and represented a wide range of ethnic backgrounds. All of the "models" were conventionally attractive, with wide, open smiles that radiated happiness and warmth. The campaign also generated enormous commercial success for the brand. For example, sales for the campaign's firming lotion exceeded sales forecasts and recorded impressive sales for the company.

In 2005, Dove kicked off the second phase of the campaign with a billboard and print ad campaign featuring "six real women with real bodies and real curves." Media sources commented on how refreshing it was to see "real" women in plain white underwear, posing for the camera and looking relaxed and joyful. The campaign was paired with a Web site that encouraged visitors to upload their own photographs and to choose their favorite among the "real" models depicted in the campaigns. This move, which gambled on the interactive role of consumers in the dialogue of "real" beauty, left many scratching their heads,

"Beauty is how you feel inside, and it reflects in your eyes. It is not something physical."

—SOPHIA LOREN

because asking viewers to choose a "favorite" still compared women to each other.

Some critics were skeptical of the ulterior motives of the corporation and commented on the fact that the campaign still promoted the sale of beauty products, including a best-selling "firming cream," to women (Johnston and Taylor 2008). Critics point out that even though the campaign relied on "real" women instead of professional models, the dress size of the women pictured in the Dove Real Beauty campaign ranged from sizes 6 to 12. This increased size represents more diversity than the average fashion model (size 4), but still presents a smaller body size than the average American woman, who is a size 14.

Critics also wonder about the transformative power of "**feminist** consumerism," which may partially disrupt gender norms, but does so in a way that reinforces and reinstates the assumptions that women should spend their resources on products that enable them to look more attractive. The notion of using "real beauty" as a marketing tactic to sell products to women reinforces the dubious logic of the so-called "beauty myth": that the women's participation in the **social construction of beauty** can serve as a meaningful source of empowerment. A more empowering tactic to promote women's beauty, critics say, would be the celebration of **body positivity** and the promotion of "fat bodies," sometimes called **BBW.**

Despite these critiques, the Dove campaign has contributed millions of dollars to transformative programming that aligns itself with feminist ideals to raise awareness for eating disorders. Since the launch of the campaign, Unilever has also sponsored the development of the Dove Movement for Self-Esteem, which sponsors educational programs and activities that encourage, inspire, and motivate girls through the Boys & Girls Clubs of America and the Girl Scouts of the USA.

In 2011, another global study by Unilever found that only 4 percent of women considered themselves "beautiful," and the researchers identified an age break during adolescence where young girls began to doubt their own self-worth as related to their appearance. This research echoed other findings by psychologists and specialists in childhood development, suggesting that the social pressures of attractiveness during adolescence contribute to a particularly dangerous time in the self-esteem of young girls (Pipher 1994).

See also: Advertising; BBW; Body Positivity; Eating Disorders; Feminism; Social Construction of Beauty; United Kingdom; United States.

Further Reading

Etcoff, Nancy, Susie Orbach, Jennifer Scott, and Heidi D'Agostino. 2004. *The Real Truth About Beauty: A Global Report*. Accessed November 20, 2015. http://www.clubofamsterdam.com/contentarticles/52%20Beauty/dove_white_paper_final.pdf.

Johnston, Josée, and Judith Taylor. 2008. "Feminist Consumerism and Fat Activists: A Comparative Study of Grassroots Activism and the Dove Real Beauty Campaign." *Signs* 33, no. 4: 941–66.

Millard, Jennifer. 2009. Performing Beauty: Dove's "Real Beauty" Campaign. *Symbolic Interaction* 32, no. 2: 146–68.

Pipher, Mary. 1994. *Reviving Ophelia: Saving the Selves of Adolescent Girls*. New York: Penguin.

Stevenson, Seth. 2005. "When Tush Comes to Dove." Slate. Accessed November 20, 2015. http://www.slate.com/articles/business/ad_report_card/2005/08/when_tush_comes_to_dove.html.

Unilever. "Campaign for Real Beauty." 2004. Accessed November 20, 2015. http://www.dove.us/Social-Mission/campaign-for-real-beauty.aspx.

Wolf, Naomi. 1991. *The Beauty Myth: How Images of Beauty Are Used Against Women*. New York: Random House.

DRAG

In American society, people tend to be raised to think of males and females and heterosexuals and homosexuals in opposite, distinct categories (Taylor and Rupp 2003). Because of the binary limitations of the English language, it can be difficult to speak with precision about the multiplicity of categories potentially present in gender identity. Drag, where a person appropriates the symbols of another gender though appearance, dress, and mannerisms, can be classified as "gender nonconforming," "gender fluid," or "gender variant" behavior. "Drag queens" are typically cis-males (meaning that they were born with the biology of a male) who perform femininity, whereas drag kings are usually cis-females who perform masculinity. Though sometimes called "female impersonators," many drag queens dislike this title for the ways it flattens out the complex negotiations of self and identity that are often at the heart of drag performances.

Until fairly recently, drag has been considered controversial because of the ways that it challenges steadfast assumptions about the primacy of a biological basis for gender and the fixed nature of sexual identity. Feminist philosopher Judith Butler, however, argues that all gender is drag. She explains that human behaviors are part of a **performance** that continually creates and reinforces an identity that exists within the context of human relationships (Butler 1990)

Perhaps the most common manifestation of "drag" in the United States features a male who dresses and behaves with exaggerated femininity. It is important to note that drag performances are viewed as a way of "playing" with gender and do not necessarily indicate the sexuality of the performer. A drag queen, for example, is not necessarily a gay man. Drag can be performed to comic effect or for more serious purposes, including self-expression, artistic expression, transvestic fetishism (those who cross-dress as part of a sexual activity or identity), or spiritual reasons (especially common in non-Western contexts).

Attention to **hair** and **makeup** is essential in order to achieve the right "look" for a contemporary drag queen performance. The ultra-feminine face of a drag queen relies on skilled contouring and shading, conveying a dramatic expressiveness that adds to the performance. A base of foundation is applied, often covering the natural eyebrows. Eye shadow is applied, along with false eyelashes in order to give the eyes a more dramatic appearance. A strong eyebrow is often added with eye pencils. Many drag queens wear wigs or hairpieces, as well as a costume. Drag shows performed in gay clubs are increasingly visible across the United States as more and more people come to accept aspects of gender fluidity in daily life.

Popular television programs like *RuPaul's Drag Race* on the LOGO network continue to introduce those who are curious to aspects of drag culture. Venues across the United States and Europe draw audiences for drag performances that range from amateur to professional. Drag shows are usually a showcase of lip-synched performances to favorite musical numbers, where audiences are encouraged to approach the stage and tip the performer.

An important feature of drag performance is allowing the experience to exist on its own terms. "There is more going on [in drag performances] than just mimicking traditional female beauty. Even the girls who are the most beautiful in drag . . . do not really look like women, because they are too tall or have muscled arms or men's waists and buttocks. They are beautiful as drag queens" (Taylor and Rupp 2003, 225). Drag performances force audience members to think differently about what it means to be a man or a woman. This is what feminist scholars mean when they talk about "troubling" gender: they are causing people to think outside of the binary of male/female identity.

It is also noteworthy that many other cultural traditions allow more tolerance and space for gender-fluid performances of identity. In India, *hijras* are often represented as a "third sex," "neither man nor woman" (Reddy and Nanda 2005). *Hijras* are cis-males who typically wear female clothing and (ideally) renounce sexual desire and practice by undergoing a castration ceremony that entails a sacrifice of the male genitalia to the goddess Bahuchara or Bedhraj Mata, one of the many incarnations of Devi in India. The *hijra* then becomes a vehicle of divine power and is symbolically sanctioned by the society to engage in the ritual work of attending births, marriages, and temple activities specific to the causes of fertility and infertility.

See also: Gender; Hair; Makeup and Cosmetics; Performance/Performativity.

Further Reading

Butler, Judith. 1990. *Gender Trouble: Feminism and the Subversions of Identity*. New York: New York University Press.

Newton, Esther. 1972. *Mother Camp: Female Impersonators in America*. Chicago: University of Chicago Press.

Reddy, Gayatri, and Serena Nanda. 2005. Hijras: An "Alternative" Sex/Gender in India. In: *Gender in Cross-Cultural Perspective*, 4th edition, 278—85, edited by Caroline B. Brettell and Carolyn F. Sargent. Upper Saddle River, NJ: Prentice Hall.

Taylor, Verta, and Leila J. Rupp. 2003. *Drag Queens at the 801 Cabaret*. Chicago: University of Chicago Press.

DREADLOCKS

Dreadlocks are a hairstyle normally associated with people of African descent whose hair is very tightly curled. In the dreadlock hairstyle, hair is washed, but not combed or brushed. The wet hair is twisted into tight braids or ringlets that hang down on all sides. Dreadlocks may be seen among groups in Africa who identify as Maasai, Fulani, Wolof, and the Mouride Brotherhood and by Sadhu holy men in India. Dreadlocks were also worn in ancient history, as seen on Greek statues, and have been dated to the fifth century, when Bahatowie priests of the Ethiopian Coptic church wore the distinctive hairstyle.

Today, the most widely recognizable wearers of dreadlocks are Rastafarians, who began wearing dreadlocks in Jamaica as part of a religious movement in the 1940s. Rastas invoke biblical teachings of the Nazirites, which include abstinence from wine and alcoholic beverages, an avoidance of corpses and graves, and a directive to refrain from cutting or shaving their hair. According to scripture: "All the days of the vow of his separation there shall no razor come upon his head . . . and shall let the locks of the hair of his head grow." Because these holy laws forbade the trimming of hair, the trademark dreadlocks are the product of continually growing uncombed, knotted locks. Dreadlocks have become a powerful marker of Rastafarian identity. The locks are symbolic

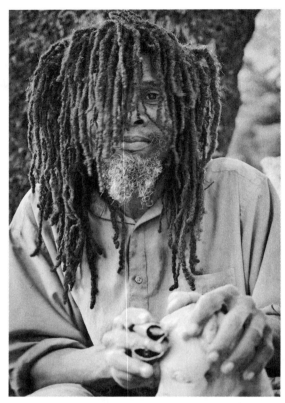

A local artisan wearing dreadlocks looks up from his work sanding a sculpture at the Old Fort in Montego Bay, Jamaica. (Lokibaho/iStockphoto.com)

of the Lion of Judah, which is sometimes seen centered on the Ethiopian flag as a tribute to Haile Selassie, who is revered within Rastafarianism.

There are two different traditions of dreadlocks, or "locks," in Jamaica (Edmonds 1998). The first, and most commonly accepted, explanation originates from guardsmen of the early days of the religious movement, who cultivated the hairstyle in an attempt to accentuate their fearsomeness. The sight of dreadlocks is meant to generate fear and anxiety on the part of the non-Rastafarian—hence the label "dread." The other tradition is connected to the activities of the influential House of Youth Black Faith movement, active from the late 1940s to the 1960s, who deliberately grew their locks in direct opposition to the social norms concerning grooming in order to accentuate their sense of alienation.

As with many religious symbols, dreadlocks can be interpreted in a variety of ways. Rastafarianism is heavily influenced by the legacy of slavery and neocolonialism that has worked to disadvantage so many peoples of African descent. Dreadlocks are symbolically powerful as an affirmation of African physical characteristics deemed to be beautiful and powerful.

Ideologically, dreadlocks also conform to the Rastafarian notion that "naturalness" is the morally superior position in all decisions. Trimming, combing, and straightening one's hair is seen as artificial and proscribed by most Rastas. Dreadlocks are also rumored to function as "psychic antenna," or a mystical link to the power of the universe which emanates from the earth. As a symbol for the connection between the Rastafarian and the earth force energy of the universe, the deliberate shaking of dreadlocks is thought to unleash spiritual energy that may bring about the destruction of Babylon.

Today, dreadlocks are a fashion statement and a matter of personal style, worn by many who are not adherents of the Rastafarian faith. Thicker or kinkier hair is best suited for growing dreadlocks, but it is possible for all hair types to develop the style, especially with the use of wax, synthetic hair extensions, and other products. Whereas religiously minded Rastafarians allow the uneven mats and ropes of hair to form through a "freeform method" of intentional neglect, some who are not of the faith prefer a more cultivated or stylized look to wear their dreadlocked hair. Typically, the style takes a long time to achieve, developing as the hair grows out naturally, though there are shortcuts to kicking off the process, including a salon service known as "dread perming." To achieve evenly sized dreads, it is necessary to plan and maintain the style. There a number of ways to achieve the look, including backcombing, braiding, and rolling the hair. There are also a wide range of dreadlock styles, including flat-twisted half-back styles, flat-twisted Mohawk styles, braided buns, and lock crinkles.

Dreadlocks remain controversial and threatening to some as a visible sign of difference. In September 2016, the 11th U.S. Circuit Court of Appeals ruled against a lawsuit filed by the Equal Employment Opportunity Commission, upholding the right of an employer to refuse to hire someone because of their dreadlocks (Gutierrez-Morfin 2016).

See also: "Black Is Beautiful Movement," or Black Power; The Caribbean; Hair.

Further Reading

Edmonds, Ennis B. 1998. "Dread 'I' in-A-Babylon: Ideological Resistance and Cultural Revitalization." In: *Chanting Down Babylon: The Rastafari Reader*, edited by Murrell, Nathaniel Samuel, William David Spencer, and Adrian Anthony McFarlane, 23–35. Philadelphia: Temple University Press.

Gutierrez-Morfin, Noel. 2016. "US Court Rules Dreadlock Ban During Hiring Process Is Legal." NBC News. September 21. Accessed September 22, 2016. http://www.nbcnews.com/news/nbcblk/u-s-court-rules-dreadlock-ban-during-hiring-process-legal-n652211.

Sobo, Elisa Janine. 1993. *One Blood: The Jamaican Body*. Albany, NY: SUNY Press.

Thomas, Deborah A. 2004. *Modern Blackness: Nationalism, Globalization, and the Politics of Culture in Jamaica*. Durham, NC: Duke University Press.

EATING DISORDERS

Social norms of body image, including both 21st-century preferences for thinness in women and lean muscularity in men, often causes unhealthy and destructive practices. The pursuit of an ideal **weight**, along with body dissatisfaction and **body dysmorphia**, can lead, in both men and women, to bingeing, purging, or self-starvation.

Eating disorders are both physical and psychological illnesses characterized by "clinical disturbances in eating behaviors and attitudes that pose very serious physiological and psychological health consequences" (Shapiro 2011). The term "eating disorder" is used generally to describe such conditions as anorexia nervosa, bulimia nervosa, and binge eating disorder, the three most common diseases (Latzer and Stein 2012).

Anorexia nervosa is a condition in which the patient refuses to maintain a healthy body weight, due to an intense fear of gaining weight or becoming fat. This condition leads patients to become dangerously thin, while still obsessing about portion sizes and/or skipping meals (Foran 2014). Bulimia nervosa is characterized by the patient's eating a large amount of food in a short amount of time and then engaging in inappropriate methods of compensating for the overeating. These methods may include self-induced vomiting or the overuse of laxatives and diuretics. Patients suffering from bulimia may also first binge and then refuse to eat for days as a way of compensating (Shapiro 2011). Both bulimia nervosa and anorexia nervosa are unhealthy ways of seeking to achieve an ideal body.

Anorexia and bulimia are serious disorders that require physical and psychological intervention. Those who suffer from anorexia nervosa may become so malnourished and underweight that they often require hospitalization. Recovery from eating disorders can be very difficult. Fewer than half of the individuals with the condition recover, and one-fifth of patients remain chronically ill from the effects of the starvation. Anorexia affects women more than men, with approximately 1 male patient for each 10 to 15 female patients (Shapiro 2011). Bulimia nervosa affects many more individuals worldwide than anorexia, but the statistics on recovery are better, with more than half of treated patients recovering from the disease (Shapiro 2011).

The final type of eating disorder, binge eating disorder, is also characterized by an unhealthy eating pattern, but does not result in extreme thinness. With binge eating disorder, patients find it hard to stop eating, eat large amounts of food repeatedly, and feel a lack of control of their ability to stop eating. People with binge eating disorder often eat secretly, ashamed of their lack of control, and eat when they are not physically hungry. Binge eaters are often obese or unhealthily overweight (Shapiro 2011).

The majority of eating disorders occur in adolescent and teenage girls, with an increasing number of young men affected every year (Latzer and Stein 2012). Low self-esteem is one risk factor that can predispose someone to an eating disorder. Patients with low self-esteem often express a high level of dissatisfaction with how they look and feel pressure to make their bodies look better. Participation in certain sports and activities is another risk factor: dancers and athletes, with their constant scrutiny of their bodies, are at higher risk for developing eating disorders. Finally, studies have demonstrated that exposure to media images of the Western ideal of thinness in models or actors causes body dissatisfaction and changes in eating habits worldwide (Shapiro 2011).

See also: Body Dysmorphia Disorder; Masculinity; Obesity; Progressive Muscularity; Weight.

Further Reading

Foran, Racquel. 2014. *Living with Eating Disorders*. North Mankato, MN: ABDO Publishing.
Latzer, Yael, and Daniel Stein. 2012. *Treatment and Recovery of Eating Disorders*. New York: Nova Science Publishers, Inc.
Pope, Harrison G., Roberto Olivardia, Amanda Gruber, and John Borowiecki. 1999. "Evolving Ideals of Male Body Image as Seen Through Action Toys." *International Journal of Eating Disorders* 26, no. 1: 65–72.
Shapiro, Colleen M. 2011. *Eating Disorders: Causes, Diagnosis and Treatments*. New York: Nova Science Publishers.

EGYPT

Judging by the archaeological evidence left behind, ancient Egyptians spent a good deal of time working on their appearance. **Cosmetics** and makeup palettes (symbolically shaped like fish or baboons) are often discovered among the grave goods of Egyptians. **Perfumes** were the key to allure for both men and women, as well as an important way to venerate the gods and negotiate a passage to the afterlife (Manniche 1999).

In love poetry and hymns to Hathor, the Egyptian goddess of beauty, writers mention the scent of the beloved, as well as the shape of her hair, her eyes, and beautiful thighs and her heavy buttocks. Dark hair was compared to the night, dark "wine-grapes," and lapis lazuli (typically a deep blue). Lovers were also celebrated for light-skinned coloring shaded as gold or white. These honey-tongued Egyptian bards also commented favorably on the voice, movement, and fertility of their beloved lady friends.

The most distinctive and instantly recognizable look of the ancient Egyptians' physical ideal is probably the iconic, thick lines of kohl eyeliner worn by both men and women, which extended a line from the outside corner of the eye almost to the ear. This striking eye treatment was mean to emulate the look of Ra, the Egyptian sun god. Traditionally, kohl was made from a mixture of lead salts derived from powdered antimony, carbon, and copper oxide. The darkening effect of the lead on the eye prevented glare in the bright sun, providing a kind of "sunglasses" effect, and is also thought to have prevented eye infections that could potentially have been caused by environmental conditions created by the annual flooding of the Nile River.

Other **cosmetics** were also commonly used. The prominent green and gray colors of Egyptian eye shadow were achieved through a combination of powders made from ground green malachite, galena, and other lead-containing minerals. The powder was then added to a base of oil or fat and stored in containers made of stone, wood, or ceramic. Mascara and eyebrow darkeners were made by burning almonds or by using kohl. Women also mixed finely ground red ochre into almond, palm, sesame, or olive oil to create blusher and lipstick. Henna was also used to accent palms, soles, and nails. Egyptians derived castor, sesame, and moringa oil to rub into the skin as an emollient to keep the face youthful and to prevent wrinkles. Women also created moisturizing facial masks made from a mixture of honey and milk.

Despite elaborate beauty rituals, Egyptian clothing was deceptively simple. Men wore kilts, and women wore simple sheaths made of linen called a "kalasaris." These simple garments could be made more elaborate through pleating, embroidery, belts, or the means to purchase higher-quality, more luxurious fabrics, including imported silk. For those of higher rank, a collar made of beads might also be worn around the shoulders. Men took great care to remove their facial hair regularly, though they sometimes wore false beards made from leather or metal as befitting their social class or role as elite. Priests who were able to wore leopard skins, which were both valuable and rare, imported from the south.

Ancient Egyptians took great care to preserve the bodies of the deceased for an afterlife, giving us tremendous insight into the styles and fashions they found attractive. Egyptian artists typically painted images of people in profile view, often with highly stylized hand gestures and elaborate **jewelry**. Circular bands made of leather or precious metals, called fillets, were frequently worn around the head in the manner of a tiara. Later, more elaborate diadems were introduced for those who could afford them, made from precious metals and set with semiprecious stones imported from around the Egyptian empire, including lapis lazuli, turquoise, agate, and carnelian. Those with more modest means often wore necklaces made of fired clay beads.

The ideal body for both men and women seems to have been a youthful, slim figure with narrow hips. Aging figures are sometimes depicted as part of funerary art and seem to be shown with a slightly drooping rear end, slightly sagging breasts, and pouching cheeks or sagging chin. Paintings of people represented a broad range of skin colors, with women typically shown with lighter-colored skin than men. Ideal skin pigmentation for women was frequently expressed in love poems as "golden," whereas men were portrayed with red or reddish-brown skin.

According to the elaborate perfume jars found in Egyptian tombs with sculpted handles shaped like animals, people, and flowers, it appears that Egyptians clearly appreciated smelling attractive. The Egyptians traded with other empires of the ancient world to acquire exotic perfumes made from herbs and flowers. Evidence has been found of myrrh, frankincense, sandalwood, cedar, and musk perfumes, often fixed to maintain the scent longer in a pear-like fruit called balanos. The Egyptians also paid great attention to personal hygiene, spending a good deal of time **bathing**. They made two versions of "soap." One contained clay or ash and was mixed with perfume. The other was a mixture of animal fats and vegetable oils, mixed with alkaline salts. Unwanted hair was removed using knives, tweezers, and the ancient **hair removal** technique known as "sugaring." Smooth skin was attended to vigorously with pumice stones to soften dry spots and remove rough skin. Sometimes, honey was applied to the skin to tighten the pores. Moisturizers for the body were also common, made from almond, palm, sesame, and olive oils.

The iconic Egyptian profile would not be complete without a mention of wigs. Wigs were fitted over shaved heads or short hair to not only beautify the appearance, but as a strategy for coping with the heat. Almost everyone in Egyptian society wore a wig, regardless of social **class**. However, Egyptian law forbade slaves to wear wigs. Expensive wigs for the elite were made of human hair, but cheaper wigs were also available made out of vegetable fibers or wool. The base for the wig was a close-fitting skull cap made from fibers in order to prevent the wig from slipping. Those who could not afford wigs sometimes augmented their natural hair with hair extensions that clipped to the underside of the natural hair, adding volume to their own styles. Both boy and girl children usually had shaved heads until adolescence, sometimes with a single lock of hair that fell down along the side of the head.

A wide range of wig hairstyles reflected hierarchical distinctions within the culture by age, gender, and status. Straight, smooth hairstyles in a blunt shoulder length with straight bangs that fell to the eyebrows was the preferred look for most wigs. Women's wigs were slightly longer than those of men. Some wigs featured asymmetrical hairstyles, so that the hair hung lower in the front than in the back. Wig styles were set with beeswax and mud in order to make the style more durable, and wigs were often adorned with additional ornaments, flowers, or ribbons. Wigs were also dyed with henna. Later, in the New Kingdom period of the Egyptian civilization, women's hair became increasingly elaborate, with styles that required long hair to be dressed in curls and braids. Only elite women and queens were eligible to wear a particularly ornate hair style called a "goddess," which was achieved by separating and curling the hair into three distinct sections, each of which was then coiled and pinned to create a striking wig headdress.

See also: Bathing and Showering; Class; Hair; Hair Removal; Makeup and Cosmetics; Perfumes and Scented Oils.

Further Reading

History Embalmed. 2015. "Egyptian Make Up and Cosmetics." Accessed November 24, 2015. http://www.historyembalmed.org/ancient-egyptians/egyptian-make-up.htm.

Jackson, Simedar. 2015. "10 Beauty Secrets from Ancient Egypt." Marie Claire. Accessed November 24, 2015. http://www.marieclaire.com/beauty/news/a14366/beauty-makeup-secrets-ancient-egypt.

Manniche, Lise. 1999. *Sacred Luxuries: Fragrance, Aromatherapy, and Cosmetics in Ancient Egypt*. New York: Cornell University Press.

McIntyre, Megan. 2015. "We Tried the Most Timeless Beauty Routine, Ever." Refinery 29. Accessed November 24, 2015. http://www.refinery29.com/famous-women-beauty-routines#.4hdn4js:4941.

Rutherford, Maggie. 2013. "The Ancient Egyptian Concept of Beauty." Tour Egypt. Accessed November 24, 2015. http://www.touregypt.net/featurestories/beauty.htm.

ELONGATED LABIA

Sometimes referred to as a "hottentot apron," elongated labia are deliberately stretched and can reach a length of four inches beyond the vulva. Labia elongation is practiced to improve the aesthetics and symmetry of female genitals. Practices of labia stretching have been noted in Burundi, Rwanda, Malawi, Mozambique, Zimbabwe, Zambia, and Uganda. Stretching begins at the early age of four or five. Young girls are usually assisted in the practice by their female adult relatives. The technique is also reportedly associated with enhanced sexual pleasure, increased intensity of female orgasm, and *kunyaza*, the Rwanda-Rundi word for female ejaculation (also called *kakyabali* in Baganda).

Ethnographic data on vaginal practices in southeastern Africa demonstrate that 65 percent of women in the area actively worked to lengthen their vaginal labia to prepare for sexual intercourse, to feel more like a woman, to satisfy her sexual partner by stimulating erection, and to feel good (Bagnol and Mariano 2012). As soon as a young girl's breasts start to grow, an older woman teaches her that in order to hold the penis of a male partner more pleasingly during sexual intercourse, she should massage and stretch the inner labia from the top to bottom with the tips of the thumb and the index finger of each hand. A girl is initially guided in this process by an older woman, but eventually takes up the practice as part of her own daily hygiene.

Traditionally, the stretching process was facilitated by the addition of an oily substance derived from the nut of a castor plant ground into a paste and added to other locally available herbs and oils. Today, women report using commercial products like Johnson's baby oil or Vaseline to achieve the necessary lubrication required for stretching the skin. The process is understood to increase sexual pleasure for both partners.

Until 2008, the practice was classified as female genital mutilation (FGM) by the World Health Organization (Bagnol and Mariano 2008). After that time, it was reclassified as genital modification because women who engage in the practice report themselves as active sexual agents who experience pleasure with their partners and reportedly suffer no ill effects due directly to the stretching. Some researchers suggest using the term "ethic genital modification" to avoid value-laden language when talking about the process of modifying genitalia (Gallo, Tita, and Viviana 2006).

See also: Body Modification.

Further Reading

Amadiume, Ifi. 2007. "Sexuality, African Religio-Cultural Traditions and Modernity: Expanding the Lens." African Research on Sexuality Research Center. 2007. Accessed November 23, 2015. http://www.arsrc.org/downloads/features/amadiume.pdf.

Bagnol, Brigitte, and Esmeralda Mariano. 2008. "Elongation of the Labia Minora and Use of Vaginal Products to Enhance Eroticism: Can These Practices Be Considered FGM?" *Finnish Journal of Ethnicity and Migration* 3(2): 42–53.

Bagnol, Brigitte, and Esmeralda Mariano. 2012. *Gender, Sexuality and Vaginal Practices.* Maputo, Mozambique: DAA, FLCS, UEM.

Crais, Clifton C., and Pamela Scully. 2009. *Sarah Baartman and the Hottentot Venus: A Ghost Story and a Biography.* Princeton, NJ: Princeton University Press.

Gallo, Pia Grassivaro, Eleanora Tita, and Franco Viviana. 2006. "At the Roots of Ethnic Female Genital Modification." In: *Bodily Integrity and the Politics of Circumcision, Controversy, and Change*, edited by George C. Denniston, Pia Grassivaro Gallo, Frederick Mansfield Hodges, 64–84. Dordrecht, Netherlands: Springer.

Khau, Mathabo. 2012. Female Sexual Pleasure and Autonomy: What Has Inner Labia Elongation Got to Do with It? *Sexualities* 15, no. 7. 763–77.

EXOTICIZE

To exoticize means to portray someone or something unfamiliar as exotic or unusual. Humans often find the unfamiliar and exotic ugly and unattractive or, alternatively, attractive and more sexually interesting.

An influential analysis by Algerian literary critic Malek Alloula investigated the trade in colonial photographic postcards of beautiful Algerian women collected by travelers during the late 19th and early 20th centuries. Alloula argued that the photographic images of Algerian "harem" women that circulated throughout Europe during this period did not accurately reflect the lives of Algerian women, but rather, a European fantasy about the non-Western woman, eroticized to fulfill the complicated sexual desires of the colonizer over the colonized (Alloula 1983). Alloula claimed that the Algerian women were not actually women of the harem, but impoverished prostitutes who were asked to pose for the photographer for a fee.

During the 19th and early 20th century, an exaggerated, sensationalized discourse centered on seemingly unique bodies of **the Other**—people from the non-Western world—especially by heightening their differences from viewers, who were rendered more comfortable and felt less threatened, by their inclusion in sideshows where admittance could be had for a small fee. Barkers at circuses tried to lure patrons into circus tents to observe "freaks," who received (sometimes dubious) identities designed to appeal to curiosity. For example, promoters told the audience that the person on exhibit came from a "mysterious" part of the world, often supplying purposefully erroneous or distorted information about the life and customs of the area of supposed origin. The "freak" being presented often was placed in a painted backdrop depicting jungle scenes or far-off geographic locations, occasionally with papier-mâché boulders, imitation tropical plants, or other touches of exotica to set the scene and fire the imagination. Exotic stories were designed to maximize audience interest in a period of intense world exploration and colonization. The so-called "savages" of the African continent were a popular motif, as were the indigenous peoples of the Philippines and the islands of the Pacific. **Skin tone** and color were important factors in the construction of exotic identity.

Perhaps the best-known figure exhibited in this shocking manner was Saartjie Baartman, a Khoikhoi woman originally from South Africa billed as the "Hottentot Venus" and displayed in both France and England (Lindors 1996). Baartman created a buzz in the media and among audiences for her distinctly generous and rounded **buttocks**, a "condition" sometimes referred to as "steatopygia" (meaning "fat buttocks"). Spectators from the audience were invited to touch her through her skin-colored dress in order to verify that she was not wearing padding.

Though slavery had recently been abolished in the United Kingdom, it is not entirely clear that Baartman was traveling with her "manager" and companion Heinrich Cesars of her own free will. Following her unhappy death at the age of 25, her body was dissected by the leading naturalist of the day, Baron Georges Cuvier.

The erasure of the black woman as a subject appears consistent with a number of (post)colonial strategies for imposing a psychological victimization on black women, suggesting that they would eventually inhibit the progress of their own race (Rowe 2009). This continual characterization of the body of the black woman as simultaneously dangerous and uncontrollable set the stage for the eventual mobilization of black femininity as a tool, such as the **Black Is Beautiful movement**.

The dangerous practice of exoticizing others serves to flatten out the identity of people with diverse histories in such a way that denies them individuality, identity, or personhood to speak for themselves. The supposedly liberating idea that there may be a "color-blind erotic democracy" such as that which persists in Brazil, actually masks racism and inequalities (Goldstein 1999) under the guise of liberating an appreciation of beauty.

See also: "Black Is Beautiful Movement," or Black Power; Butts and Booty; Orientalism; The "Other"; Performance/Performativity; Skin Tone.

Further Reading

Alloula, Malek. 1983. *The Colonial Harem*. Minneapolis: University of Minnesota Press.

Bogdan, Robert. 1996. The Social Construction of Freaks. In: *Freakery: Cultural Spectacles of the Extraordinary Body*, 23–27. New York: New York University Press.

Goldstein, Donna. 1999. "Interracial Sex and Racial Democracy in Brazil: Twin Concepts?" *American Anthropologist* 101: 563–78.

Karp, Ivan, and Steven D. Lavine. 1991. *Exhibiting Cultures*. Washington, D.C.: Smithsonian Press.

Lindors, Bernth. 1996. "Ethnological Show Business: Footlighting the Dark Continent." In: *Freakery: Cultural Spectacles of the Extraordinary Body*, 207–18. New York: New York University Press.

Rowe, Rochelle. 2009. "Glorifying the Jamaican Girl." *Radical History Review* 103: 36–58.

Thomson, Rosemarie Garland. 1996. Introduction: From Wonder to Error—A Genealogy of Freak Discourse in Modernity. In: *Freakery: Cultural Spectacles of the Extraordinary Body*, 1–19. New York: New York University Press.

EYE COLOR

Eye color is composed primarily of two factors: the pigmentation of the eye's iris and the frequency of the scattering of light (called Tyndall scattering, an optical phenomenon similar to Rayleigh scattering, which causes the sky to look blue) by the stroma of the iris. Eye color is genetically linked to skin color; the amount of melanin in the iris allows the eye color to range from brown to green to blue. However, eye color is not dictated by a single gene like many other genes, which allows for a blending to create many shades of color (Frost 2014). Eye color can be measured and compared by physical anthropologists using the Martin–Schultz scale, which assigns twenty distinct eye colors a value from 1 to 16 (Sturm and Larsson 2009).

Brown and black eyes are the most common eye colors. These have the highest concentration of melanin and are found all over the world, especially in Asia, Oceania, Africa, the Americas, and southern Europe. Amber eyes have a strong yellowish/gold or russet/coppery tint. Eyes that are so brown that they appear to be black are among the rarest eye color.

Today, between 20 and 40 percent of people of European descent have blue eyes, but originally, all humans had brown eyes. Using new technology designed to study mitochondrial DNA, scientists have tracked down a single genetic mutation in the OCA2 gene that occurred between 6,000 and 10,000 years ago in Europe, which gave rise to all the blue eyes in the world today (Bryner 2008). Gray eyes are a variation of blue eyes and will often show a yellow ring around the pupil. Gray eyes are prominent among the Shawia people of the Aures Mountains of northeast Algeria. Deeply blue eyes will occasionally photograph or appear in certain lights to be violet.

Although green eyes may occur in people of any race, only about 2 percent of the world's population has green or hazel eyes. Green eyes tend to appear in places where blue-eyed people came into contact with brown-eyed peoples, often due to exploration or warfare. Outside of Europe, the highest rates of green-eyed people occur in **Iran**, Pakistan, Afghanistan, Central Asia, Spain, northern Africa, and **Brazil**. Green eyes spread to Europe when the Moors invaded Spain (Rhodes 2016). In Ireland and Scotland, 14 percent of people have brown eyes, whereas 86 percent of the population has blue or green eyes. Another study found green eyes to be more prevalent in women than in men among Icelandic and Dutch populations (Frost 2014). Hazel eyes consist of a combination of green and brown/gold colors, which may appear to change according to different lights as a result of the Rayleigh scattering.

Very rarely, a person may be born with two different colored eyes or they may display "mosaic" eyes, which show different colors on the same iris, and babies are often born with lighter eye colors than they eventually have. The process of eye darkening in children usually happens within the first three years as melanin is produced.

Eye color may also appear to "change" based on the conditions of the light. These changes are often attributed to changes in mood, which may be influenced by pupil dilation, which tightens the iris and makes the eyes look darker and brighter. Hormonal changes during puberty, pregnancy, and after serious trauma may cause impermanent, temporary gradations to eye color. Crying can also change the appearance of the eyes by creating bloodshot pupils, exaggerating the color of the iris when contrasted with the pinkish color. Wearing certain clothing or eye shadow colors such as blue, yellow, or green will also affect the way that light is reflected by the eyes, allowing the color more prominence. Eye color can also change with age. Dramatic changes to eye color should be checked out by a doctor, as this may be a sign of certain serious, vision-threatening diseases such as Fuch's heterochromic iridocyclitis, Horner's syndrome, or pigmentary glaucoma.

See also: Brazil; Eye Shape; Iran.

Further Reading

Bryner, Jeanna. 2008. "One Common Ancestor Behind Blue Eyes." *LiveScience*. January 31. Accessed October 14, 2016. http://www.livescience.com/9578-common-ancestor-blue -eyes.html.

Frost, Peter. 2014. "The Puzzle of European Hair, Eye, and Skin Color." *Advances in Anthropology* 4, no. 2: 78–88.

Sturm, Richard A., and Mats Larsson. 2009. "Genetics of Human Iris Colour and Patterns." *Pigment Cell and Melanoma Research* 22, no. 5: 544–62.

Rhodes, Courtney. 2016. "Learn about the Origins of Green Eyes." *Owlcation*. July 16. Accessed October 14, 2016. https://owlcation.com/stem/The-Origins-of-Green-Eyes.

EYE SHAPE

People of Asiatic descent show a tendency toward more prominent epicanthal folds in the lid area that hoods the upper eyelid, especially at the inner corner of the eye. The effect may make the eyes look "small"; however, human eyes are the same size. Differences in eye shape come from the ways that the eyelids are oriented. Evolutionary biologists speculate that the tendency toward the so-called "monolid eyes" common to Asians may have been an adaptation to environmental conditions, which favored people whose eyes were provided more protection against glare and harsh winter conditions. This type of eye shape is sometimes referred to as an "almond "shape, with a natural lift at the outer corner. In order to affect a more Western, "open" eye appearance, some people with this eye shape opt for epicanthoplasty (also referred to by the more general term, "blepharoplasty," which means surgery of the eyelid), an **eyelid surgery** that reduces the appearance of the fold. The procedure is especially popular in **China** and **South Korea**.

More open, "round" eye shapes are popular in contemporary Western standards of beauty, in particular for the way they appear to be more **youthful.** "Round" eye shapes feature highly curved upper and lower lids, which make the eyes appear larger. The perception of large eyes, as measured by the height and width of the eye, correspond closely with appraisals of attractiveness (Cunningham 1986). Symmetry of the eyes is also valued when assessing standards of beauty.

Cosmetics may be used to enhance the natural eye shape. Deep-set eyes, typically large and set deeper into the skull, create the illusion of more prominent brow bone and can be brightened and softened with neutral colors flecked with metallic. Stylists usually treat monolid eyes, which are almost flush against the face with very little crease, by using a gradient of eye shadows from dark to light to add dimension to the eye. So-called "hooded eyes," which feature an extra layer of skin that drops over the crease and causes the eye to appear smaller, can be accented with the addition of a dark eye shadow that draws the focus upward. Protruding eyes, where the natural shape of the eye creates the appearance of projected lids in the eye socket area, opens up a great deal of lid space and is well suited to a "smoky eye" treatment, a dramatic look that features dark, slightly smudged liner close to the lash line.

"Upturned" and "downturned" eyes are both classic almond-shape eyes with natural lift or a slight drooping at the edge closest to the ear—both look more striking with a "cat's eye" shape, which uses a dark liner on the top lid to extend and emphasize the eye shape. Eyes that are close set or wide set (measured by the distance between the two eyes) can also be maximized by shading light eye shadow on the inner corners to make eyes appear farther apart or lining with a dark color to the tear duct in order to make the eyes appear closer together.

See also: Body Modification; China; Eyelid Surgery; Makeup and Cosmetics; South Korea; Youth.

Further Reading

Cunningham, Michael R. 1986. "Measuring the Physical in Physical Attractiveness: Quasi-experiments on the Sociobiology of Female Facial Beauty." *Journal of Personality and Social Psychology* 50, no. 5: 925–35.

EYEBROWS

Eyebrows add expressiveness to the face and prominently frame the eyes, which are sometimes referred to as the "windows to the soul." Because of the ways that eyebrows create and enhance facial expressions, the shape and size of the brows may be key to beauty standards in a number of cultures around the world. Arches that are too pointy create a look of surprise, or even anger. Overextending the tail of the brow can create a droopy effect, drawing the face down. Brows that are overly darkened can appear stern or masculine.

Proper grooming of the brows can enhance the appearance of youth, femininity, and polished good looks in a variety of cultures. Removing hairs to create the desired shape or adding the illusion of a thicker hair on the brow can be done with **cosmetics** such as pencils, brow powders, colored eyebrow gels, or brow tints. Stencils are also available to create an ideal brow line.

As part of a beauty standard, women have historically been encouraged to culti-vate and groom a distinct eyebrow shape through cutting, shaving, plucking, or wax-ing. During the 18th century, when women often used caustic potions containing lead on their faces to whiten their skin, they also inadvertently lost their eyebrows. Fre-quently, mice would be trapped and cultivated for their short silky fur. Mouse hide was cut and glued into place on the natural brow line to create temporary eyebrows (Downing 2012).

Today's perfectly shaped eyebrows begin directly above the center of the nostril and the arch falls over the back third of the eye. Eyebrows may also be enhanced or added to the face through the use of pencils, darkening substances like soot or ash, and eyebrow stencils. In some cases, the natural eyebrow hairs are removed completely, and the brow line is reapplied to achieve the desired aesthetic effect, as is sometimes the case with the eyebrows of transgendered women.

Plucked eyebrows are pulled out individually, directly from the follicle, with the assistance of tweezers. In general, it takes about 64 days for eyebrow hair to grow back in after it is plucked, although if the area has been overplucked, the follicle may be damaged, which prevents the hair from ever growing back again.

Waxing also works by pulling the hair out from the follicle. Typically, there should be some hair growth present so that the wax has something to adhere to. Brow waxing may be done at home with the assistance of wax strips, which are heated and then pressed on the eyebrow in small sections against the direction of hair growth, then pulled quickly to remove unwanted hairs. Waxing can also take place in a salon in consultation with an esthetician who can recommend an ideal shape and size for the brow line. Heated wax is applied around the desired shape of the brow, topped with a piece of cloth or muslin, and then removed quickly, leaving a new shape to the brow.

Sugaring is a similar hair-removal technique that has been practiced for centuries in North Africa, **Greece**, and the Middle East. A paste-like gel composed of sugar, lemon, and hot water is prepared; applied to the area where hair removal is desired; and then strips of cloth are secured to the top of the drying solution and quickly pulled off to remove the unwanted hair. Unlike wax, the sugaring solution residue can be easily removed from the skin with water after the procedure and reportedly provides less irritation.

Threading, also called epilation, is an ancient practice for removing small stray hairs from the brow line or the upper lip that comes from **India**. A think cotton thread is doubled, then twisted, and rolled over the stray hairs, deftly removing several shafts of hair in a simultaneous line to achieve a precise shape. The thread is sometimes anchored between the teeth of an experienced practitioner, increasing the speed of the procedure. This efficient practice of threading has spread so that today it is common throughout Asia, the Middle East, and North Africa. Though not completely free of side effects (Litak, Krunic, Antonijevic et al. 2011), threading is said to be less painful and creates less skin irritation than plucking.

Hair may also be permanently removed with the use of lasers. This process is more expensive than the others, but is frequently recommended for the area between the brows, which can create the illusion of the so-called "unibrow," which refers to a pair of eyebrows that appear to be connected so that they are not easily seen as two distinct brows and form a seemingly continuous line across the upper third of the face. However, the unibrow look is considered attractive in some parts of the world, including Central Asia, **Iran**, and ancient Greece, where women used soot to darken and enhance their natural brow. Mexican artist Frida Kahlo is also famous for cultivating a unique and distinctive unibrow, making her self-portraits instantly recognizable.

Standards of shape and size of eyebrows change over time and according to culture. For example, the fashion icons of the World War era preferred a thin brow line, whereas thick eyebrows were popular in the **United States** during the 1980s, when Brooke Shields popularized the natural brow look. Later, thick, prominent brows were also a part of the sex appeal of a young Madonna.

The "power brow" popular in the United States today typically features a dark color and a high arch, which make the face look younger. One of the most frequently performed cosmetic surgeries is the eyebrow lift, which stretches the skin upward to enhance the illusion of youth.

See also: Greece; Hair Removal; Iran; United States.

Further Reading

Cosio, Robyn, and Cynthia Robins. 2000. *The Eyebrow.* New York: Harper Collins.

Downing, Sarah Jane. 2012. *Beauty and Cosmetics 1550–1950.* Oxford, England: Shire Publications.

Litak, Jason, Alkesandar L. Krunic, Sasha Antonijevic, Pedram Pouryazdanparast, and Pedram Gerami. 2011. "Eyebrow Epilation by Threading: An Increasingly Popular Procedure with Some Less-Popular Outcomes." *Dermatologic Surgery* 27, no. 7: 1051–54.

Schreiber, Jeffrey E., Navin K. Singh, and Stanley A. Klatsky. 2005. "Beauty Lies in the 'Eyebrow' of the Beholder: A Public Survey of Eyebrow Aesthetics." *Aesthetic Surgery Journal* 25, no. 4: 348–52.

Taylor, English. 2014. "Eyebrows, Why?," *The Atlantic.* July 24. Accessed November 24, 2015. http://www.theatlantic.com/health/archive/2014/07/eyebrows-why/374479/.

Valenti, Lauren. 2014. "The History of Women and Their Eyebrows." Marie Claire. Accessed November 24, 2015. www.marieclaire.com/beauty/makeup/a9381/eyebrows-through-the-years.

EYELID SURGERY

Surgery on the eyelids, known to surgeons as blepharoplasty, is a procedure designed to "rejuvenate the upper and lower eyelids by removing excess fat, skin and muscle" and to tighten "drooping upper eyelid skin" while reducing "puffy bags below the eyes" (ISAPS 2015a). Although this procedure can be performed on any individual, the biggest consumers of this surgery are Asians and Asian Americans seeking to create the double eyelid held as a social norm of Euro-descended beauty. The surgery is common for both men and women, and worldwide is the number-one cosmetic surgery procedure undertaken by men (ISAPS 2015b).

In 2014, blepharoplasty was the most commonly performed cosmetic surgical procedure performed worldwide, with 1.4 million surgeries being reported in that year alone (ISAPS 2015b). The nations that reported the most blepharoplasty procedures were **Brazil,** Japan, the **United States**, and **South Korea**, each nation recording more than 100,000 surgeries in that year (ISAPS 2015b).

In general, blepharoplasty is undertaken by individuals of various ethnic backgrounds who seek to reverse the signs of aging around their eyes, to reduce bags and excess skin under the eyes, and to tighten the sagging skin of aging eyelids. Some young people, notably in the United States, have experimented with nonsurgical methods for lifting and changing the shape of the eye. These methods include the use of theatrical glue or even Scotch tape on the eyelid. Blepharoplasty remains, however, the only permanent technique (Pak 2007).

In Asian populations, however, the procedure is commonly understood to be a method of looking "more white" or appearing "more awake and alert." Worldwide, approximately half of people of Asian descent are born with eyelids that are naturally smooth and flow down to the eye without a crease in the skin above the eye. Blepharoplasty (sometimes referred to as the more specific term "epicanthoplasty," which refers to surgical removal or reduction of the epicanthal fold which can cover the opening of the inner corner of the eye) creates or exaggerates the crease above the eye in the eyelid, creating what is commonly known as a "double eyelid" (Lin 2001).

This physical feature is then often seen as promoting a "sleepy" appearance that communicates lack of interest and intelligence. Many Asian and Asian Americans seeking this procedure for themselves and their children are looking to create a wide-awake and capable image. Indeed many parents in the United States, Taiwan, Japan, and South Korea opt to have the procedure performed on infants, with the understanding that the improved appearance of the eye will help the child succeed in life (Oulette 2009).

Beyond the notion of open eyes communicating intelligence and attentiveness, another reason cited by patients seeking the procedure is the desire for a solution to the reported problem among Asian women in applying eyeliner, as in women without a double eyelid, the eyelid is covered by skin obscuring the area where eyeliner would be applied (Jesitus 2004).

In the United States, eyelid surgery first became popular in both Asian and Asian American populations after World War II. Scholars propose that the American occupation of Japan and the conflict in Korea in the 1950s had the effect of both familiarizing Asian citizens with Western models of beauty and reinforcing the status and social power of Western nations in Asia. The first medical research and publication on the procedure was performed and written by U.S. surgeons stationed in Korea who found that although surgeons in Seoul, Hong Kong, and Tokyo were already performing these procedures, there was no extant research or medical literature to support their work (Haiken 1999).

In the 21st century, one of the biggest national increases in eyelid surgery has been in **China** and among Chinese citizens seeking surgery in South Korea. Although plastic surgery to create the double eyelid is available in China, South Korean procedures are considered by Chinese visitors to be safer and more hygienic (Stevenson 2014).

As with rhinoplasty, many social critics complain that blepharoplasty is a way of erasing Asian identity, promoting cultural assimilation and teaching nonwhite people to internalize racism (Jones and Heyes 2009). The link between the kind of racial miming engaged in by some non-Asians as an insult (making "slant-eyes" by pulling the skin by the sides of their eyes taut) and the understood need to change eye size and shape to avoid prejudice can be seen as both a cause for the popularity of blepharoplasty and a signal of racist social norms (Lin 2001).

Blepharoplasty surgery itself takes approximately two hours and is done under general anesthesia. Most patients can have the surgery done as an outpatient procedure, and the risks are minimal. After the surgery, excessive tearing, light sensitivity, and itching are normal, but rare. Some temporary risks include blurred vision, infection, bleeding, swelling at the corners of the eyelids, dry eyes, or difficulty in closing the eyes completely. Although rare, risks associated with the procedure may require further surgery (ISAPS 2015a).

See also: China; Eye Shape; Nose Jobs; Plastic Surgery; South Korea; United States.

Further Reading

Haiken Elizabeth. 1999. *Venus Envy: A History of Cosmetic Surgery*. Baltimore: Johns Hopkins University Press.

ISAPS. 2015a. "Blepharoplasty." Accessed August 27, 2015. http://www.isaps.org/procedures/blepharoplasty.

ISAPS. 2015b. "Global Statistics." Accessed August 27, 2015. http://www.isaps.org/Media
/Default/globalstatistics/2015%20ISAPS%20Results.pdf.

Jesitus, John. 2004. "Eyelid Surgery Can Preserve Asian Identity." *Cosmetic Surgery Times* 7,
no. 5: 15.

Jones, Meredith, and Cressida Heyes. 2009. *Cosmetic Surgery: A Feminist Primer.* Farnham,
England: Ashgate.

Lin, Shirley. 2001. "In the Eye of the Beholder?: Eyelid Surgery and Young Asian-American
Women." Accessed August 27, 2015. http://www.alternet.org/story/10557/in_the_eye_of
_the_beholder%3A_eyelid_surgery_and_young_asian-american_women.

Oulette, Alicia. 2009. "Eyes Wide Open: Surgery to Westernize the Eyes of an Asian Child."
The Hastings Center Report 39, no. 1(Jan.—Feb): 15–18.

Pak, Suchin. 2007. "Erasing Ethnicity." *Marie Claire (US Edition)* 14, no. 10(October): 56.

Stevenson, Alexandra. 2014. "Plastic Surgery Tourism Brings Chinese to South Korea." *The
New York Times.* December 24. Accessed August 27, 2015. http://www.nytimes.com/2014
/12/24/business/international/plastic-surgery-tourism-brings-chinese-to-south-korea
.html?_r=0.

FACELIFTS

Perhaps one of the most common of **plastic surgery** procedures, a rhytidectomy, or "facelift," is defined by the International Association of Aesthetic and Plastic Surgeons as a procedure that "improves the skin and tissues of the lower two-thirds of the face, from the ears, across to the cheeks, and down to the jaw line, by removing excess fat, tightening muscles and re-draping skin" (ISAPS 2015b). Most patients undergoing a facelift do so in order to seem more youthful and to counteract the sag in facial skin that accompanies age.

There are two types of facelifts: a full facelift that tightens the skin and muscles of the bottom two-thirds of the face, and mini, or midface, facelifts that focus on the area from below the lower eyelid to the top of the patient's upper lip (ISAPS 2015c). A last, nonsurgical method for tightening facial skin also exists, called "barbed suture lift," commonly known as a "thread lift": a procedure popularized in the 1990s in which sutures, or threads of surgical line, are sewn through the midface, jowls, brows, or neck of the patient to create a lifting and tightening effect (ISAPS 2015a). Although initial criticisms of the procedure included the number of threads that eventually broke, causing infection, as well as general unhappiness with the result, in the 21st century, the practice of thread lifts is gaining popularity (Prince 2015).

Facelift procedures, as with many plastic surgeries, gained popularity in the period after World War II. Battlefield surgeons and doctors on the home front, performing seemingly miraculous transformations on disfigured veterans, helped shape popular perceptions about what plastic surgery could achieve. Many began to envision equally miraculous changes in their own appearance. A postwar period of affluence and stability then helped fund more widespread demand for cosmetic surgery in general, and facelifts in particular (Haiken 1999).

Facelifts in the United States were once among the most commonly recognized, and criticized, plastic surgery procedures. Celebrities who were believed to have undergone too many facelifts were often considered to have worsened, not improved, their appearances. Perhaps for this reason, the number of facelifts performed in the United States has fallen significantly over the last decade (Galloway 2012). In the United States more patients are seeking less invasive thread lifts or solutions linked to **cosmetics** and lotions as well as injectables such as **Botox**, which has often been touted as the "no facelift, facelift miracle" (Hagloch 2003).

This trend away from the facelift can be seen in global statistics as well. In 2014, the **United States** and **Brazil** led the world in the number of facelift procedures performed (77,000 and 74,000, respectively), but that number was dwarfed by the number of patients receiving Botox injections: 1.3 million in the United States and 355,000 in Brazil (ISAPS 2015d).

A facelift is a significant medical procedure that lasts approximately four hours. It may be done as an outpatient surgery, but many patients require a hospital stay. After the surgery, some side effects include a "tight feeling" in the skin and the need for men to start shaving behind their ears, as the beard-growing skin has been repositioned there. Some patients' hairlines may be changed as well. Risks associated with facelifts include injury to the nerves in the face, infection, bleeding, and permanent scarring (ISAPS 2015b).

See also: Botox; Brazil; Injections; Plastic Surgery; United States.

Further Reading

Galloway, Lindsey. 2012. "No-Surgery Face-Lifts." *Natural Health* 42, no. 5: 42.
Hagloch, Susan B. 2003. "The Botox Miracle: Get "Face-Lift" Results—Without Painful Surgery or Recovery Time." *Library Journal* 128, no. 10: 85.
Haiken, Elizabeth. 1999. *Venus Envy: A History of Cosmetic Surgery*. Baltimore: Johns Hopkins University Press.
ISAPS. 2015a. "Barbed Suture Lift." Accessed November 16, 2015. http://www.isaps.org /procedures/barbed-suture-Lift.
ISAPS. 2015b. "Face Lift - Full." Accessed November 16, 2015. http://www.isaps.org /procedures/facelift.
ISAPS. 2015c. "Facelift - Mini/Midface." Accessed November 16, 2015. http://www.isaps .org/procedures/mini-facelift.
ISAPS. 2015d. "Global Statistics." Accessed November 16, 2015. http://www.isaps.org/Media /Default/global-statistics/2015%20ISAPS%20Results.pdf.
Prince, Jessica. 2015. "The New No-Knife Face Lift." *Harper's Bazaar* no. 3638: 292.

FACIAL HAIR

Facial hair is hair that is grown on the face and consists of three main parts: a beard, sideburns, and moustache. These may be styled in a variety of ways.

A beard is a growth of hair on the chin and cheeks. The average man has 25,000 hairs on his chin. The hormone dihydrotestosterone triggers the growth of facial hair during adolescence; the same hormone also promotes balding later in life for some men. Facial hair can provide warmth to keep the face safe from elements. Facial hair also creates the appearance of a thicker, stronger-looking jaw line. The presence or absence of a beard can signal important information about a man within a culture, including membership to religious organizations, marital status, social status, virility, sexual prowess, cultural sophistication (or lack thereof), and wisdom. Today, about one-third of American men have facial hair, and 55 percent of men worldwide have facial hair (Offenhartz 2015).

Removing facial hair requires specialized tools. Stone Age paintings show men plucking out facial hair with sea shells (Peterkin 2002). During the Neolithic era, shaving was possible with sharpened stone tools or obsidian glass. The earliest record of shaving is a portrait of a shaved Scythian (**Iranian**) horseman with a moustache dating to BCE 300 (Offenhartz 2015). Professional **barbers** were available to attend to men's shaving needs because they had these necessary tools and were able to keep them sharp. Ancient Egyptians used razors made of flint and bronze to remove hair from the cheeks, but many elites preferred to allow beard growth on the chin, sometimes even dying the beard or braiding it with gold threads. Egyptian men of some periods also sometimes wore artificial beards to indicate maturity or elite status. Mesopotamian leaders cultivated long, curling beards that were specially oiled and groomed.

In BCE 345, Alexander the Great decreed that soldiers should not have beards because he was afraid that enemies would grab or pull beards in battle (Voakes 2012). Men of the Roman Empire shaved their facial hair to conform to the clean-cheeked look of the emperor.

In some cultures, age or accomplishment of life course rituals entitles a man to begin wearing a beard. Religious customs also dictate appropriate standards for facial hair. Beards and moustaches must be groomed and trimmed in order to show group membership. In Sikhism, a practice in India since the 15th century, a full beard is considered an absolutely essential marker of membership to the faith for all adult males. The Prophet Muhammad advised men to grow beards and moustaches, but to cut longer hairs so that they did not cover the upper lip. Long beards and short, trimmed beards are preferred by adult men in many Muslim communities. Mormon men, on the other hand, are expected be clean shaven. Amish men continue to wear long beards. However, Amish men do shave their upper lips, in part because of their explicit rejection of the German military tradition of moustaches, continued since their relocation to the United States in the 1700s.

During the Elizabethan period in the United Kingdom, men paid a great deal of attention to the proper grooming of their facial hair, prompting historians to continue to use the nickname "The Peacock Age." Those who were able to afford it spent resources on keeping their beard short and well trimmed, in vogue with the new trends. Perhaps the most iconic beard style of the era was a tidy, medium-length pointed beard, known as a "Van Dyke" style. Elizabethan-era beards were also cut into square, round, oblong, or T-shapes. Men often matched their hair to the length of their beard; periodically, they would find a barber to dress the hair, curling it under with a hot iron rod in a style known as "love locks." Men with longer beards required less regular maintenance: they slept with their beards confined in a specially designed wooden press, and they routinely brushed out their beards.

Some beard styles incorporate sideburns, another type of facial hair that joins the hair on the cheeks and chin with the hair worn on the head alongside the ears. The beard style known as "mutton chops" (also known as "burnsides") combines a full beard and moustache through the sides of the face and above the upper lip, allowing the hair at the sides of the face to be very prominent and the chin to be bare. This style of beard was worn extensively during the Victorian era in England and the Civil War era in the United States. Sideburns worn without beards are also part of some hairstyles. Following the Civil War, men in the United States began to wear full beards with mutton chops. A man's whiskers were believed to show wisdom, trustworthiness, and maturity. It was during this era that a bearded "Uncle Sam" began appearing in political cartoons as a symbol of the United States (Sherrow 2006). During the 1970s, many men wore long sideburns, alone or with moustaches.

A renewed acceptance of beards in the United States and Europe has attracted men who wear beards to competitive bearding events. Competitive bearding, inviting "weirdos and beardos," allows bearded men to celebrate the attractiveness of their facial hair in a large, sometimes televised venue (Rolling Stone 2015). Events feature a wide variety of competitive categories, including moustaches (natural, English, Wild West, handlebar, Dali, Fu Manchu, and imperial), partial-beard categories (musketeer, goatee, and sideburns), and full beard categories (natural, full, Garibaldi, and Verdi). Each competitive group also included a category known as "freestyle."

Some men wear their beard as "stubble," which allows hair growth for a few days before trimming or shaving. Depending on the speed at which hair growth occurs, the stubble style can be maintained for up to a week using a trimmer attachment on a commercial shaver. Some men prefer to shave the hair just below the cheekbone. A "circle beard" is worn with a moustache, framing the mouth, but without any hair on the cheeks or sideburns.

A goatee features hair grown just below the lower chin. A smaller version of the goatee is sometimes known as a "soul patch," also known as a "jazz dab." This beard style is often paired with a moustache, and features a small, triangular area of beard beneath the lower lip.

The Garibaldi beard style, named for a key leader in the foundation of modern **Italy**, is a large beard, about six to eight inches long, merged seamlessly with the moustache and with a wide rounded base at the bottom and featuring a slightly "unkempt" look. Another beard style, named after Italian composer Giuseppe Verdi (1813–1901), is a full beard, shorter than the Garibaldi, which is paired with a well-groomed, slightly curled moustache distinct from the beard. A very long, very full beard, usually attached to a full untrimmed moustache, is

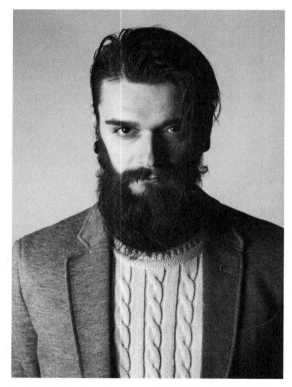

A Bandholz beard, named for pioneering "urban beardsman" Eric Bandholz. The renewed popularity of beards in the United States and Europe has even led to competitive bearding events. (Vladimir Floyd/ Dreamstime.com)

known as the Bandholz style, named for Eric Bandholz, who initiated what he called the "urban beardsman lifestyle." This movement gave rise to a new category of metrosexual consumer, sometimes labeled the "lumbersexual," a man who wears a large (usually well-groomed) beard paired with rugged, outdoors-wear, including plaid shirts and leather boots.

Hair growth on the upper lip is called a moustache. Moustaches can be worn with beards or alone. A "chevron" moustache covers the area between the nose and the upper lip to the edges of the upper lip, but does not extend farther than that. This style was popularized in the 1970s by singer Freddie Mercury of the band Queen, race car driver Richard Petty, and heartthrob star of the television program *Magnum P.I.*, Tom Selleck.

Since ancient times, Asian men have worn moustaches, both with and without beards. The legendary warlord Genghis Khan wore a distinctive full, straight, long moustache without a beard called a "Fu Manchu" style. The distinctive feature of this style is that the Fu Manchu is grown exclusively from the corners of the upper lip, which creates two long tails that hang below the chin area. A thicker version of this moustache is sometimes called the "Pancho Villa" style.

A similar style, often confused with the Fu Manchu and Pancho Villa moustache, is called the "horseshoe moustache." The horseshoe moustache is also called a "biker" or a "cowboy" moustache. In this style, the hair also falls straight to the chin but involves hair that begins growing over the top of the lip. This style was famously worn by pro-wrestler Hulk Hogan. A very bushy version of this moustache hanging down over the lips, often covering the entire mouth, is called the walrus style. This moustache was made famous by writer Mark Twain.

The Dali-style moustache also involves narrow, long strands of hair, but rather than falling over the lips, the hair is waxed and bent to curve steeply upward, usually not past the corner of the mouth. The style is named after Spanish artist Salvador Dalí. Another narrow form of moustache is called the "pencil moustache," closely clipped, which outlines the upper lip with a wide gap shaved between the nose and the moustache. This style was made famous by 1940s movie star Clark Gable and counter-culture filmmaker John Waters.

An English moustache is narrow and begins at the middle of the upper lip. The hair of the moustache is very long, and styled to pull to the side with a slight curl, pointing slightly upward. A thicker version of this moustache is called the Hungarian, which can be quite big and bushy, extending beyond the end of the lips. When the whiskers of the cheeks are also incorporated into the moustache style (without a beard), it is called an Imperial moustache.

Moustache grooming includes trimming, waxing, combing, setting, and styling with waxes or pomades. Some men also wear moustache protectors at night to keep the shape and style of their moustache. A moustache binder, made of silk with small leather straps, was invented in Germany and worn by Kaiser Wilhelm II. This device was pressed over the moustache and then strapped to the head for sleeping. Moustache cups feature a raised lip guard around the rim in order to protect the hair of the moustache while a man drinks.

Recently, in the United States, men have begun embracing facial hair by participating in "No-Shave November" to raise cancer awareness, asking participants to donate their monthly hair-maintenance expenses to the cause. The movement's Web site states, "The goal of No-Shave November is to grow awareness by embracing our hair, which many cancer patients lose, and letting it grow wild and free" (Matthew Hill Foundation 2016). Companion sites have popped up on Facebook and Instagram, celebrating the bearded beauty of men. (Women are also encouraged to participate by foregoing shaving and waxing during the month of November.)

Generally speaking, beards are only considered attractive on men. Some women with heightened levels of testosterone may be able to grow beards. In general, in most cultures, women are encouraged to remove facial hair in order to appear more feminine. Women go to great lengths and use a variety of hair removal techniques to prevent hair from appearing on their faces. During the **aging** process, some women notice thicker or more frequent facial hair growth after the onset of menopause.

See also: Aging; Baldness; Barbershop; Hair Removal; Iran; Italy; United Kingdom; United States.

Further Reading

Corson, Richard. 1965. *Fashions in Hair: The First Five Thousand Years*. London: Peter Owens Publishing.

Hou, Kathleen. 2014. "The Best Way to Get Rid of Your Chin Hair." *New York Magazine*. Accessed February 6, 2017. http://nymag.com/thecut/2014/11/best-way-to-get-rid-of -your-chin-hair.html.

Markey, Sean. 2005. "Whiskers Go Wild at World Beard, Mustache Games." *National Geographic World*. March 25. Accessed October 11, 2016. http://news.nationalgeographic .com/news/2005/03/0325_050325_beardmustache.html.

Matthew Hill Foundation. 2016. "No Shave November." Accessed October 11, 2016. https:// www.no-shave.org.

Offenhartz, Jake. 2015. "The 8 Most Important Mustaches Through History." *History Buff,* November 6. Accessed October 11, 2016. http://historybuff.com/the-8-most-important -moustaches-through-history-kbxeD8OlA6OL.

Oldstone-Moore, Christopher. 2015. *Of Beards and Men: The Revealing History of Facial Hair.* Chicago: University of Chicago Press.

Peterkin, Alan. 2002. *One Thousand Beards: A Cultural History of Facial Hair*. Vancouver, British Columbia: Arsenal Pulp Press.

Real Men, Real Style. 2016. "20 Beard Styles." Accessed October 11, 2016. http://www .realmenrealstyle.com/20-beard-styles.

Rolling Stone. 2015. "Inside the Weird World of the Hairiest Sport: Competitive Bearding." June 4. Accessed October 11, 2016. http://www.rollingstone.com/culture/videos/inside -the-weird-world-of-the-hairiest-sport-competitive-bearding-20150604.

Voakes, Greg. 2012. "The Amazing History of Beards." *Huffington Post*. April 4. Accessed October 11, 2016. http://www.huffingtonpost.com/greg-voakes/the-amazing-history-of -be_b_1398008.html.

FEMINISM

One of the earliest feminists of the modern era to critique the ways that culture continually conditions young women to perform femininity was French existentialist

Simone de Beauvoir. In her landmark book *The Second Sex*, published in 1949, de Beauvoir pointed out that during adolescence, a girl becomes aware of the physical changes in her body and she notices how these changes significantly alter her freedom to do things that her male companions from childhood are still able to do. Women's appearances, too, become more heavily scrutinized than those of their male counterparts, and an expectation to experiment with clothing, makeup, and manners emerges in a way that has no parallel for men in Western culture. The cultural assumption is that women can look good if they apply themselves with enough care and effort to their appearance. With regard to this **beauty myth**, women are judged by different, sometimes unattainable, standards, contributing to a double standard that has been written about by a great many feminists.

In *The Beauty Myth* (1988), Naomi Wolf critiqued the role of beauty in women's oppression. Western women are expected to accommodate themselves as often as possible to patriarchal standards of female beauty, even if this accommodation involves regarding her own body as an enemy or as a failure, or learning to mistrust their own bodies during the transformations of adolescence. Women routinely mold, squeeze, and even starve themselves through a variety of **eating disorders** to conform to the expectation of the social **male gaze**.

Some feminist theorists borrow from the work of French critical theorist Michel Foucault to comment upon the ways that power acts upon the gendered body. For Foucault, the shift to Enlightenment models of social control emphasized more routine, individualized ways of regulating social groups. Feminist philosopher Sandra Bartky applied Foucault's theory to the ways in which modern women experience patriarchal power, particularly the "tyranny of slenderness," and the constraints of feminine presentation, which rely upon constant self-vigilance from women. Social beauty norms place significant demands on women's time and self-mastery so that women should appear groomed and attractive or suffer the consequences of being denigrated, alienated, or marginalized. Women themselves internalize these high standards of attractiveness and subject themselves to preventive self-policing so that they do not transgress the various rules associated with femininity. Women are also raised to judge each other through informal sanctions. Ultimately, Bartky notes, all of these complex negotiations of the beauty imperative are naturalized so that they do not seem unusual or oppressive to those who enact them.

Many contemporary feminists raise five main critiques against beauty practices. The first critique is often known as the "double standard" of beauty. Physical attractiveness simply makes more of a difference in how women are treated than it does for men. Women are often strictly evaluated and given access to options based on how they look, and when they do not look a particular way, they may be excluded from opportunities that they are otherwise qualified to do. In order for women to appear more "beautiful," in many cultures it is essential to subscribe to time-consuming and resource-intensive beauty regimens. These same requirements are not made for men.

Related to the first criticism about beauty practices is the second criticism: cost. When women are required to spend more time and more resources on seeking beauty, the cost for these things must be shouldered at the expense of something else. Overwhelmingly, women are asked to bear the costs of appearing beautiful to men, often in systems where men continue to make more money or have more access to wealth than women do.

The third criticism of beauty practices from the perspective of feminists is the issue of choice and control. The standards of beauty that are set for women are often arbitrary and guided by the pharmaceutical, fashion, and cosmetic industries and influenced by the commercial entertainment media such as television, movies, and celebrities. Women have a choice to make their own decisions, but there can be severe limitations on how women are able to exercise their choices given the overwhelming pressure to follow industry-created directives about how to look and how to present themselves. Often, women's beauty decisions are less about their own desires to look a particular way and more about the ways in which they capitulate to look the way others want them to.

Potentially most importantly, feminists critique the ways beauty practices involve potentially negative physical and mental health effects on women. Some women's beauty practices are merely uncomfortable or inconvenient, including high heel shoes or tightly cinched waistbands or belts. However, many beauty practices sacrifice women's health and may even be dangerous or life threatening. These include toiletries or cosmetics with toxic ingredients and some weight loss or beauty aids that can make the user sick. In the case of eating disorders, some women literally kill themselves in the pursuit of beauty. Additionally, research shows that the standard of an unattainable beauty ideal can cause women to become depressed or feel self-loathing and contribute to low self-esteem among women of all ages.

Finally, feminists express concerns about the ways that beauty standards are used to enforce other forms of inequality between people, including on the basis of class, race, or age. Western standards of beauty, for example, are making unsettling inroads to many places around the world (Rossini 2015), and in turn, many ethnic forms of beauty are co-opted and appropriated in ways that reinforce and reinscribe ethnic stereotypes in patronizing or dehumanizing ways.

See also: Body Dysmorphic Disorder; Disciplinary Practices/Disciplinary Power; Eating Disorders; Male Gaze.

Further Reading

Bartky, Sandra. 1988. "Foucault, Femininity, and the Modernization of Patriarchal Power." In: *Feminism & Foucault: Reflections on Resistance*, edited by Irene Diamond and Lee Quinby. Boston: Northeastern University Press.

De Beauvoir, Simone. 2011 [1949]. *The Second Sex: Woman as Other*. Translated by Constance Borde and Sheila Malovany-Chevallier. New York: Vintage.

Foucault, Michel. 1995. *Discipline and Punish: The Birth of the Prison*. New York: Vintage Books.

Jackson, Linda A. 1992. *Physical Appearance and Gender: Sociobiological and Sociocultural Perspectives*. Albany, NY: SUNY Press.

Rossini, Elena. 2015. The Illusionists. Film. http://theillusionists.org/

Wolf, Naomi. 1988. *The Beauty Myth: How Images of Beauty Are Used Against Women*. New York: Harper Perennial.

FETISH

The idea of a "fetish," a strong preference or obsession for certain elements of the body, is a psychological term that has increasing relevance in the area of beauty and fashion. Psychologically, the term "fetish," describes an intense need or desire for an object, body part, or activity as a key element of a person's sexual excitement. Increasingly in the 21st century, however, the word "fetish" is also used as a way of identifying a certain kind of apparel or costume often associated with bondage and sadomasochistic sexual activity.

The term "fetish" originally comes from the writing of 19th-century French psychologist Alfred Binet, who introduced the notion of sexual deviance as part of his larger work on practical intelligence. He argued that fetishism has its roots in childhood and is frequently associated with the nostalgic feelings of first sexual awakening (Binet 1888). Later, the idea of fetishism was picked up and developed by other important thinkers, including Sigmund Freud and Lacan (Caprio 1967). In the 21st century, there is much debate about how fetishism should be understood, either as a normal variation on human sexuality or a "harmful dysfunction" (Singy 2012).

Whether or not an individual considers fetishism to be a disorder or a normal part of being human, what is clear is that the concept of placing particular importance and desire on one certain element of appearance is not limited to European cultures. Both the concept and the experience of sexual excitement from one object or body part are global phenomena from Asia to the Americas (Jing 2014).

Fetishized attributes are valued in a similar way that beautiful attributes are valued: the existence of a given type of physical attribute ultimately creates desire. More technically, a fetish is an object or idea that compels a person's sex impulse or libido to become attached to or fixated on that object or idea as a sexual symbol of the love object. A fetishist (or person with a fetish) may be erotically attracted to a woman's shoe, stocking, glove, handkerchief, corset, undergarment, hair, type of fabric (like velvet, silk, or fur), or some other item.

One example of the crossover from fetish to fashion is the rise of high-end, designer clothing made of latex rubber. Latex, as a material, is a fetish item for some, and is often associated with nontraditional sex practices. As a material for clothing, it can be more difficult to wear, especially if the item is very tight. As celebrities like Kim Kardashian, Rita Ora, and Taylor Swift began to wear latex designs made famous by Japanese designer Atsuko Kudo, the style gained popularity and acceptance, and other designers from Marc Jacobs to Balenciaga began offering clothing made of latex (Fetish 2016).

Latex dresses, skirts, and leggings are not the only items of "fetishwear" that have increasingly shown up in the fashion mainstream. Glossy, thigh-high vinyl boots, corsets, and petticoats are all elements of fashion that have moved from ladies' fetishwear to fashion wear (Freeborn 2002). The trend does not only pertain to women, however. Leather menswear, for example, in pants, vests, underwear, and harnesses, although often associated with bondage sex, also has made its way onto fashion runways. Men's underwear designer Andrew Christian, in particular, in addition to his traditional offerings, has an entire line of fetish underwear for men (Christian 2016).

See also: Burlesque; Corsets, Shapewear, and Waist Trainers; High Heels.

Further Reading

Binet, Alfred. 1888. *Études de Psychologie Expérimentale*, Paris: Octave Doin.
Caprio, Frank S. 1967. "Fetishism." In: *The Encyclopedia of Sexual Behavior*, edited by Albert Ellis and Albert Abarbanel, 435–38. New York, Hawthorn Books.
Christian, Andrew. 2016. "Andrew Christian Bio." Accessed July 11, 2016. http://www.andrewchristian.com/about-us.
"Fetish Fashion Dominating the High Street." 2016. *The Times (United Kingdom)* (January 9): 18–19.
Freeborn, Amy. 2002. "It's Back! A Sexy Item to Leave You Breathless." November 9. Accessed July 11, 2016. *The Advertiser (Adelaide)*: *Newspaper Source*, EBSCOhost.
Jing, Jiang. 2014. "From Foot Fetish to Hand Fetish: Hygiene, Class, and the New Woman." *Positions* 22, no. 1: 131–59.
Kudo, Atsuko. 2016. "About Us." Accessed July 11, 2016. https://www.atsukokudo.com/About-Us/.
Singy, Patrick. 2012. "How to Be a Pervert: A Modest Philosophical Critique of the Diagnostic and Statistical Manual of Mental Disorders." *Revista De Estudios Sociales* no. 43: 139–50.

FOOTBINDING

Ancient Chinese stories offer a variety of origins for the practice of footbinding. One set recounts the tragic story of Yang, a well-known consort of the Tang emperor Xuanzong, who ruled from 712–756. Following a mutiny, Xuanzong's military leaders held Yang responsible for the fall of the capital city and demanded her death. Yang was legendary for her arched and small feet. Upon her death, her tiny silk socks (*luowa*) remained a potent legacy of her astounding beauty, inspiring others to regret her untimely death (Ping 2000).

Another set of stories heralds the fame of Yaoniang, a dancer in the court of Li Yu, the Buddhist ruler of the Southern Tang dynasty who was in power from 969–975. Inspired by his love for her, the ruler made a six-foot-tall golden lotus covered in jewels, ribbons, and garlands of pearls and gems. He encouraged Yaoniang to wrap her feet with silk (*yibo raojiao*) so that they would be slender and small (*xianxiao*), curling up like the new moon. When she danced, her arched and slender feet (*gongxian*) allowed her to look like she was soaring into the clouds. She inspired others to emulate her lotus-shaped feet (Ping 2000).

Lotus feet conformed to the Chinese ideal of feminine beauty as a model of selfless devotion to others. The ideal woman was supposed to be at once cheerful and bashful. Footbinding added an embodied dimension of two qualities that were admired in women: passivity and serenity. Bound feet, called *chanzu*, began at about the age of four or five while the bones in the foot were still fairly pliable. To accomplish the unique and painful shape of a bound foot, the feet were first softened in hot water. Dead skin was scrubbed off, and the toenails were clipped as short as possible. Long cotton bandages soaked in hot water were then wrapped around a young

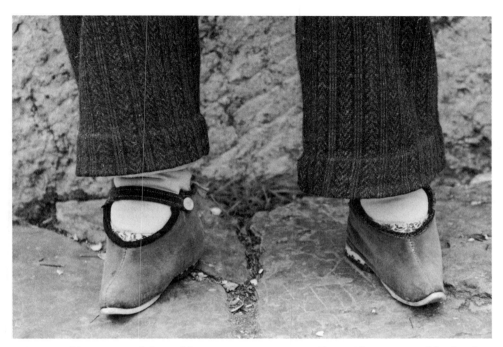

A 90-year-old woman with bound feet in Yunnan Province, China. The practice of footbinding in China was outlawed in 1912 but continued in rural areas well into the 1940s; it was banned again in 1949 when the Communists came to power. (Torsten Stahlberg/iStockphoto.com)

girl's foot, which was forced into an arched position so that the four small toes were folded under the ball of the foot. The goal of the binding was to keep the big toe and ball of the foot intact while exaggerating the foot's arch to bring the heel forward toward the front of the foot. The girl was then forced to walk on her folded-over toes. Over time, the bones in the arch and the foot would weaken and break, allowing them to be tied together more tightly. The process was extremely painful and took place over the course of many years, with daily attention paid to unbinding, bathing, and rebinding the foot to avoid infections. A tightly bound foot was shaped like a crescent moon and could measure only three inches in length. Unbound feet were seen as ugly and lewd. Small feet were prized as a beautiful feature, though footbinding limited women's mobility, forcing them to stay close to home (Levi 1966).

There are four main theories about why footbinding continued for nearly 1,000 years. Perhaps the most popular explanation comes from Freudian interpretations of **fetishism**, wherein the projection of a man's castration anxieties upon the body of the women produces acutely eroticized meanings. In this scenario, footbinding serves as a symbol of the castration of a woman and places her in a less powerful, less dominant role than that of the male partner. Small feet were also seen as highly sensual and erotic. Ancient sex manuals instructed men on how to sensually fondle feet and how to use them to enhance sexual encounters. The Chinese believed that because the binding forced women to take small steps, their vaginal muscles were strengthened, making sexual intercourse more pleasurable (Ping 2000).

A second popular theory about the durability of footbinding as a beauty technique for certain women suggests that conspicuous leisure time can be connected with ideas of wealth and success. When a family reaches a stage where they no longer need to rely upon the labor of their daughters or wives, they are able to engage in practices of "conspicuous consumption," thus constricting the movement and productivity of women members of the household in such a way that the wasted or mutilated bodies of women are eroticized and considered beautiful. The ridiculously small, corseted waists of women of means in the Western world provides a parallel example of how the appeal of family wealth can produce an unrealistic aesthetic about feminine beauty that constrains the ability of the woman to be a productive member of the household (Ko 2005).

The "mystification of female labor" (Ko 2005, 2) offers a third explanation for footbinding from a Marxist-**feminist** perspective. Some anthropologists suggest that whereas the binding of women's feet severely limited their mobility, peasant women were still required to conduct valuable work such as spinning, weaving, food processing, and harvesting tea, which required skill and strength in a woman's hands but not her feet. Despite the fact that the labor of these women as daughters and wives was key to the production and functioning of the household economy, the mechanism of footbinding allowed the work of these women to be masked by the patriarchs of the economic system. Women remained uncompensated in this "petty capitalist" mode of production, subsidizing the family without adequate acknowledgement of their contributions. Homemade textiles, for example, were standard in all Chinese homes until 1925, when factory-made textiles replaced home-based weavings. After this time, footbinding became redundant, as bound women were no longer required by the economic system. The new factory-based economy demanded women who could perform such heavy labor as porterage, mining, road construction, and rice faming. Footbinding no longer made economic sense, and so the practice was abandoned.

Finally, the "marrying-up" thesis argues that women with bound feet were considered more beautiful and would be more likely to be chosen as brides if their families were able to begin the process very early. "Marriage constituted the best if not the only avenue for female self-advancement. Bound feet, a ticket to a brighter future for the bride and her family, translated into 'good destiny' or social prestige" (Ko 2005, 3). Women with especially small feet resembling lotus petals commissioned finely embroidered silk shoes, called "lotus shoes," which were considered intimate apparel. Lotus shoes were an important part of a bride's trousseau, and wedding shoes were always red and the most ornate, sometimes featuring erotic embroidery on the inside (History of Footwear 2015).

Of course, no single economic, social, symbolic, or psychological factor is likely adequate to explain why the custom of footbinding endured in such a widespread way for such a long period of time. Even trying to determine a direct linear progression that points to when the practice ended is a difficult proposition for historians, as footbinding was phased out over a period of time ranging from the 1880s to the 1930s. The invention of the term "natural feet" (also called "heavenly feet," or *tianzu*) in 1875 marked a distinct change in the way that the "lotus" feet were thought about across China. English missionaries, many of whom came to China during the Opium Wars, which directly served their country's economic interests, introduced the phrase to show that the doctrine of heavenly feet was predicated on the **social construction** of a God-given natural body that did not yield to modifications decided by men. However, it is also important to note that indigenous reformers were also active in the campaigns to ban footbinding; educated women attempted to "liberate" their counterparts from the lower **classes**, with mixed success. After 1916, *chanzu* became criminalized by the nationalist government. Young girls under the age of 15 began to *jiefang* (to unwrap) and release their feet, and parents were forbidden to allow their young daughters to start binding under penalty of a fine.

In her 2005 history of footbinding, Dorothy Ko argues that for the women between the 12th and 20th centuries for whom footbinding was a lived reality, the practice of binding was an ongoing experience that required daily maintenance and care of the feet, which were often painful and distracting. The embodied experience of footbinding as a **body modification** was much more than an aesthetic statement; it was also a commitment to an ideology about gender and identity. The prototypes of Chinese womanhood were scripted by the history of the nation itself, and both economic and cultural transformations were involved in the eradication of the practice.

See also: Body Modification; China; Class; Feminist; Fetish; Social Construction of Beauty.

Further Reading

Foreman, Amanda. 2015. "Why Foot Binding Persisted in China for a Millennium." *Smithsonian Magazine*. [Web site]. Accessed July 12, 2016. http://www.smithsonianmag.com/history/why-footbinding-persisted-china-millennium-180953971/?no-ist.

History of Footwear. 2016. "Lotus Shoes." Accessed July 12, 2016. http://www.footwearhistory.com/lotus- shoes.

Hong, Fan. 1997. *Foot Binding, Feminism, and Freedom: The Liberation of Women's Bodies in Modern China*. London: Frank Cass.

Ko, Dorothy. 2005. *Cinderella's Sisters: A Revisionist History of Footbinding*. Berkley, CA: University of California Press.

Kunzle, David. 1982. *Fashion and Fetishism: A Social History of the Corset, Tight-Lacing, and Other Forms of Body Sculpture in the West*. New York: Rowman and Littlefield.

Levi, Howard S. 1966. *Chinese Footbinding*. New York: Walton Rawls.

Ping, Wang. 2000. *Aching for Beauty: Foot Binding in China*. Minneapolis: University of Minnesota Press.

GEISHA

The unique tradition of **geisha** (meaning "one who lives by art") found in Japan centers on a highly stylized woman who is accomplished in the art of entertaining men. The arts of the geisha were performed in special venues for exclusively male audiences, with the intent of creating an atmosphere of luxury and tranquility.

Typically, a geisha would begin her training as a young girl at an *okiya*, or geisha house. During training, a geisha is called *maiko*. While in training, a *maiko* may be identified by the style of her kimono, as well as her hairstyle, which is frequently arranged by pulling hair from both the front and the back of the head and then rolling it so that there is an attractive overlap of hair on either side of the face.

Training would include attention to speech and graceful movements. Geisha were also trained to play a three-stringed instrument called a *samisen* to accompany poetry recitations or songs. Geisha were also given extensive training in the classical arts of femininity, which included mastery of refined conversation, as well as *sado* (the Japanese tea ceremony), *ikebana* (flower arranging), calligraphy, and perfumery.

Geisha are identifiable by their dramatic makeup, which features very light skin and very dark eyes and hair, complimented by a pop of red color at the lips. First, the face was prepared to appear as white as possible with an application of rice powder followed by an application of white pancake makeup covering the face and the neck. White is considered a sign of purity in Shintoism (a religion in Japan) and was both beautiful and desirable. The lips are colored a shade of very rich red and are shaped to resemble the bud of a flower. Sometimes,

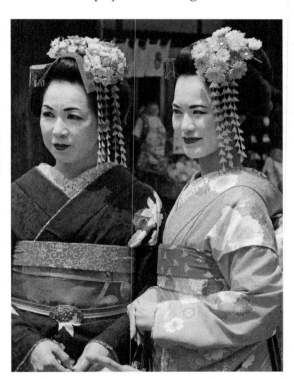

Geisha in the old town Geisha district of Kyoto, Japan. In Japanese culture, the geisha embodies the essence of femininity. (Dreamstime.com)

a red color may also be added to the cheeks. The natural brow is either plucked or shaved, and a strong, dramatic brow line is added with black pencil. Historically, there were a variety of styles for the shape and placement of the brow. The arch of the brow could, for example, indicate marital status and other important information.

White teeth were considered unattractive and even vulgar. Geisha often blackened their teeth with a dye made from soaking a powdered nut in tea or vinegar, a custom known as *o-haguro*. Some speculate that by rendering the teeth less visible, the geisha was better able to control her presentation of emotion and not be seen to smile in a way that might be considered unbecoming.

The stunning kimono costume worn by geisha begins with T-shaped robes with wide sleeves that ideally fall to the ankle. Kimonos are secured with a wide, belt-like sash called an *obi*, which is tied at the back. Kimonos were traditionally made from a single bolt of fabric measuring about 36 centimeters in width and 11.5 meters in length. A finished kimono typically is made of four main strips of fabric and requires that the wearer be fairly slim to fit the dimensions available within the bolt of fabric. The most expensive kimonos are made of silk, silk brocade, or silk crepe, but today, it is possible to buy kimonos in a variety of less expensive, easier-to-care-for fabrics. A kimono may also be layered with an under-kimono, called a *hiyoku*. An accomplished *maiko* or geisha may use this layering technique to emphasize the back of the neck in order to add a subtle erotic suggestion to her costume by discreetly displaying something that is meant to remain unseen.

Kimonos are also highly formalized and quite difficult to put on, requiring the assistance of a professional dresser. The level of formality of women's kimonos is reflected in the weight and pattern of the fabric and the predominant colors. Usually, unmarried women's kimonos have longer sleeves than kimonos for married women. The *uchikake* is a highly formal, heavily brocaded kimono in white or red, usually only worn by a bride, with a train that is supposed to trail along the floor. Less formal "visiting" kimonos are known as *homongi* and may be worn by both married and unmarried women. There are also specific types of kimonos suited for mourning. The typical kimono geisha are expected to wear is called a *susohiki* or *hikizuri* and are a bit longer than the standard ankle length. They also typically feature an elaborate underskirt, which is designed to be displayed. A geisha would typically wear a kimono with *geta* (similar to flip-flops, but with an elevated heel platform at the front and the back of the shoe) and split-toe socks (*tabi*). Depending on their quality, kimonos can easily cost tens of thousands of dollars.

In addition to the luxurious kimono worn by geisha, special care and attention were paid to the dressing of the hair. The traditional hairstyle of an accomplished geisha comprises an elaborately arranged high bun, called *shimada*. Throughout their training period, the geisha would have a variety of hairstyles, each signifying her occupational role. Traditionally in Japan, long hair was elaborately arranged by specialists into traditional styles called *nihongami*, which was then sometimes set with specially made combs, ornaments, and hot wax (*bintsuke*) in order to stay in place. Additional hair jewelry, sometimes made of crane bones or tortoiseshell, called *kansashe*, were sometimes added to the hairstyle to increase the drama. In order to prolong the effect of elaborate coiffures, geisha slept on special pillows or wooden props (*takamakura*) that allowed them to keep their head elevated while they slept.

It is important to note that the beauty and the elegance of the geisha were intended to mark her as an ideally feminine hostess. Geisha do not typically engage in sex work. Courtesans, called *oiran* in Japanese, rose to prominence during the Edo period (1600–1860) in the pleasure quarters of the exclusive closed districts available to important men. Courtesans of this era were prostitutes (called *yūjo*) who shared some training in the traditional feminine arts with geisha. The status of an *orian* was based upon her beauty and her mastery of the traditional arts.

See also: Japan; Makeup and Cosmetics; Teeth Blackening.

Further Reading

Dalby, Liza. 2001. *Kimono: Fashioning Culture.* Seattle, University of Washington Press.
Downer, Lesley. 2001. *Women of the Pleasure Quarters: The Secret History of the Geisha.* New York: Broadway Books.
Golden, Arthur. 1999. *Memoirs of a Geisha: A Novel.* New York: Vintage.

GENDER

Sexual dimorphism refers to the biological differences between males and females. Not just primary sex characteristics (like genitalia), but also secondary sexual traits, including height, weight, distribution of body hair, and relative proportions of the body. In general, for example, the pelvis is wider in females to accommodate the birth of the relatively large-headed infants of our species.

Gender is also, however, a **social construction** that ascribes qualities of masculinity and femininity to people often based on biological, or perceived biological, gender. Beyond the construction of social norms of gender, or the rules we create about what males or females "are like," is a way in which we organize our societies. Through these rules, we create acceptable and unacceptable identities and enforce customs, laws, and practices that govern citizenship and participation in our culture (Sheppard and Mayo 2013). Looked at like this, "a person's gender is not simply an aspect of who one is, but more fundamentally it is something that one does, recurrently, in interaction with others" (West and Zimmerman 1987, 126).

Many of the rules and norms of gender are intrinsically tied to sexual identity. Some cultures, such as the Native American Diné, recognize more than one gender or sexual identity (Sheppard and Mayo 2013). However, many societies, such as those in 20th- and 21st-century United States or Europe function under a binary, "either/or" heteronormative framework that assumes the heterosexual interest of men for women and women for men.

Because the idea of gender is one of the central organizing principles around which societies revolve, many of the rules and standards governing acceptable or ideal appearance are tied to ideas of what men and women "should" look like (Berkowitz, Namita and Tinkler 2010). Looking at it this way, to be beautiful is to conform to the ideal version of an individual's biological gender, assuming that the individual is seeking the sexual attention of a member of the opposite biological sex.

Evolutionary psychologists argue that as individuals seek the attention of potential mates, what they find attractive about members of the opposite sex are the traits that are most likely to produce viable and healthy offspring, as well as the elements of physical appearance that indicate the individual's ability to care for the children (Etcoff 2000). In this view of beauty, preference for the wide hips of a woman (to more easily bear children) or large breasts (to feed the children) are biological adaptations that drive men to seek women who look like they can have and care for more babies (Etcoff 2000). The preference of women for men who look both muscular and wealthy can be seen similarly as a product of women's search for men who will care for and protect them.

In both sexes, the smooth skin and shiny hair that signify good genes and good health are attractive for all of these reasons, and recent studies conducted globally confirm that women from healthier nations prefer more "feminine-looking" men, whereas women from nations whose mortality rates are higher prefer the "manlier" look of men who seem strong and healthy (Pinchott 2010).

The theories of evolutionary psychologists about the differences of beauty standards being linked to reproductive capacity also then may help explain the different attitudes toward appearance and aging. In general, women are considered "old" and unattractive at an earlier age than men. This is possibly linked to the fact that women's ability to bear children ends as she ages, whereas men's reproductive ability lasts for a much longer time (Cantwell and Barrett 2006).

The differences in societal expectations for men and women when it comes to attractiveness, beauty work, and age are evident in many situations. Some research has found that "beauty is beastly" for women seeking leadership roles, for example. Scholars speculate that the devaluing of highly attractive female candidates for leadership roles may be linked to the underlying social rules about gender. Men, generally, are "supposed to be" more active agents, task completers, and leaders. Women are generally asked to be nurturers and guarders of communal peace. When a woman is highly attractive and engages in beauty work, she may be drawing attention to her femininity. "Attractiveness fuels femininity perceptions and thereby increases the perceived lack of fit between female gender role and leader role" (Braun, Peus and Frey 2012).

This linkage between traditional roles and traditional preferences for appearance also leads researchers to speculate that women who are more educated and have more financial means may prefer the man who looks less masculine, and therefore less aggressive or contentious. A woman who feels less dependent on her mate, both financially and for physical protection, may prefer a man whose more "feminine" looks signal a "cooperative, communicative and caring" personality (Pinchott 2010).

See also: Hair; Metrosexual; Social Construction of Beauty.

Further Reading

Berkowitz, Dana, Namita N. Manohar, and Justine E. Tinkler. 2010. "Walk Like a Man, Talk Like a Woman: Teaching the Social Construction of Gender." *Teaching Sociology* 38, no. 2: 132–43.

Bickmore, Kathy. 2002. "How Might Social Education Resist Heterosexism? Facing the Impact of Gender and Sexual Ideology on Citizenship." *Theory and Research in Social Education* 30, no. 2: 198–215.

Braun, Susanne, Claudia Peus, and Dieter Frey. 2012. "Is Beauty Beastly? Gender-Specific Effects of Leader Attractiveness and Leadership Style on Followers' Trust and Loyalty." *Zeitschrift Für Psychologie* 220, no. 2: 98–108.

Cantwell, Laura, and Anne Barrett. 2006. "Undergraduate Students' Perceptions of Aging: Gender Differences." Accessed October 6, 2016. http://research.allacademic.com/meta /p_mla_apa_research_citation/1/0/2/9/8/p102985_index.html?phpsessid=4lgkd46eri 7f9jus6ncgjq8c63. *Conference Papers—American Sociological Association* 1. SocINDEX with Full Text, EBSCOhost.

Etcoff, Nancy. 2000. *Survival of the Prettiest: The Science of Beauty.* New York: Anchor.

Frayer, David W., and Milford Wolpoff. 1985. "Sexual Dimorphism." *Annual Review of Anthropology* 14: 429–73.

Pinchott, Jena. 2010. "Why Women Don't Want Macho Men." Accessed October 6, 2016. http://www.wsj.com/articles/SB10001424052748704100604575145810050665030.

Sheppard, Maia, and J. B. Mayo. 2013. "The Social Construction of Gender and Sexuality: Learning from Two Spirit Traditions." *Social Studies* 104, no. 6: 259–70.

West, Candace, and Don H. Zimmerman. 1987. "Doing Gender." *Gender & Society* 1(2): 125–51.

GOTH AND GOTHIC

Characterized by a preference for black clothing, dramatic makeup, tattoos, and multiple piercings, goth fashion has been a notable global subculture of fashion and style since the late 20th century. Goth culture and aesthetics give participants an avenue to challenge social norms of beauty and appearance by overtly rejecting the standards of gender, image, and power in their respective cultures.

Contemporary "goth" culture takes its name from an aesthetic movement of the 19th century, known as the "Gothic." Gothic style originated in the European ghost and vampire stories of the 1800s, using the fantastical and dark themes to explore issues and ideas that would otherwise have been taboo under the strict rules of behavior of the Victorian era (Wisniewska and Lowczanin 2014). Although Gothicism began as a literary movement, it has always had a strong visual element; the way a scene or setting looks is as important as what happens in it. This visual strength of the genre made the later transition to painting, theater, and film a logical outgrowth.

Famous literary examples of British Gothic literature from the 19th and early 20th centuries include Mary Shelley's original 1818 novel *Frankenstein*, as an exploration of the dangers of science, and Bram Stoker's 1897 novel *Dracula*, which added extreme emotional distress to the supernatural (Mullan 2016). In the United States, Edgar Allen Poe and H. P. Lovecraft continued this trend of dark, emotionally charged horror in their 19th-century short stories (Wisniewska and Lowczanin 2014).

As the visual aesthetic of the original Gothic literature continued to be developed in the 20th century, the visual element of the body became increasingly important for followers and fans. Gothic, and later, "goth," aesthetic became a way for participants to reimagine their image and their appearance as transgressive: monstrous, ungendered, or gender-flipped (Wisniewska and Lowczanin 2014). Clothing, jewelry, and makeup all helped a subculture of men and women seeking to explore darker and less accepted elements of identity find space and freedom. By 1972, the "goth" subculture had been recognized (Wisniewska and Lowczanin 2014).

Participants in the goth culture and aesthetic often reject global social norms of beauty. For women, this means the opportunity to be powerful rather than submissive; to show age, decay, or ill health; and to portray decadence instead of innocence. For men, goth subculture also allows experimentation with less accepted gender roles, being submissive instead of dominating, weak instead of strong, and visually more "feminine." In the 20th and 21st centuries, one example of this aesthetic is found in the music and visual performance of the artist Trent Reznor of the band Nine Inch Nails, who regularly explores sexual submission and the performance of femininity in his music and videos (Siegel 2005).

Goth fashion and style are particularly notable for the way in which participants design their appearances to make blending into the mainstream social norm impossible. Using multiple facial piercings, highly visible tattoos, and cosmetics that seek to portray death (corpse-white makeup and deeply shadowed eyes), goth fashion is highly visible and stands out (Siegel 2005).

The aesthetic is also a critique of capitalistic celebrations of consumption and development. Whereas most cultures celebrate and practice social norms of beauty that showcase the health, vibrancy, and wealth of an individual, goth culture presents a sickly image that often includes ripped or stained clothing, suggesting both poverty and decay, and rejects the ideas of health, prosperity, and progress (Siegel 2005).

One artist well known for working with the goth aesthetic in film is the director Tim Burton, who has been called the architect of "goth-cool," by mainstream media, but has been rejected by some in gothic subculture (MX 2010). In films such as *The Corpse*

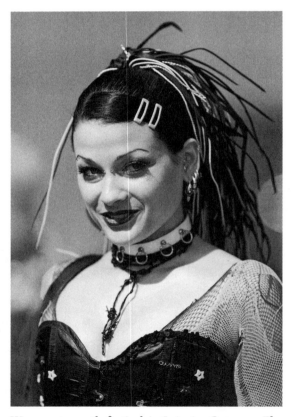

Woman at a goth festival in Leipzig, Germany. The "goth" aesthetic actively rejects social norms of beauty in favor of a more "transgressive" appearance which challenges traditional standards of gender. (Markus Kammerer/Dreamstime.com)

Bride, *The Nightmare Before Christmas*, and *Sweeney Todd*, Burton shows the same interest in images of death and decay, dark imagery of circuses and the supernatural that are associated with the goth subculture.

Some goth adherents, however, object to the highlighting of Burton as an instructive example of the style. Because goth subculture originated and continues as a way to challenge mainstream, socially accepted practices of consumerism, corporate power, and social class, many individuals who consider themselves goth object to the "manufactured," processed, and corporate type of expression of the aesthetic that comes from a Hollywood production (TheGothAlice 2014).

Because much of goth subculture, including in fashion, decoration, and practice privileges the use of found items (such as furniture made from junkyard finds), thrift store purchases of clothing, and a preference for do-it-yourself art and crafting, there is something deeply dissonant for goths when they see major fashion designers such as Alexander McQueen embrace the "goth" style. A key component to the goth aesthetic is to "avoid looking store-bought" and to embrace imperfection, age, and decay, an idea antithetical to the concept of a multinational fashion house making a profit from the style (Carlson 2007).

See also: Burlesque; Corsets, Shapewear, and Waist Trainers; Fetish; Piercing.

Further Reading

Carlson, Peter. 2007. "A Piercing Look at Goth Culture and Fashion." *The Washington Post*. January 23. Accessed July 12, 2016. http://www.washingtonpost.com/wp-dyn/content /article/2007/01/22/AR2007012201448.html. *Newspaper Source*, EBSCOhost.

Mullan, John. 2016. "The Origins of the Gothic." Accessed July 12, 2016. http://www.bl .uk/romantics-and-victorians/articles/the-origins-of-the-gothic.

MX. 2010. "A Look Back at the Bounties of Burton." *Mx 2*. Accessed July 12, 2016. www .acmi.net.au. *Newspaper Source*, EBSCOhost.

Siegel, Carol. 2005. *Goth's Dark Empire*. Bloomington, IN: Indiana University Press.

TheGothAlice. 2014. "Tim Burton and Gothic Subculture." YouTube Video. Accessed July 12, 2016. https://www.youtube.com/watch?v=YdRKooCzE2k.

Wisniewska, Dorota, and Agnieszka Lowczanin. 2014. *All That Gothic*. New York: Peter Lang AG.

GREECE

Ancient Greek civilization remains an important measure of culture in the contemporary West for the ways that society was marked by reason, balance, avoidance of excess, and the absence of most mystical and ascetic ideals. Greeks believe the mind and body were fused and expressed this ideal in the term *kalokagathia*, meaning a harmonious and symmetrical development of the body and the soul. One of the tendencies that contributed to this belief was an emphasis on physical beauty, including an idealization of the naked body of both men and women (Ellis and Abarbanel 1967, 119). Nakedness played a role in Greek life, and Greeks understood the erotic use of clothing and ornament to enhance the beautiful body. Public nakedness was a standard in wrestling matches between boys and girls, activities carried out in the gymnasia, beauty contests, and performances of dancers from Thessaly and Crete (Ellis and Abarbanel 1967, 122).

The Greek ideal of beauty was uniquely masculine, and male beauty was highly prized in the ancient world. The phallus was revered as a sacred organ of generation, and representations of the male sexual organ were carried in processions and emblazoned on art of the era. In addition to maintaining wives and concubines, adult men sought to establish homoerotic relationships with attractive male youths who were considered beautiful. To properly judge male beauty, there were competitions linked to particular cults and deities held throughout Greece known as *kallisteia*. Young male contestants competed in athletic feats and then received weapons as prizes. The winners were frequently celebrated with ribbons and honored to lead a procession to the temple of a cult where they were crowned with a wreath of myrtles. Crowther (1985) identifies two additional "beauty" contests for men known as the *euandria* and the *euexia* which required extensive athletic training and were associated with militarism. The most famous *euandria* was held in Athens and was a competition emphasizing size and strength for the tribes of Athens whereupon the winning team received an ox for a feast and individual members received shields. The *euexia* was a more individualistic competition for men under the age of thirty documented in several Greek cities which emphasized bodily beauty and a well-formed masculine physique that demonstrated symmetry, definition, tone, and a generally fit and healthy appearance.

Physical beauty was also highly prized for girls and women. Beauty competitions for women were known to be held at Basilis, Lesbos, and Tenedos sanctioned by Aphrodite, the Greek goddess of love, beauty, pleasure, and procreation. Aphrodite was born when she rose from the foam of the sea near Cyprus. There are no stories of Aphrodite's childhood: she was born as a fully sexual adult and often depicted nude. Her beauty threatened that the other gods would resort to violence in their rivalry to possess her, so Zeus married her to Hephaestus, who was not viewed as a threat because of his ugliness and deformity. Regardless, Greek mythology reports that Aphrodite took many lovers who were captivated by her radiant beauty. Her most prominent lover was the legendary beautiful man, Adonis. Aphrodite's infamous beauty (and jealousy) also intersects with the origins of the Trojan War in a story that begins at the wedding of Achilles. All the gods were invited, except Eris, the goddess of discord. Eris conjured a golden Apple of Discord with the inscription "To the Fairest One." As revenge, she threw the apple among the goddesses Aphrodite, Hera, and

Phryne the Beautiful

One of the world's most famous beauties was the Greek courtesan Mnesarete, who used the name "Phryne" professionally. Histories indicate that Phryne's beauty led her to pose for several famous artworks as the goddess Aphrodite, including the Cnidian Aphrodite currently on display at the Vatican. Phryne lived in Athens, where she was so successful in her work that she had enough money to offer to rebuild the walls of the city of Thebes, which had been destroyed by Alexander the Great. She was proud enough, then, to insist that the walls carry the message, "destroyed by Alexander, restored by Phryne the courtesan." History reports that when charged with blasphemy, and in the moment when it seemed she would lose, she ripped her dress and the beauty of her body swayed the jurors to spare her.

Athena. Zeus delegated a mortal named Paris to judge between the three goddesses and determine which was the most beautiful. The goddesses each offered him a bribe of immense value to be chosen the winner. Hera offered him supreme power. Athena offered him wisdom, fame, and military victory. Aphrodite offered him the famed Helen of Troy, the most beautiful mortal woman in the world. Unfortunately, Helen was already married to King Menelaus of Sparta, and when Paris kidnapped her for his own, it was Helen's "face that launched a thousand ships."

To intensify a fashionably pale complexion, Greek women often used white face paints, which were derived from a lead-based or a mercury-based source. The Greek physician Galen wrote, "Women who often paint themselves with mercury, though they may be very young, they presently turn old and withered and have wrinkled faces like an ape." Greek women of the Bronze Age rimmed their eyes with thick lines of kohl, and they frequently painted or tattooed small red suns onto their cheeks. Greek women also shaved the sides of their heads, allowing the rest of their hair to grow long and be styled into rolls piled on the top of the head. A fuller figure was preferred for Greek women, and women typically allowed their breasts to be exposed or covered with a diaphanous cloth of gauze. Greeks also described beauty with the term "golden" or "tawny" (*xanthos*), and women also prized **red hair.**

See also: Breasts; Makeup and Cosmetics; Red Hair/Ginger; Skin Whitening; Wrinkles.

Further Reading

Crowther, N. B. 1985. "Male 'Beauty' Contests in Greece: The *Euandria* and *Euexia*. *L'antiquité classique* 54, no. 1: 285–91.

Ellis, Albert, and Albert Abarbanel. 1967. *The Encyclopedia of Sexual Behavior*. New York: Hawthorn Books.

Hughes, Bettany. 2015. "Would You Be Beautiful in the Ancient World?." BBC Magazine. January 10. Accessed November 24, 2015. http://www.bbc.com/news/magazine-30746985.

Sandbeck, Ellen. 2010. *Green Barbarians: How to Live Bravely on Your Home Planet*. New York: Scribner.

GRILLZ (GRILLS)

In 2004, when Destiny's Child collaborated with Lil' Wayne and T.I. on the international hit "Soldier," they invited fans to admire men with "street credibility," who "open their mouth their grill gleamin'." The following year, St. Louis rapper Nelly released his ode to gold- and diamond-studded teeth in his hit single, "Grillz." After a decade or so of underground bling in the hip-hop community, lavish dental ornamentation as a status symbol entered the American pop culture mainstream. As expensive and elaborate symbols, grills embody the definition of wealth, social status, and masculine virility in the contemporary U.S. urban landscape (Schwartzberg 2014). Later, women celebrities like Kylie Jenner and Lady Gaga also began wearing grillz (Roberts 2015).

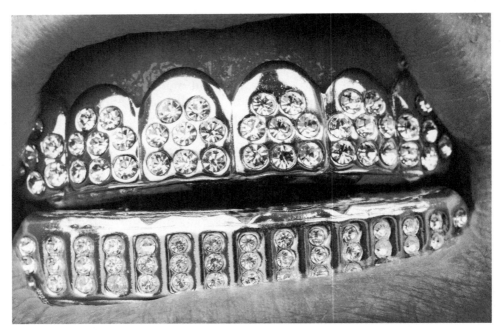

Gem-inlaid silver grillz are worn to symbolize wealth, status, and masculine virility. (spxChrome /iStockphoto.com)

"Grillz," also called "fronts" or "golds," are a type of jewelry worn over the teeth. The accessories are typically made of precious metals, like silver or gold, but may also feature gems or semiprecious stones. Grills are usually customized for the fit of the mouth of the wearer by first making a tooth mold. Designed to dazzle with the status of "bling," grillz can be extremely expensive: Lil' Wayne reportedly paid $150,000 for his famous gold smile (Roberts 2015). Less costly, ready-to-wear options are also available for those who wish to spend less on the look.

Decorated teeth are not a recently invented phenomenon, but actually have roots in ancient history. A commonly held perception is that grills originated in ancient Egypt, based on an archaeological finding at Giza from the early 20th century of front teeth that were held together with thick gold wire (Holloway 2014). However, it is unclear whether the wire was added before or after death. Although it's likely that dental fillings have existed at least 6,500 years, the procedure was not intended to enhance beauty but to address the pain and swelling associated with a dental cavity.

Dating to the middle of BCE seventh century, archaeologists have found evidence of flat gold bands worn by Etruscan women over their teeth, probably to keep false teeth in place or to stabilize teeth loosened by periodontal diseases (Becker 1999). It appears that these dental devices were worn by women of means only, suggesting that the gold bands were worn on the teeth for cosmetic purposes. According to most archaeological evidence, wealthy Etruscan women appear to have spent a disproportionate amount of household resources on public presentation. Another variation on the flat gold band was "the Van Marter appliance," a technique for wrapping the front of the base of a false tooth made of ivory or bone in precious metal in order to anchor it into the gum by attaching to other teeth on either side and wrapping them from the back. The effect would appear as three consecutive teeth, wrapped in gold for the bottom third of the tooth. Later, a similar, though more elaborate and secure, process was achieved using a technique called "the Copenhagen appliance." The procedure would have been necessitated by aging, as many adults lose molars to tooth decay after the age of 40, but archaeologists suspect that some wealthy Etruscan women had teeth pulled to deliberately place gold "grills" in their mouths for effect. The Etruscan practice of gilding teeth seems to have waned under Roman occupation. Neighboring Phoenicians of the era also appear to have had similar dental appliances fashioned from gold or silver wire, called "a Gaillardot appliance." These were wrapped around groups of three to five teeth, likely to anchor a loose or false tooth into place and to provide an aesthetic detail to the mouth. It seems, however, that these devices were worn only by men (Becker 1999).

Ancient Maya decorated their teeth with notches, grooves, and semiprecious stones before 1500 (Roach 2009). Holes were skillfully drilled into the enamel of the front of the tooth with a drill-like device, likely made of obsidian, and then set with an inlay of colorful stone like jade, turquoise, or hematite. The stones were permanently fixed in place using a natural resin, such as plant sap, mixed with crushed bone. This dental procedure appears to have been limited to men only. Because the teeth augmentation is found in 38–65 percent of burials and not only in the graves of the elites, archaeologists suspect that the practice was not a mark of social class, but rather, for some other reason, perhaps for beautification (Neiburger 2002). Jade was invested heavily with cultural symbolism in ancient Central American societies and central to a number of body modification practices. Because of its close relationship to the supernatural Breath Spirit, jade was central to rituals for conjuring the gods and the ancestors for the Olmec and the Maya (Taube 2005). Placing jade within the mouth makes sense when one considers that the breath was considered an essential factor for establishing a passageway for communication with supernatural forces. The Maya also frequently filed their teeth. Later, gold became the standard both for repairing teeth and for adding status. Embellished teeth continue to be popular in Central America today as a signifier of wealth and virility. Dentist E. J. Neiburger estimates that about 65 percent of men in urban Guatemala today wear some sort of gold dental decoration (Neiburger 2002).

"Waterloo teeth" refer to teeth collected as grisly tokens from the youthful dead during the 19th century, especially after combat in the Crimean and Civil Wars (Fitzharris 2014). The stolen teeth were sold to dentists and surgeons of the era for a high profit in order to create dentures for wealthy patrons, which were often held together with metal wire and might have given the appearance of "grills," though they would not have had the same appearance while the tooth owner was alive.

In some parts of the world, embellished teeth also mask a history of neglect for dental hygiene. Drakulić (1996) documents how teeth do not necessarily represent an index of one's social status in her native Croatia, but rather, represent a metaphor for a social and economic system that failed to develop a strong sense of personal responsibility for one's own life. In neighboring Tajikistan, commentators note that young people have turned away from the previously common practice of repairing tooth damage with flashy (and expensive) gold treatments as the price of gold has risen, though consumers in Uzbekistan still replace healthy teeth with gold ones (Fergusson 1997).

See also: Dental Hygiene and Cosmetic Dentistry; Egypt; Jewelry; Maya; Mexico.

Further Reading

Becker, Marshall Joseph. 1999. "Etruscan Gold Dental Appliances: Three Newly 'Discovered' Examples." *American Journal of Archaeology* 103: 103–11.

Drakulić, Slovenka. 1996. *Café Europa: Life After Communism*. New York: WW Dutton.

Fergusson, J. J. 1997. "Gold Loses Its Shine Among Young Tajiks." The Independent. May 15. Accessed July 13, 2016. http://www.independent.co.uk/news/world/gold-loses-its-shine -among-young-tajiks-1261758.html.

Fitzharris, Leslie. 2014. "Dead Men's Teeth: A History of Dentures." *The Chirugeon's Apprentice*. Accessed July 13, 2016. https://thechirurgeonsapprentice.com/2014/03/28/dead -mens-teeth-a-history-of-dentures/.

Holloway, April. 2014. "From Jewel Capped Teeth to Golden Bridges: 9000 Years of Dentistry." *Ancient Origins*. Accessed July 13, 2016. http://www.ancient-origins.net/human -origins-science/jewel-capped-teeth-golden-bridges-9000-years-dentistry-001427?page =0%2C1.

Neiburger, E. J. 2002. "Jaded Smiles: Ancient Mayan Dental Inlays and Today's Central American Patients. *Journal of the Massachusetts Dental Society* 60, no. 4: 36–39.

Roach, John. 2009. "Ancient Gem-Studded Teeth Show Skill of Ancient Dentist." *National Geographic* Accessed July 13, 2016. http://news.nationalgeographic.com/news/2009/05 /090518-first-dentists.html.

Roberts, Brian. 2015. "A Brief History of Grillz: 4500 Years of History." *Huffington Post* August 28. Accessed July 13, 2016. http://www.huffingtonpost.com/brian-roberts/a-brief -history-of-grillz_b_8055030.html.

Schwartzberg, Lauren. 2014. "The Ancient History of Grills." *Vice*. December 15. Accessed July 13, 2016. http://www.vice.com/read/the-ancient-history-of-grills-456.

Taube, Karl A. 2005. "The Symbolism of Jade in Classic Maya Religion." *Ancient Mesoamerica* 16, no. 1: 23–50.

H

HAIR

Hair, for both men and women, is a significant measure of beauty and attractiveness. Around the world and over the course of centuries, how healthy hair is, how it's styled, what color it is, and how long it is have all played key roles in assessments of beauty and status. From the powdered wigs of the 18th century to the weaves and waxing of the 21st century, hair has been an essential part of social norms of beauty.

Hair, for some scholars, is a particularly interesting element of beauty to study, for it is of great importance as a frame for the face, another key measure of beauty. Hair is also one of the easiest parts of appearance to change and control. Hair can be worn up or down, cut short or allowed to grow long, made big and obvious or hidden under clothing. Hair can be colored and have its texture changed, and hair can be adorned and decorated (Rich and Cash 1993). Hair also naturally replenishes itself, growing constantly and growing back if cut off. This element of hair has lent it magical or mythical powers in many cultures. Fairy tales such as Rapunzel or the Old Testament tale of Samson are examples of the symbolic value of hair (Koppelman 1996). Beauty prescriptions for hair appear in the Bible. 1 Corinthians 11:14–15 states: "Doth not even nature itself teach you that if a man have long hair, it is a shame unto him? But if a woman have long hair, it is a glory to her."

Some scholars speculate that humans prefer big hair or long hair on potential mates because the health and quality of a person's hair can tell us so much about that person's affiliations, taste, gender, age, and wealth (Etcoff 2000). Hair serves as a way of identifying who might be an attractive husband or wife, or who is of the same religion, social class, and age as ourselves. Men with very short "buzz-cut" hair are assumed to be soldiers or police officers, for example, and women who cover their hair with shawls and scarves are understood to be devout Muslims or Jews. In some African cultures, a shaven head can be associated with humiliation, renunciation, or mourning. Heads are often shaved to mark initiations, such as the passage to adulthood or, more generally, admission to a new social category.

The importance of hair as an identifying element of appearance goes beyond style, however. Hair is also a reliable indicator of the health of a person. The strength, sheen, and length of hair are influenced by diet and a person's well-being—not only of their body in the moment, but also of their genetics. A full, thick head of hair can be an indicator of healthy genes as well as lack of disease or parasites. During the Medieval period and the Renaissance, a wide variety of hair care remedies were devised to keep hair pest free, including a concoction of myrtle berry, broom, and clary seeped in vinegar. Noblewomen were also encouraged to wear musk or clove oil in their hair to cover the odor of vinegar (Zajaczkowa 2016).

Hair is also an indicator of wealth and prosperity, making it a status symbol. At a basic level, the appearance of hair is determined by how well a person eats. Lack of copper, zinc, iron, and vitamins A or E will result in thin and damaged hair. Therefore, healthy hair is a sign of enough prosperity to eat a healthy diet (Etcoff 2000). Similarly, the amount of care, treatment, and beauty work that one can afford to spend on hair is indicative of wealth. Hair work like permanents, highlights, hair weaves, or straightening are indicators of the amount of money a person has and their class status. In African societies, hair is often the most time-consuming part of a person's beauty regimen. Hair may be perfumed, oiled, dyed, coated with clay or red ochre, and decorated with feathers, cowrie shells, combs, or hairpieces. There is nothing random about the arrangement of hair: the patterns

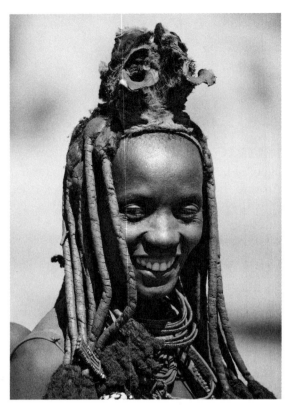

The striking traditional hair styles of Himba women have led to frequently exoticized visual representations within the global media. For the Himba themselves, the meaning of a person's hairstyle references lineage membership, age, and gender. (Dmitry Pichugin/ Dreamstime.com)

of braids or the adornments worn within the hair often symbolically transmit a subtle social language that can yield information about an individual's lineage, social or marital status, age, accomplishments, and personality.

Wigs are another way in which humans display both wealth and position. In 17th- and 18th-century Europe, for example, wigs were symbols of power and status, marking the difference between aristocracy and commoner and pointing to the wealth and "high birth" of the wearer. Wigs were expensive, and wearing a wig meant that the owner did not need to engage in physical labor (Kwass 2006). Even still in the 21st century, wigs can be indicators of both economic power and personal power and confidence. Both men and women wear wigs to express themselves, change their appearance to suit their mood, and show the amount of money they have to spend on such items (Shepheard 2015). For those undergoing treatments that cause hair to fall out, such as chemotherapy, wigs can also replace the self-esteem of a patient who has lost such an important element of their physical appearance and beauty.

The wig worn by indigenous Mbukushu women of Namibia, Angola, and Botswana is made of leather, fiber, and beads to imitate the *thihukeka* hairstyle of adult women. Long sisal fibers are twisted to create the illusion of long hair in elaborate styles, ornamented with decorative patterns of glass beads, cowrie shells, and copper buttons, and finished with a **pomade** of animal fat, grass, tree resins, and ochre pigment. The wig provides a more practical and convenient technique for wearing the hairstyle associated with married women of the area (Smithsonian 2014).

Hair also makes important social and political statements. In many cultures around the world, those in mourning shave their heads as a symbol of their grief. As the **Black Power/Black Is Beautiful movement** in the United States shows, certain hairstyles can be appropriated to register strong sentiments about power relationships. Long, natural, and unrestrained hair was a symbol of the "Free Love" movement in the 1960s in the United States. The Broadway production (later a movie) "Hair: The American Tribal Love-Rock Musical" (MacDermot 1966) protested the Vietnam War and celebrated hippie counterculture with a joyful musical ode to "long, beautiful hair. Shining, gleaming, steaming, flaxen, waxen. Give me down to there hair, shoulder-length or longer."

The so-called "Chinese queue" was a style of male haircutting mandated by the 1645 Manchu Qing order for all Han men to signify submission to Manchurian rule in **China.** The hair on the top of the head was grown long and the front and the sides of the head were shaved. Sometimes, the queue was braided and could reach lengths to a man's waist. Citizens were required to conform to the Manchu hairstyle for more than three centuries. After the collapse of the Qing imperium, some continued to wear the queue style as a symbol of political resistance.

In the same way that hair is an indicator of wealth and power, a person's locks are also an indicator of race. Indeed, in many cultures, hair can be the main indicator of the racial background of an individual. Black, tightly curled, "kinky," or "nappy" hair is associated with African descent. Very straight black hair is assumed to be of Native American or Asian descent, and blonde hair carries the assumption that the person is of northern European origin. Many cultures, especially those with populations that are of mixed racial origin, spend a great deal of time categorizing the racial background of citizens based on their hair. In the Dominican Republic, for example, researchers have found that people identify nine separate hair colors and fifteen different hair textures to be used when identifying other people (Kunsa 2013).

Finally, hair has deep and important ties to gender norms. Many societies use the norms for length, style, or covering of hair to help identify who is male or female. Generally, however, worldwide, long hair is the accepted standard for beauty in women, a preference that goes back to the Christian Bible, which identifies long hair as "a woman's glory" (Massey 2011). Hair must frequently be covered by pious women in the formal religious settings of a variety of world religions. Studies demonstrate that even in the 21st century, men worldwide prefer long hair on women (Etcoff 2000).

Marcel Wave

In 1872, Marcel Grateau was a hairdresser in a small, dingy salon in Paris's Montmartre neighborhood, catering mostly to prostitutes and chorus girls. By experimenting with a new way of holding a curling iron (upside down), he invented a new technique for creating a head full of crimped, natural-looking waves similar to "finger waves" that would last for up to a month. The wealthy Madame Gaston Menier, wife to the famous chocolatier, "discovered" Grateau's technique. She was reluctant, however, to visit his "exceedingly uninviting" salon in the disreputable neighborhood, and so she paid him well to come dress her hair on her yacht. Grateau's fame spread and he was soon able to buy a salon in the upscale Théâtre française district. One famous wearer of his style was the notorious Josephine Baker. By 1884, Grateau only accepted clients who competitively bid for his services. When he died in 1936, Marcel Grateau was a celebrity of the Parisian beauty world and a very rich man.

This emphasis on the length and appearance of hair for women creates a specific set of issues for women of all races and classes. Ideas and ideals of hair and beauty can be particularly problematic for women of African descent. Whereas the global norm of beauty privileges long, soft, straight, or wavy hair, women (and men) who have inherited elements of Afro-textured hair often battle what scholars call the "kink factor" (Robinson 2011). Centuries of global racial mixing have meant that there is a wide variety of "black hair," from very tightly curled and short, to wider, fuller curls. Africans and people of the African diaspora discuss hair with a great deal of specificity, less concerned with hair color than with hair texture, hair grades, and length.

Mid-century European and American women of means needed to maintain their hairstyles with regular visits to the **salon** to have their hair coiffed into elaborate styles, which required teasing (a way of "backbrushing" the hair to make it stand up), rollers, forms, and a great deal of hairspray. These styles needed to be carefully maintained until the next salon appointment, requiring accommodations to sleep, wear hats, and go out into the rain. In the 1960s, London-based hairstylist Vidal Sassoon revolutionized the haircut for the average woman. He pioneered the wash-and-go "five-point cut" for the woman on the go. This style, made famous by Mia Farrow, featured easy bangs worn low over the eyebrows, with a pixie point in front of each ear and at the nape. After a haircut, Sassoon asked the client to stand up and shake her head with the logic that a "good cut" would fall back into place (McCracken 1995, 48). In 1963, Sassoon struck again with the introduction of the geometric bob cut, worn a bit longer than the earlier pixie cut, which featured shaping by the stylist to add swing and fall to the hair without any fussy styling. Sassoon's hallmark "wash-and-wear" freedom of style resonated strongly with women of the era, many of whom wanted to experience mobility, self-expression, and freedom of choice. Hair was meant to "swing," which also carried strong sexual connotations in the decade (McCracken 1995, 54).

For women with Afro-textured hair, the choice to leave their hair "natural" is often seen as a radical political statement. Women, especially, but also men in the United States and other nations, have been taught that the social norm of hair is to have straight, soft locks. When people of African descent choose natural hairstyles such as dreadlocks, Afros, or braids, they often face professional and legal discrimination. The U.S. military prohibits those hairstyles, the Transportation Safety Administration was recently sued for disproportionately "patting down" Afros on travelers, and workers have been fired for wearing natural hairstyles, as these do not fit with workplace rules of grooming (Brown 2015).

See also: Baldness; Blondes and Blonde Hair; Burqa; China; Hair Extensions and Weaves; Hair Straightening; *Hijab*; Pomade.

Further Reading

Brown, Stacia L. 2015. "My Hair, My Politics." *New Republic* 246, no. 11 (Fall): 16–17.

Etcoff, Nancy. 2000. *Survival of the Prettiest: The Science of Beauty*. New York: Anchor.

Koppelman, Connie. 1996. "The Politics of Hair." *Frontiers: A Journal of Women's Studies* 17, no. 2: 87–88.

Kunsa, Ashley. 2013. "History, Hair, and Reimagining Racial Categories in Junot Díaz's The Brief Wondrous Life of Oscar Wao." *Critique* 54, no. 2 (April): 211.

Kwass, Michael. 2006. "Big Hair: A Wig History of Consumption in Eighteenth-Century France." *American Historical Review* 111, no. 3: 630.

Lester, Neal A. 2000. "Nappy Edges and Goldy Locks: African-American Daughters and the Politics of Hair." *The Lion and the Unicorn* 24: 201–24.

MacDermot, Galt. 1966. *Hair: The American Tribal Love-Rock Musical*. Broadway soundtrack.

Massey, Preston T. 2011 "Long Hair as a Glory and as a Covering Removing an Ambiguity from 1 Cor 11:15." *Novum Testamentum* 53, no. 1 (January): 52–72.

McCracken, Grant. 1995. *Big Hair: A Journey into the Transformation of Self*. Woodstock, NY: Overlook Press.

Rich, Melissa K., and Thomas F. Cash. 1993. "The American Image of Beauty: Media Representations of Hair Color for Four Decades." *Sex Roles* 29, no. 1/2 (July): 113–24.

Robinson, Cynthia L. 2011. "Hair as Race: Why "Good Hair" May Be Bad for Black Females." *Howard Journal of Communications* 22, no. 4: 358–76.

Shepheard, Sherri. 2015. Wig Out This Spring. *USA Today Magazine*. (March) 143, no. 2838: 74.

Smithsonian. 2014. "Wig. Mbukushu Peoples." Smithsonian. Accessed October 5, 2016. https://africa.si.edu/collections/view/objects/asitem/items$0040:16674.

Zajaczkowa, Pani Jadwiga. 2016. "Hair Care Recipes from Medieval/Renaissance Sources." Gallowglass. Accessed October 5, 2016. http://www.gallowglass.org/jadwiga/SCA/Hair.html.

HAIR DYE

Around the world, a variety of naturally occurring botanicals or organic materials can assist in changing the color of hair or beards. Saffron and alfalfa have been used on light-colored hair to add shine. In the Middle East and Iran, men often treated their **facial hair** with henna first to condition it, then topped it with an indigo dye to make the color blue-black (Cordwell 1973). Ancient Romans made a black dye formula by fermenting leeches for two months directly inside a lead vessel (Guenard 2015). Women across North Africa, India, and the Middle East use **mehendi** (henna) to tint their hair shades of red. **Tuareg** women in Mauritania use camel urine to lighten their hair (Beholding Beauty 2016). In Germany, a combination of beechwood ash and goats' fat can bring up the red highlights natural to the hair color (Guenard 2015). Natural dyes, however, do not produce vivid colors and lack the staying power of non-natural dyes produced in laboratories.

There is an important distinction between coloring hair, which typically consists of adding pigments that will eventually wear out, and dying hair, which chemically transforms the color of the hair. Dyes, combined with ammonia, initiate a chemical change that transforms the color of the hair by penetrating the protein shaft and accessing the melanin pigment beneath, which gives hair its color. Individual dye molecules need time to work on the hair in order to reach the desired color, and the dye and its ammonia base must then be quickly removed. Peroxide, a bleaching agent, may also be added to hair dye and ammonia when the desired effect is to lighten the hair color. Typically, the reaction takes at least thirty minutes (Guenard 2015).

Over the years, there have been a number of concerns about the harsh chemicals used in hair dying. These chemicals can cause allergic reactions, creating discomfort, and they can also burn the skin of the scalp and the face. The Food and Drug Administration (FDA) has banned a number of ingredients used in hair dyes that are also found to cause cancer in laboratory animals (Guenard 2015).

The first non-natural hair dye was introduced in the mid-1800s by a British chemist named William Henry Perkin. Hoping to create a quinine-like antimalarial drug, he began with a black coal tar and ended up with a mauve substance that was suitable for use as a durable dye. The result, paraphenylenediamine (PPD), was the first synthetic hair dye and was influential in the products that launched the enormous success of the L'Oreal company in 1907 (Hopp 2015).

Many women and men decide to begin dying their hair or their **beards** with the appearance of grey hairs. Greying hair can be the first and most obviously visible sign of **aging**. Estimates suggest that 70 percent of American women dye their hair at some point in their lives (Guenard 2015).

Highlighting is a popular technique for adding appeal to the hair color and also for "covering" grey. Highlighting uses both dye (lightener) and hair color to create a more complex color effect on the hair than dying it one color alone. Often, some parts of the hair remain the original color and other sections are color-treated. The technique, known as "foil highlights," separates a section or strand of hair that will be treated with color from the other hairs, which remain the natural color. Chunking is a similar technique for adding bold, natural colors to the existing hair, especially those used to create contrast. Hair painting uses a brush to add highlights of color to the hair. The results are more subtle than foil treatments or chunking. The technique known as balayage (from the French "to sweep") is preferred by many women because dye is "painted" on to create a graduated, natural-looking highlight effect. There are no demarcations between the hair colors.

Frosting is another highlighting technique, often used on shorter hair and in men's highlighting. Frosting is a free-hand technique that uses dye to lighten the tips of the hair and create the illusion of "sun-kissed" texture.

Another popular hair dying technique similar to balayage is known as "ombré," borrowed from the French term to refer to the shading effect of hair colors. The ombré technique leaves hair darker at the roots, gradually lightening through the mid shaft and lightest at the ends. Unlike traditional dying, which shows at the roots as the hair grows out naturally and needs regular maintenance, the versatility of the ombré technique allows the wearer to remain stylish for a longer period. Graduated ombré styles are also becoming popular in **makeup** applications and **manicures**.

See also: Facial Hair; Makeup and Cosmetics; Manicures; Mehendi; Tuareg.

Further Reading

Beholding Beauty. 2016. "Five Beauty Rituals from the Saharan Aristocrats." Accessed October 1, 2016. http://www.beholdingbeauty.com/tuareg-women-five-beauty-rituals-from -the-saharan-aristocrats.

Cordwell, Justine. 1973. "The Very Human Arts of Transformation." In: *The Fabrics of Culture: The Anthropology of Clothing and Adornment*, edited by Justine Cordwell and Ronald A. Schwartz, 47–76. Chicago: International Congress of Anthropological and Ethnological Sciences.

Corson, Richard. 1965. *Fashions in Hair: The First Five Thousand Years*. London: Peter Owens Publishing.

Guenard, Rebecca. 2015. "Hair Dye: A History." *The Atlantic*. January 2. Accessed September 11, 2016. http://www.theatlantic.com/health/archive/2015/01/hair-dye-a-history /383934/.

Hopp, Deven. 2015. "From 1500 BC to 2015 AD: The Extraordinary History of Hair Color." *Byrdie*. December 9. Accessed September 11, 2016. http://www.byrdie.com/hair-color -history.

Sherrow, Victoria. 2006. *Encyclopedia of Hair: A Cultural History*. Westport, CT: Greenwood Press.

Stenn, Kurt. 2016. *Hair: A Human History*. Seattle: Pegasus Books: Amazon Digital Services.

HAIR EXTENSIONS AND WEAVES

The global beauty norm of long, wavy, thick hair of the type seen on candidates for the Miss Universe pageant has created an industry of hair extensions. Hair extensions and weaves both describe the practice of adding either artificial or natural hair to a customer's own existing hair through a variety of processes. First popularized by women of African descent who sought to conform to a globalized social norm of beauty that sought long, soft, flowing locks, hair extensions are increasingly popular around the world and across racial lines.

Hair extensions, from individual strands to long fringes of hair, may be made of artificial substances or be the human hair of another person. Extensions may be as inexpensive as twenty dollars or run into the hundreds of dollars for the hair, with additional hundreds necessary for the application and maintenance of the extensions.

In the world of hair extensions and weaves, the most expensive, most prestigious, and most sought-after hair is known as "Remy Hair"—the product of an Indian tonsuring (or head shaving ceremony) that forms part of a Hindu tradition practiced by many in India. Extensions for weaves are most commonly sold in cheaper, lower-quality "packets" or more expensive, higher-quality "bundles" of hair (Jones 2013).

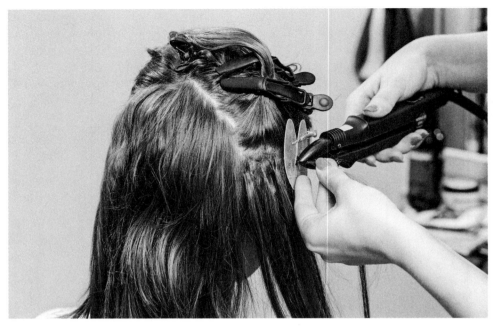

Hair extensions applied at a salon. Extensions range in price and quality, and are often sought to achieve the illusion of a globalized beauty norm favoring long, soft, flowing locks. (Stas Tolstnev/Dreamstime.com)

Both men and women in India follow a traditional ritual known as tonsure, the shaving of one's head, in honor of the Hindu God Venkateswara (also known as Vishnu). Pilgrims travel every year to the Indian town of Tirupati to give their hair to the god in thanks and praise. This act is also seen as a way of humbling the person before the god, effacing the ego (Tirumala Tirupati 2016). The temple then collects the hair and sells it on the international market, where the long, silky locks can fetch huge prices. This practice has made the Temple of Venkateswara the richest in India (Coppen 2003). As Indian women traditionally wear their hair very long, the hair makes for highly prized extensions. Women in India also rarely dye or treat their hair with chemicals, making the hair "virgin hair."

Although hair weaves for women of non-European descent are one major use of hair extension products, other customers purchase hair extensions to add fullness or a different color. These products often do not need to be woven and sewn onto the scalp, but may be clipped in or applied with adhesives. Customers who might already have hair that is long and straight or wavy might purchase extensions to add thickness, add layers, or add highlights or areas of another natural or vibrant color (USA Today 2014).

Hair weaves are most common among women of African descent who are seeking to replicate the global norm of long, silky hair, sometimes known as "good hair" (Rock 2009). As some scholars note, although "natural" hairstyles for black women are increasingly common and tolerated, the choice for women with curly, coarse

"African" hair to leave their hair unstraightened or natural is still criticized by many as rebellious or "political." Women who leave the natural texture in their very curly hair are often perceived as making a radical, race-based political statement (Prince 2009). Therefore, it is most common for black women, especially those in high-profile positions, to straighten their hair or use hair weaves.

A hair weave is a form of hair extension in which a person's own hair is braided tightly against the skull in a circular pattern. Long fringes of hair extensions, then, are laid against and woven or sewn onto the braids, affixing them firmly. This process costs hundreds of dollars, in addition to purchasing the hair, and is very time consuming. The resulting extensions, however, will last about three months (Waldron 2011).

Several different types of nonweave hair extensions are available on the market in the 21st century. On the smallest scale, strand-by-strand extensions can be bonded to thinning areas like the temples using adhesive micro-bonds. Keratin-bonded extensions of very small amounts of hair are applied to the customer's existing hair with heat and a matching color adhesive. Larger portions of hair, bonded in wefts, may also be applied using adhesives.

U.S. and world celebrities are leading the way in extensions, both by reinforcing the norm of thicker, longer, and more voluminous hair, and by using hair extensions in increasing numbers. Some credit the early rise in popularity of extensions in the United States to the celebrities Paris Hilton, Jennifer Anniston, and Jennifer Lopez (Chadwick 2006). Reports from 2013 have indicated that many female actresses and performers use hair extensions on a permanent basis and that any famous woman with long hair on a red carpet runway is wearing hair extensions (Fifield 2013). The pop star Beyoncé is rumored to travel on tour with up to three trunks full of custom extensions made by her personal stylist and has one weave made from Swedish hair that was rumored to cost more than 100,000 dollars (102.5 KSFM.com 2014).

The rise in both adhesive technologies and desire to manage hair has lead in 2016 to the creation of new products as well, including hair extensions for eyebrows, for those who have overplucked their natural brows or want a more dramatic look (InStyle 2016).

See also: Hair; India; Pageants—International, National, and Local Contests.

Further Reading

Chadwick, Alan. 2006. "Indian Hair: The Next Hot Beauty Trend?" Day to Day (NPR). Accessed January 27, 2016. http://www.npr.org/templates/story/story.php?storyId=5173974.

Coppen, Luke. 2003. "India's Wealthiest Hindu Temple." *The Times (United Kingdom)*. July 5. Accessed June 18, 2016.

Fifield, Kathleen. 2013. "Hollywood's Best-Kept Hair Secret." *InStyle* 116.

InStyle. 2016. "The Buzz." 23, no. 4: 225.

Jones, Latoya. 2013. "Bundles or Packs? How to Choose Your Hair When Getting Weave." Accessed June 18, 2016. http://www.latoyajonesblog.com/2013/08/bundles-or-packs-how-to-choose-your.html.

102.5 KSFM.com. 2014. "Beyonce's New Weave Cost How Much? Over $100K." Accessed
    February 6, 2017. http://ksfm.cbslocal.com/2014/03/19/beyonces-new-weave-cost-how
    -much-over-100k/
Prince, Althea. 2009. *The Politics of Black Women's Hair.* London: Insomniac Press.
Rock, Chris. 2009. *Good Hair.* Film. Directed by Chris Rock. HBO Films.
Tirumala Tirupati. 2016. "Offering Hair." Accessed June 18, 2016. http://tirumala-tirupati
    .com/offering-hair/.
USA Today. 2014. "What's New?" 142, no. 2828: 67.
Waldron, Clarence. 2011. "The Right Weave." *Jet* 120, no. 14: 34.

HAIR REMOVAL

Humans have been removing their hair as a way to be more attractive for thousands
of years and around the globe. Although some forms of hair removal, such as shaving
of the face, are practiced regularly by men, most forms of hair removal are practices that focus on women. Worldwide, hair removal is practiced on every part of
the body and in almost all world cultures.

Hair—and lack of hair—have, over time, played a significant role in the categorization of people, from race and ethnicity to gender and social class. Early European
settlers wrote extensively about the differences in the facial and chest hair between
themselves and the Native Americans they encountered and linked those differences
directly to intelligence and work ethic. The early 1700s Swedish scientist Carl Lin-
naeus even went so far as to say that the lack of body and facial hair on "the American
savage" reflected a lack of "will and motivation" in those men (Herzig 2014). This
visible body difference was used to justify the categorization of the native peoples
as feeble and uncivilized.

Hair and body hair differences are not only perceived as a dividing line between
races, however. Women are more often expected to remove hair from their bodies,
and have been through history. The ancient Roman poet Ovid advised women that
their legs should not be "rough with bristling hair" (Etcoff 2009). One possible reason
for the pressure on women is the desire to make the dividing line between genders
clear. Women have less body hair than men generally, but the removal of what hair
they do have accentuates the difference between male and female in a way that may
appeal to each as they seek a partner and mate (Etcoff 2009). Especially in Europe,
but also in Asia and North America, through the 19th century, the norm of beauty for
women was skin that looked like porcelain—without spots or blemishes, and also
without hair or fuzz (Herzig 2014).

Another possible reason that women are expected to remove more hair is that
women typically display more skin than men. Because the expectation is for a
woman's skin to be hairless and "without blemish" (including hair), whatever skin
fashion and culture dictate she display should be hair free (Herzig 2014). This idea
would explain why the advent of shorter skirts that bared the leg coincided with more
products for leg shaving and why the bikini came with the invention of the bikini wax.

A wide array of beauty practices and products are designed to remove hair on
women, and not all are designed to only amplify the difference between male and
female. In the example of eyebrow removal, for example, women's eyebrows are

plucked in order to make her eyes appear larger, an element of global beauty preferences (Etcoff 2009). Additionally, the modern trends of hair removal in the pubic area for women, first popularized in Brazil, and the removal of back and chest hair for men, have more to do with changing aesthetics than differentiation between male and female.

Hair removal, however, as the example from ancient Rome demonstrates, is not a new phenomenon. In the 14th and 15th centuries in Europe, women covered the hair on their heads with a cloth and then plucked the small hairs of their forehead that peeked out of the covering to only display smooth, hairless skin (Etcoff 2009). By the 1800s, plucking and shaving for women were joined by a wide variety of packaged products designed to remove hair, some of which contained such dangerous and damaging chemicals as arsenic or thallium (Herzig 2014).

Most women in the United States did not remove hair from their underarms or their legs prior to World War I, though any visible hairs may have been removed from the upper lip and chin thought to be undesirable. Hair removal was thought to be a vain practice that dealt with body parts that should best remain hidden and was practiced primarily by "bad girls," such as those who performed as chorus girls. However, between 1914 and 1945, the rise in commercially available depilatory products designed specifically to remove female body hair is clear by examining advertisements in print media, including "wholesome" publications like *Harper's Bazaar* and *McCall's* (Hope 1982). Before 1919, American women were encouraged to remove visible hair from underarms in order to improve hygiene and comfort. Women were also persuaded through **advertising** that removing "superfluous" and "ugly" body hair would allow them to feel less self-conscious and avoid embarrassment. In 1922, the first safety razor was invented, designed especially to fit the curve of the underarm. From the 1920s to the 1940s, hemlines revealed the leg below the knee, and hair removal came into fashion as a way to preserve sheer stockings and also for going bare-legged at the beach or swimming pool. By 1930, famous beauty consultants like Helena Rubenstein were arguing that regular removal of hair from the underarms and legs should be as much a part of a routine for every woman as washing her hair or manicuring her nails (Hope 1982, 96). Hemlines continued to rise in the early 1940s. Women were not so much told by advertisers to shave their leg hair as they were told to consider their legs fashionable, with the rise in leg makeup and hosiery with patterns or seams. In 1964, a survey found that 98 percent of American women between the ages of 15 and 44 removed their body hair (Hope 1982, 97). From this era on, female body hair in the United States has been treated as "disgusting" or linked with potential uncleanliness. The emphasis on female hair removal seems to revolve around a cultural idea that hairlessness is "neat" and feminine, not in the sense of "womanly," but in the sense of more childlike. Some have speculated that Caucasian American women are thought to be more desirable when they manifest nonadult personality characteristics and remove certain, potentially threatening signs of bodily adulthood, like hair (Hope 1982, 98).

In the late 19th and early 20th century, after the discovery of x-rays, the Austrian scientist Leopold Freund recommended the use of radiation for permanent hair removal, causing thousands of women to suffer illness and damage in x-ray hair removal clinics (Collins 2007). In this same time period the use of electrical current, applied with a thin needle to the hair follicle, a practice known as electrolysis, became widely used and continues in some places today (Herzig 2008).

Although many of these practices are no longer common, the idea of hair removal as desirable continues into the 20th and 21st centuries, targeting men's and women's faces, but also legs, underarms, and the public region. And in the modern era, hair removal is not limited to women. Men not only shave their faces, but when baring chests and backs, men in some cultures are using hair removal techniques, sometimes called "manscaping," to achieve the look of smooth skin. This hair removal allows for the definition of the muscles in the chest and back to be more obvious and mimics the look of an armored chest piece (Etcoff 2009).

Whether practiced on men or women, in the 21st century, an even wider variety of products and practices for hair removal are available to consumers worldwide than ever before. Techniques such as shaving, hair removal creams, waxing, laser hair removal, and IPL (intense pulsed light) are the most common for men and women.

Modern hair removal, or depilatory, creams are composed of acids that gradually dissolve hair just below the surface of the skin. Waxing, or the process of applying hot wax to the skin and letting it cool long enough to grab onto the hair, can be a painful process, as the technique ends with the wax, and the hair, being ripped out. Shaving, waxing, and depilatory creams are the less costly options for those seeking to get rid of unwanted hair in the 21st century, with prices in only the tens of dollars. These three techniques, however, are not permanent, though hair often grows in finer and less noticeable after waxing (Nishi 2002).

The more high-tech hair removal techniques of the current century, however, can cost thousands of dollars per treatment. Laser hair removal and IPL both use different strengths of laser light to target hair follicles, eliminating hair with nearly permanent results (Nishi 2002).

Although these techniques are the most common hair removal techniques in Europe and the United States, other practices, such as threading, have been used for hundreds of years in other parts of the world. Threading, in which rows of hair are twisted in cotton string and yanked forcibly out of the skin, is an ancient, and still popular, method of hair removal in the Middle East.

See also: Advertising; Brazil; Eyebrows; Eyelid Surgery; Hair; Manscaping.

Further Reading

Collins, Paul. 2007. "Histories: The Perils of X-ray Hair Removal." *New Scientist* 195, no. 2620: 68.

Etcoff, Nancy. 2009. *Survival of the Prettiest: The Science of Beauty.* New York: Anchor.

Herzig, Rebecca M. 2008. "Subjected to the Current: Batteries, Bodies and the Early History of Electrification in the United States." *Journal of Social History* 41, no. 4: 867.

Herzig, Rebecca M. 2014. *Plucked: A History of Hair Removal.* New York: NYU Press.

Hope, Christine. 1982. "Caucasian Female Body Hair and American Culture." *Journal of American Culture* 5, no. 1: 93–99.

Nishi, Dennis. 2002. "Bald by Choice." *Men's Fitness* 18, no. 9: 52.

HAIR STRAIGHTENING

The practice of hair straightening is a common beauty practice among those men and women who seek to conform to global norms of soft, straight, long hair. Those who have the tightly curled hair that is associated with African descent use a variety of products and techniques to straighten their hair. The straightness of hair, however, is a continuum, and people of both genders and a variety of racial backgrounds practice hair straightening. Styles and trends often lead people with all textures of hair to seek straighter locks.

Tightly curled "African" hair, sometimes called "nappy" hair, is naturally dry, absorbs moisture easily, and must be oiled or conditioned regularly to prevent breakage. This type of hair also grows very slowly and is often much shorter than that of people who have the straighter hair associated with a Euro-descended lineage (Robinson 2011). For people with Afro-textured hair, there are three main ways to achieve straight hair: chemical treatments, a pressing comb, a ceramic flat iron of a "Brazilian blow-out" (ABCs 2006).

Chemical treatments for very curly hair are often known as "perms" or "relaxers." These treatments are strong chemicals, often acids, that break bonds in the outside shaft of very tightly curled hair to allow the hair to "relax." These chemicals strip off the coating of the hair that gives the hair its shape, permanently straightening it. Chemical relaxers are often criticized because of the strong chemicals that are used and the potential to damage both the scalp and the hair itself, as well as other potential health risks including burns and baldness. Relaxers use acids in the form of hydroxides to break hair bonds and carry the potential to injure skin and cause such health problems as uterine fibroids (Thompson 2014).

An early form of chemical treatment for straightening short hair, especially on men, was called "conking," a trend from the early to mid-20th century and popular among performers such as Nat King Cole and Fats Domino (Dash 2006, 29). The process used dye, which could cause burns and even blisters on the scalp.

Beyond, or in addition to, relaxers, the two main tools of hair straightening are the pressing comb and the flat iron. A pressing comb, or "hot comb," is a traditional tool that uses heat, in conjunction with a hair treatment or pomade, to achieve straight and silky hair. Developed in France in the 1800s by women seeking to emulate their perception of "Egyptian" hair, and popularized in the United States by **Madam C. J. Walker**, the hot comb is still in use today (Uwumarogie 2011).

A hot comb is a wide-bristled comb made of metal that is heated to high degrees and passed through hair to straighten it. In the past, hot combs were heated on the stove and could reach temperatures that actually burned instead of straightening hair. The risk of burning skin, and not just hair, is also high with the traditional type of hot comb. Although the stove-heated types of combs are still used in the 21st century, many people prefer electric hot combs, which let the user control the amount of heat and lower the risk of burns (Uwumarogie 2011).

Another tool used for hair straightening is the flat iron. Many 21st-century professional stylists prefer ceramic flat irons for hair straightening because of the lower risk of burns to skin and hair. The ceramic surface of the comb transfers heat to hair with less risk of burns to skin and is electric, with variable temperature gauges to allow the user to control the level of heat (ABCs 2006). When straightening either with a hot comb or ceramic flat iron, hair stylists insist on the necessity of protecting hair from the heat with an oil or serum. Because tightly curled hair is often very dry, these products protect the hair from breakage when exposed to high heat.

Although hair straightening is most often associated with women of African descent, women with wavy or frizzy Euro-descended hair sometimes also use ceramic flat irons to achieve a stick-straight look. Women with less kinky or tightly curled hair, however, may also seek a "Brazilian" keratin blowout.

Unlike a chemical relaxer, in a keratin blowout, hair is treated with a chemical that weakens and softens, but does not break, the bonds that give each strand of hair its shape. The hair is treated and then styled with a blow dryer on medium to low heat and a ceramic flat iron (Bailly 2016). The result is straighter hair for approximately two to four months. After that time the treatment wears off, the bonds reassert themselves, and hair regains its curl. Although this treatment is increasingly popular, scientists warn that the formaldehyde used in it may be dangerous for the customer (InStyle 2011).

Whatever method they might have used, almost all black women in the United States straightened their hair from the late 1940s to the early 1960s (Walker 2007, 129), when the **Black Is Beautiful movement** gained prominence and created opportunities for women to wear "natural" hairstyles.

See also: "Black Is Beautiful Movement," or Black Power; Hair; Walker, Madame C. J.

Further Reading

"The ABCs of Straightening Natural Hair." 2006. *Jet* 109, no. 19 (May 15): 34.
Bailly, Jenny. 2016. "O Investigation: Hair Straightening Treatments." Accessed June 29, 2016. http://www.oprah.com/style/The-Truth-About-Hair-Straightening-Treatments.
Corbin, Nicola A. and James F. Hamilton. 2012. "Black Women's Hair and the Postcolonial Practice of Style." Presented to the Feminist Studies Division, International Communication Association Convention, May 24–28, Phoenix.
Dash, Paul. 2006. "Black Hair Culture, Politics, and Change." *International Journal of Inclusive Education* 10, no. 1: 27–37.
InStyle. 2011. "The Straightening Controversy." *InStyle Special* (April 10, 2011): 36.
Robinson, Cynthia L. 2011. "Hair as Race: Why "Good Hair" May Be Bad for Black Females." *Howard Journal of Communications* 22, no. 4: 358–76.
Thompson, Cheryl. 2014 "Black Beauty Products." *Herizons* 28, no. 1 (Summer): 20.
Uwumarogie, Victoria. 2011. "Five Things You Should Know about Hot Combs." Accessed June 29, 2016. http://madamenoire.com/48084/five-things-you-should-know-about-hot-combs/3.
Walker, Susannah. 2007. *Style and Status: Selling Beauty to African American Women, 1920–1975.* Lexington, KY: University of Kentucky Press.

HEADBINDING

Headbinding, also called "headshaping," is a form of **body modification** that transforms the "normal" shape of the skull in order to conform to a culturally appropriate standard of beauty. Deliberate cranial deformation can be produced by applying tightly wound bandages to the head or, in some cases, binding the head to a board in order to produce a flatter surface to the forehead or to create exaggerated flat, elongated, conical, or round head shapes. Even regular head massaging can alter the natural growth trajectory of cranial bones (Brown 2010). The procedure is usually done on infants before the skull bones are fully fused and while the cranium is still fairly malleable; however, the process could take several years to achieve the desired results. Modifications made to the shape of the skull in infancy and childhood remain visible into adulthood. These modifications are considered beautiful, or possibly more masculine (Barras 2014), within the cultures that practice headbinding. The transformed shape might also be augmented to greater effect with particular hairstyles or other accessories.

Archaeological and ethnographic evidence indicate that headbinding has been practiced by many cultural groups around the world, possibly as a way to distinguish certain groups of people from others or to indicate the social status of individuals (White 2015). Such practices have been recorded on every continent, including the Maya of Central America; the Chinook and the Choctaw of North America; the Minoans of the Mediterranean; ancient Egyptians; several Oceanic cultures; and by some groups in some parts of Africa, most notably the Mangbetu people of Central Africa.

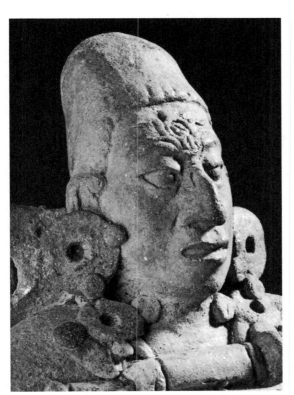

Figurine of a Maya ballgame player, ceramic, Guatemala, Maya, 550–850 CE. The high, flat forehead—a result of headbinding—was considered a mark of beauty and status in Maya culture. (Los Angeles County Museum of Art)

The first evidence of intentional cranial shaping comes from the famous archaeological remains at Shanidar Cave, Iraq, dating to BCE ninth century (White 2015). Skull elongation can also be seen in art and mummies from classical Europe and from ancient **Egypt**. The best known Egyptian figures, Queen Nefertiti and King Tutankhamen, are both often depicted with what appear to be unnaturally elongated skulls, accented with tall headdresses to maximize the illusion of a longer head.

For the **Maya**, who frequently accentuated high, broad foreheads as a mark of beauty in their iconographic art, the skulls of children were deliberately molded to accentuate a more pleasing plane of flatness and slope from the nose to the top of the head. Head shaping was also a way that elite members of the society defined themselves. A high, pointed head shape was viewed as a sign of noble birth (Barras 2014). Within a few days of birth, the parents of a child would tie a flat wooden board to the back of the baby's head and another to the forehead. The two boards would then be lashed together as tightly as possible. The boards prevented the child's head from expanding outward, and instead it would grow upward in a kind of a "loaf shape." Typically, the boards were removed from the child after a few days, but the skull would remain flattened for the rest of his or her life. The Maya also found crossed eyes to be beautiful. A mother would attach balls of resin and other small objects to a child's hair and allow them to dangle between the eyes (Ackerman 1994, 300). The movement would attract the child's gaze and train the eyes to look inward in a becoming way. Both of these deliberate modifications of the body may have been inspired by a religious devotion. Head deformations among the Maya have been explained by archaeologists as an effort to imitate the jaguar's skull, which would also show prowess, and the head of the indigenous maize god, whose presence indicated fertility (White 2015).

The Chinook of the Pacific Northwest (and other Salishan people of the area) fashioned specially made cradles for babies that would be influential in shaping the baby's skull. Babies were swaddled and laid flat in the cradle. Another board was attached, protruding at forty-five degrees from the top of the cradle, and designed to gradually flatten the forehead of a child into a pleasing shape. Flattened skulls were a biological marker of freedom among Pacific coastal peoples: children born into slavery continued to have rounded foreheads (Barras 2014). In this way, the social hierarchy of the cultural group was embodied within the faces of individuals.

The Mangbetu people, who live in the northeastern region of the Democratic Republic of Congo, practiced "*lipombo*," the art of skull modification, until the 20th century (Afritorial 2013). The heads of infants were bound by tight cords made from animal hides, resulting in a characteristic head elongation that was thought to increase the brain cavity and to increase the intelligence of the child. A tribe in Papua New Guinea also modified the skull shapes of infants because they believed that the new shape boosted intelligence (Barras 2014). In addition to being more attractive to members of the group, the resulting head shape denoted majesty, nobility, and status (Afritorial 2013). Specially braided hairstyles in the shape of a tall funnel tube were interwoven with straw in order to emphasize the elongated shape of the head. At the very top of the tube, a small "halo" was braided into the style to symbolize social status. The style was often pierced by decorative pins made of ivory to emphasize the shape and the intricacy of the resulting hairstyle. The distinctive head shape is immortalized in art and sculpture of the region. Although the practice was outlawed by the Belgians during the colonial era, the hairstyles are still worn for ceremonial occasions, and the Mangbetu cultural appreciation of the form remains intact.

See also: Body Modification; Egypt; Maya.

Further Reading

Ackerman, Diane. 1994. *A Natural History of Love*. New York: Vintage.
Afritorial. 2013. "The Mangbetu: The Head Elongation Fashionistas of Central Africa." Accessed July 17, 2016. http://afritorial.com/tribe-the-mangbetu.

Australian Museum. 2010. "Headshaping." Accessed July 17, 2016. http://australianmuseum
.net.au/headshaping.

Barras, Colin. 2014. "Why Early Humans Reshaped Their Children's Skulls." BBC Earth.
Accessed July 17, 2016. http://www.bbc.com/earth/story/20141013-why-we-reshape
-childrens-skulls.

Brown, Peter. 2010. "Nacurrie 1: Mark of Ancient Java, or a Caring Mother's Hands, in Ter-
minal Pleistocene Australia." *Journal of Human Evolution* 59, no. 2: 168–87.

Dingwall, Eric John. 1931, *Artificial Cranial Deformation: A Contribution to the Study of Ethnic Mutilations*. London: John Bale, Sons and Danielson.

White, Chris. 2015. "Head Space: Behind 10,000 Years of Artificial Cranial Modification.
Atlas Obscura. Accessed July 17, 2016. http://www.atlasobscura.com/articles/head-space
-artificial-cranial-deformation.

HEIGHT

In many nations around the world, height is considered a key element of a good physical appearance. For both men and women, height is associated with confidence, power, desirability, and beauty. In both national and international studies, people from around the world pick taller men and women as the most beautiful in any group (PTI 2011). Men and women who are taller are considered to be more attractive in most cultures.

In the United States and Canada, studies dating back to 1980 track the direct correlation of height to a person's perception of their own beauty and self-worth. Taller people feel more beautiful, attractive, and more able to make friends, find jobs, and have influence in social groups (Adams 1980). More recent studies find that, especially among men, height is such an important indicator of attractiveness and desirability that men exaggerate their height substantially when talking about it to others. This tendency is understandable, given that taller men in North American and European nations have been demonstrated to be more successful in their professional and financial achievements, but also, have greater dating and reproductive success in their personal lives (Bogaert and McCreary 2011). Studies have shown that both heterosexual and homosexual people use height as a significant determining factor when choosing a partner. Heterosexual women, for example, prefer men who are taller than they, and heterosexual men prefer women who are shorter (Valentova, Stulp, Třebický, and Havlíček 2014).

These preferences and the correlation between height, attractiveness, and success are equally true in China. In China, many opportunities, from dating, to driving, to school and work, are directly dependent on the height of the individual. Citizens must be at least five foot three inches tall to even take a driver's test, and many universities and professional schools have minimum height requirements for applicants (Watts 2004). Job applications and advertisements in China also routinely specify minimum height requirements, with a common cutoff being 1.6 meters for women (five feet four inches) and 1.7 meters (five feet seven inches) for men (Hua 2013). Even China's government admits to having unwritten height requirements for its employees, seeking to recruit the "tallest or the prettiest people, because it makes them (the government departments) look good" (Hua 2013, 92).

International preferences for taller men and women are also evident in the worlds of beauty pageants and modeling. Global modeling agencies often peg the absolute minimum height for female models to be five foot six or seven inches tall and the minimum height for male models to be five foot ten inches tall, with models shorter than these minimums taught to understand that their "chances of success are very limited in comparison to taller models" (Models 2015). Indeed, to be at the top of the profession and do the most internationally sought-after fashion runway shows, agents report that the true minimum height for women is five foot nine inches tall, and for men, five foot eleven inches (Effron 2011).

These guidelines for height are then also reflected in national and international beauty pageants. In Venezuela, widely regarded as the leader in the arena of beauty contests, the minimum height for participation in the national pageant is five foot nine inches, and young women fearful of not achieving that height at times resort to the use of human growth hormone (Roper 2014). In the 2014 Miss Universe competition, where the contestants' height is reported alongside their age and country of origin, the average height of the contestants was five foot eight inches, with no contestant being shorter than five foot five inches tall. The 2014 winner of the pageant, the Colombian Paulina Vega, was herself five foot nine inches (Miss Universe 2015).

See also: China; Leg Lengthening Surgery; Pageants—International, National, and Local Contests; Venezuela.

Further Reading

Adams, Gerald R. 1980. "Social Psychology of Beauty: Effects of Age, Height and Weight on Self-Reported Personality Traits and Social Behavior." *Journal of Social Psychology* 112, no. 2: 287.

Bogaert, Anthony, and Donald McCreary. 2011. "Masculinity and the Distortion of Self-Reported Height in Men." *Sex Roles* 65, no. 7/8: 548–56.

Effron, Lauren. 2011. "Fashion Models: By the Numbers." September 19. Accessed September 15, 2015. http://abcnews.go.com/blogs/lifestyle/2011/09/fashion-models-by-the-numbers/.

Hua, Wen. 2013. *Buying Beauty: Cosmetic Surgery in China*. Hong Kong: Hong Kong University Press.

Miss Universe. 2015. "Contestants 2014." Accessed September 15, 2015. http://www.missuniverse.com/members/profile/661314/year:2014.

Models. 2015. "Question: What Are the Requirements of Being a Model?" Accessed September 15, 2015. https://models.com/help/005-what_are_requirements.html.

PTI. 2011. "Youthful Looks, Height Define Beauty." Accessed September 15, 2015. http://timesofindia.indiatimes.com/life-style/beauty/Youthful-looks-height-define-beauty/articleshow/6664623.cms.

Roper, Matt. 2014. "Butt Implants Aged 12." *Daily Mail*. December 12. Accessed September 15, 2015. http://www.dailymail.co.uk/news/article-2868260/Butt-implants-aged-12-waists-crushed-painful-straps-weeks-intestines-removed-16-Inside-extreme-Venezuelan-beauty-factories-lengths-pump-Miss-World-winners.html.

Valentova, Jaroslava Varella, Gert Stulp, Vít Třebický, and Jan Havlíček. 2014. "Preferred and Actual Relative Height among Homosexual Male Partners Vary with Preferred Dominance and Sex Role." *Plos ONE* 9, no. 1: 1–9.

Watts, Jonathan. 2004. "China's Cosmetic Surgery Craze. Leg-Lengthening Operations to Fight Height Prejudice Can Leave Patients Crippled." *Lancet (London, England)* 363, no. 9413: 958.

HENNA. *See* Mehendi.

HIGH HEELS

Although high-heeled shoes are nearly synonymous with fashionable modern femininity, the practice of wearing shoes with heels is a centuries-old tradition associated with high status for both men and women. Sixteenth-century ladies in Venice, for example, wore high platform shoes of embroidered cloth attached to wooden pedestals ranging from six to twenty inches in height called "*chopines*" to elevate themselves above earthly triviality (and the soupy terrain of flooded Venice). During the Renaissance, upper-class European men wore wigs and stacked heel shoes, most likely inspired by Persian riding boots, as an integral symbol of male privilege and support for the hierarchy of dynastic monarchies.

The earliest known high heels were worn by the most stylish residents of ancient Greece. Known as the *korthonos*, these lace-up shoes featured a built-up elevated sole along the length of the foot (including the heel, arch, and ball) made from exaggeratedly thick cork soles. Wealthy Etruscan women during this period also wore a type of platform sandal with hinged soles and golden laces. During the Roman Empire, these shoes were worn by actors and courtesans and came to be known as *cothurni*. During the Ottoman Empire, women wore wood stilt-clogs with two heels balanced beneath the heel and the ball of the foot, called *qabâqib*, to balance on the slick floors of the steamy *hammam*, or public **baths**. Elite women wearing these impractical, elevated, slip-on shoes would almost certainly have needed assistance from a servant, maid, or slave to prevent dangerous slipping or falling. Trade routes spread the influence of stylish shoes back and forth from Europe to the so-called "Orient," giving rise to a market for luxurious shoes that marked social status. Although many Europeans wore clog overshoes to protect their feet in nasty weather, during the 14th and 15th centuries, the *chopine*, a slip-on, mule-style shoe with an elevated heel and embellished with velvet or embroidery, became popular in Italy. Despite not being visible beneath a long gown, *chopines* were made specifically for women to elongate their silhouette and were designed to be worn in public. In the Far East, Ottoman influences inspired the "Manchu *chopine*," a clunky, oversized shoe with an elevated sole that compelled the wearer to take dainty, mincing, feminine steps and was seen by some as an alternative to the practice of **footbinding.** Later, this dual-pedestaled style of shoe appeared again as a thong variation in Japan as a *geta*, worn by the **geisha** to embody women's fragile, delicate grace.

In the 15th century, the *chopine* shoes that had become so fashionable for women in Europe came under fire of the Venetian Major Council, who fined women for wearing shoes that were "excessively high" in accordance with a new set of sumptuary laws designed to reinforce modesty and respectability among the wealthy citizens of Europe. During this period, elevated shoes became associated with prostitutes and vice, though they continued to be worn into the 17th century.

Historically, men also appreciated the way that heels augmented their stature. In the 16th century, the "high heel" was adopted across Europe from Persia as a part of equestrian military wear, initially designed to keep the foot securely in the stirrup while riding. In the 1590s, new construction techniques allowed stacked leather heels to become possible with a flat sole at the front of the shoe, allowing the wearer more stability than the elevated sole styles of the *chopine*. New materials were also used for creating innovative styles of shoes: Persian "shagreen" became wildly popular as a durable material for boots and was in great demand as a luxury export. Shagreen was made using horse hide, dyed a green color and featuring mustard seeds that were embedded into the wet leather that left a rough, patchy appearance that reduced the look of wear. (Today, shagreen is made from the skin of sharks or rays.) The "breasted heel" was a technique in which the leather of the sole followed the curve of the heel to become the front-facing surface, thus enhancing and supporting the natural arch of the wearer. Later, metal was added to shoes in the heel and also in the form of eye-catching buckles. When King Louis XIV of France (1643–1715) held court at Versailles, he elevated the status of fancy shoes to a type of political tool. In the early 1670s, he declared that only aristocrats wearing red heels would have access to his court (Semmelhack 2008).

Men's heels were typically squared at the toe and more sturdy than women's shoes. High-heeled shoes for women were higher and more tapered to the toe, providing less support, and designed primarily to be noticed as they peeked out from under the edge of a long skirt. As men's fashions gradually became more subdued and men abandoned high heels as daily dress by the 1730s, women's clothing styles continued to incorporate lavish and extravagant details, confining women's movements at the same time that public sentiment agreed that women were inherently deficient in reason, unfit for education, citizenship, and control of property (Semmelhack 2008). Elite women were encouraged to look good and to enhance the reputation of the men in their lives.

Gradually, heel heights decreased to make way for the so-called "cult of domesticity" in the United States and Britain, which directed women to concentrate on sentimental emotions of homemaking and motherhood, less concerned with matters of physical adornment. High heels went out of fashion in favor of practical, side-lacing ankle boots, which preserved modesty by covering the ankle and the lower part of the leg. In the 19th century, a revival of the high heel accompanied new ideas about industrialization and the commodification of fashionable display across Europe. High heels, especially those that could be easily slipped on and off, came to be associated with prostitution and the new technology of photographic pornography (Semmelhack 2008). Women who adopted the newer high-heeled styles were often considered at high risk for moral corruption and the inevitable doom of women's independence and agency. The eroticization of the high heel in the contemporary era can be traced directly to this period and the explosion of imagery that featured women mostly undressed except for very high-heeled shoes. High heels also came to be associated with fetish objects, which charge routine, everyday activities with a subtext of sexuality. Images of "pin-up" women wearing little more than swimsuits and heels heightens the voyeuristic appeal of pornography, suggesting both demure femininity and frank lasciviousness (Semmelhack 2008).

Undeniably cramped, impractical, and uncomfortable, high heels made a resurgence in 1947 to complement Christian Dior's "New Look," which demanded an hourglass figure. Heels are designed to artificially transform the physical posture of the wearer to appear both precarious and imperious by extending the length of the leg and transferring the center of gravity to accommodate an exaggerated posture with breasts pushed forward and derriere arched to the back (Vartanian 2011). High heels continue to be endured by women around the world for the alluring ways that they make the foot appear more delicate and accentuate the sensual curve of the foot's arch. The stiletto ("little knife" in Italian) was invented by Roger Vivier, Dior's shoemaker, thanks to postwar industrial innovations that allowed shoes to be manufactured with a strong metal rod to support needle-thin heels. The newly strong heel supported women's weight and allowed women of the era to rebalance their posture in ways that emphasized the breasts and the buttocks. Heel sizes flattened out again for women in the free-wheeling 1960s era, but "the peacock revolution" opened up new possibilities for men to wear more colorful clothing and jewelry, as well as a return to men's high heel shoe styles. In the urban United States, African American men wore high heel styles, and in the UK, garish platform shoes became fashion standards for glam rock stars like Elton John and David Bowie, who used spectacle to project a unique take on gendered identity and fame. Higher heels crept back into women's fashions, too, in the "power dressing" of the 1980s era of professional women in the workplace. Women were encouraged to dress as much like men as possible, with the exception of heels. Later, a consumer-oriented wave of "girl power" encouraged women to indulge themselves in luxury items, including finding ways to consume fashion to promote self-actualization. Popular culture sources like HBO's hugely successful *Sex and the City* celebrated the ability of regular women to buy and wear expensive heels from designers like Manolo Blahnik and Jimmy Choo as a way to proclaim their newly found equality.

Some feminist scholars argue that wearing of high heels in contemporary culture carries ambiguous, contradictory, and contested messages. Many professional women view the wearing of high heels in the workplace and in social settings as a way to communicate good taste, elegance, luxury, and power. In this sense, women perform their wealth and status through purchasing expensive high-heeled shoes and by literally "elevating" themselves, making themselves taller and giving them the feeling of self-confidence, authority, and control. Men, however, do not commonly view high heels on women as either natural or transgressive markers of wealth and authority. Rather, for many men, high heels are erotic and seductive tools that communicate power, but the specific erotic power of seduction. In this way, for many men, high heels on women, especially in the workplace, are sometimes interpreted as tools designed to distract men through sex appeal (Wobovnik 2013).

See also: Bathing and Showering; Fetish; Footbinding; Geisha.

Further Reading

Semmelhack, Linda. 2008. *Heights of Fashion: A History of the Elevated Shoe.* Toronto: Periscope Press.

Small, Lisa, editor. 2014. *Killer Heels: The Art of the High-Heeled Shoe.* Brooklyn, NY: Brooklyn Museum Press.

Tonchi, Stefano. 2014. "This Is Not a Shoe." In: *Killer Heels: The Art of the High-Heeled Shoe*, edited by Lisa Small. Brooklyn, NY: Brooklyn Museum Press.

Vartanian, Ivan. 2011. *High Heels: Fashion, Femininity, and Seduction.* London: Thames & Hudson.

Weber, Caroline. 2014. "The Eternal High Heel: Eroticism and Empowerment." *Killer Heels: The Art of the High-Heeled Shoe,* edited by Lisa Small. Brooklyn, NY: Brooklyn Museum Press.

Wobovnik, Claudia. 2013. "These Shoes Aren't Made for Walking: Rethinking High-Heeled Shoes as Cultural Artifacts." *Visual Culture & Gender* 8, 82–92.

HIJAB

"*Hijab*" refers both to the convention of modesty in Islamic cultures, especially covering the **hair** but leaving the face uncovered, and the garment used to do so, sometimes referred to as "the veil." The *hijab* is a headscarf that covers a woman's head, hair, neck, and ears, but leaves her face uncovered.

Two distinct discourses are present in conceptions of female beauty in the Islamic world today, correlating with the "modern," Westernized, or globalized world and the "traditional" notions about the intensely held values of the Islamic world. Many also comment that this binary distinction is overly simplified: that there are a great many variations in style and taste between these two seemingly incompatible positions about women's physical appearance in public space.

In Arabia, standards of beauty illustrate the great differences experienced by Islam in its expansion and contact with other cultural traditions in the Middle East (Sonbol 1994, 57). The earliest societies of pre-Islamic Arabia were organized along a social structure known as tribalism, where men joined with their other male relatives to organize raiding parties and to be well organized defensively. Ideal characteristics celebrated for the men of the tribal society included loyalty, agility, endurance, courage, chivalry, generosity, physical strength, and strong character. Women's physical beauty is not described by any specific physical attributes within the Koran, the holy book of Islam. Rather, ideals of womanhood are seen as part of an overall allure, according to moral, religious, social, and spiritual standards. Women are compared to the full moon, a symbol that represents beauty, purity, and brightness. The poetry of the seventh century recalls the sensuous poetry of pre-Islamic Arabia, describing the sweetness of a woman's breath and her "sultry" walk (Sonbol 1994). In the tenth century, poets catalogued descriptions of various parts of a woman in order of importance: hair, temple, cheeks, brows, eyes, nose, teeth, scent, saliva, conversation ability, voice, complexion, face, skin color, physique, neck, neck ornaments, breasts, hips, thighs (which should be full and firm), and clothing. Beauty was also measured according to elegance of manners, symmetry, proportionality of build, and general roundness of the body. The poets also enjoyed the opportunity to comment on the contrast of a woman's appearance: they note a dark beauty spot

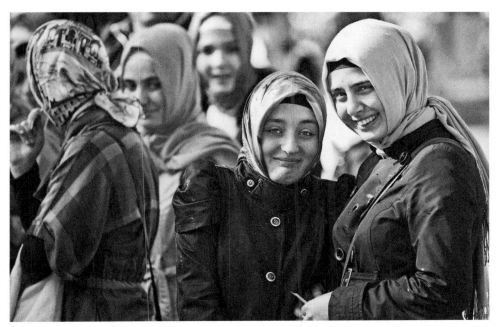

Muslim women wearing *hijab* in Istanbul, Turkey. The practice of wearing *hijab* has become increasingly controversial in the era of globalization. (Scott Griessel/Dreamstime.com)

in a fair face, a fair face framed by long dark hair, the contrast between dark eyes with the white of the eyes, and the use of dark black kohl next to pinkened cheeks. Eyes in particular are described by poets in great detail. They should be lively, large, and "liquid, with a long, dark, curved, precise eyebrow." The eyes themselves should show the promise of coyness, but also be accomplished in appearing to be aloof.

A pointed emphasis on the facial beauty of a woman in a region that covers much of the body for modesty purposes is no accident. The movement and timing of a woman's walk was considered important for revealing femininity and sexuality. The manner of walking invokes a number of metaphors about the gliding movement of clouds and the swaying motion of graceful horses.

Male physical desires are poetically expressed though idioms of "hotness" and sexual pleasure, once tolerated more openly in pre-Islamic times, but now frequently downplayed and admonished in the Koran. For Islamic faith, but also importantly for Islamic culture, the integration of marriage, love, and sex into one legally recognized relationship remains central to establishing one's identity relative to others. Despite expectations that women wearing *hijab* are more servile than their "modernized" counterparts, women wearing Islamic garb are as insistent on husband loyalty, fidelity, and monogamy as are women who do not choose to veil (Sonbol 1994, 63).

In her autobiographical study of veiling, Egyptian television personality Kariman Hamza wrote candidly in Arabic about her decision to veil as the result of a personal exploration about a rejection of the imposed standards of "modernity" and revisiting her own self-worth and the "liberation" to return to a set of neotraditional ideals about purity and respectability (Sonbol 1994). The return to the veil today can be viewed as a self-creation for women in a new image that is being informed and structured by the experiences of women themselves (Zuhur 1992). College students and graduates opt to wear Islamic garb even if they come from a social class that was at one time seemingly "becoming Westernized." For many women, adopting *hijab* must be seen as a form of empowerment.

In the contemporary United States, over one-third of the estimated 700,000 Muslim women living in the country report wearing a headcover or observing *hijab* in public (Williams and Vashi 2014). For each woman, there is a personal or familial process by which she negotiates two competing cultural discourses about the veil: a liberal discourse that emphasizes individual choice, liberty, and equality and a second discourse that critiques materialism, individualism, and rapid social change.

See also: Burqa; Hair.

Further Reading

Sonbol, Amira. 1994. "Changing Perceptions of Feminine Beauty in Islamic Society." In: *Ideals of Feminine Beauty*, edited by Karen A. Callaghan, 53–65. Westport, CT: Greenwood Press.

Williams, Rhys H., and Gira Vashi. 2014. "*Hijab* and American Muslim Women." In: *The Politics of Women's Bodies: Sexuality, Appearance, and Behavior*, 4th ed., edited by Rose Weitz and Samantha Kwan, 331–45. New York: Oxford University Press.

Zuhur, Sherifa. 1992. *Revealing Reveiling*. Albany, NY: State University Press of New York.

HIMBA OF NAMIBIA (HERERO, OVAHIMBA)

The Himba are an indigenous people of northwest Namibia. Pastoralists, the Himba live in an arid border region called Kaokoland, still deeply affected by the memories of apartheid under the South African occupation from 1918–1990, a civil war between 1666 and 1988, and international conflict that began in the mid-1970s and continued until 2002 (van Wolputte 2004). In recent years, the Himba, especially Himba women, have become a focus of the international media gaze. Visual images of Himba women, often represented as "savage beauties," have become icons of a romanticized and estheticized Africa within the global discourse (Bollig and Heinemann 2002).

Most Himba practice herding as a way of life, and as such, their culturally experienced notions of "the self" do not refer to a psychological or biological identity in the same way as a Euro-American person might consider their "self." Instead, Himba learn from childhood to consider their "self" as an identity that also references "outer" fields of meaning that are constitutive of their material world, the animals they live with, and the social and kin-based relationships they have with other people. The individual sense of fragmentation of the body-self can be partly or temporarily overcome during rituals and other emotionally charged events, such as giving birth or at a death bed.

Images of the Himba presented as an archaic people, body conscious, beautifully adorned, erotically appealing, and peaceful drive a curiosity for their traditional lifestyle. The skin of Himba women is often quite striking, treated with a preparation of a distinctive skin emollient, a paste called *otijize* from butterfat and red ochre mixed with an aromatic resin from the omazumba shrub (*Commiphora multijuga*). The paste is then rubbed into the skin of women and children, applied to untreated goatskin clothing, and spread through elaborately braided hairstyles (Cole 2013). In addition to providing a shiny, deep, rusty-red color to the skin, the emollient offers protection from the skin and insects. They famously use resins and barks to scent the smoke of the fire, which they use to "bathe" themselves in aroma.

Himba women traditionally wore cloth around their waist and hips, but their **breasts** were exposed in daily life. They also wore **jewelry** made of beads, shells, and copper pieces. Their hair was dressed in elaborate braided styles, which are then coated heavily with a mixture of ashes, clay, ochre, and animal hair. Girls begin to wear the traditional heavily coated hairstyle at the time of menarche. The skin of Himba women shines with a distinctive red color paste that signified the age and marital status of the wearer. On her wedding day, a bride is given a small headdress to wear. Known as *ekori*, these small leather pieces are handed down through generations. After the first month of marriage, married women trade in the *ekori* for a larger leather headdress, known as *erembe*, to add to the top of her distinctive plaited and pasted hairstyle. Women also highly prize fine white shells that have been traded from the coast: these treasures are part of a woman's wealth and estimated to be valued at about the same cost as a young goat or sheep. Women wear these white shells between their breasts as a symbol of fertility and beauty.

Garments and finery are important markers of individual and group identity. Aprons, bracelets, scarfs, flags, and uniforms can embody belonging, and they legitimize the individual who wears them as part of a larger social and moral community (Van Wolputte 2004, 258). Herero women were converted to Christianity by European settlers and taught to sew by German settlers. They made Victorian-style dresses out of local cloth and goat leather in order to work as domestics in the homes of the European women (Cole 2013).

As mentioned earlier, the main metaphors that govern Himba lives typically refer to the traditional culture, including the dominant ideologies regarding human relationships that govern authority, power, gender, seniority, and the ideal notion of the "self." For example, the meaning of a person's body and the ways in which it might be decorated or displayed are always associated with lineage membership, relative age, and gender (van Wolputte 2004, 254). The meanings of the objects in one's life are not just representational; they are also embodied. Ancestors are remembered by the particular diet of each lineage. There are taboos on speaking the given names of one's father, and later, one's husband. Garments, hairstyles, and finery are particular items that may be worn or displayed according to the lineage identity. In other words, the range of beauty practices open to an individual depend heavily on who that person is, who she is descended from, and how she is related to others.

Today, tourism factors heavily into the way that the Himba make a living. Like other marginalized African groups, they "perform" cultural authenticity for tourists in order to preserve their autonomy, prompting some critics to comment on the Disneyfication of the Himba image (Bollig and Heinemann 2002, 299). During the rapid economic growth of Namibia during the 1990s, tourism became the nation's fastest-growing sector, and Himba settlements were strategically positioned as prime sites for cultural tourism. The Himba became "the predominant cultural branding tool" of Namibia as a tourist destination (Cole 2013, 155). Himba display **mannequins** are used at the international airport to welcome tourists alongside other displays of the neighboring San shown foraging and the neighboring Okavango shown fishing (Bollig and Heinemann 2002).

In part because of the ways that the media represents a continually bare-**breasted**, **exoticized** version of their lives, the Himba are widely recognizable as the "**other.**" The South African branch of the British-based Land Rover automobile company drew criticism in 2000 when they worked with an advertising company and digital special effects crew to create a campaign where a Land Rover speeding through the desert actually caused the breasts of a Himba woman to sway and extend in the direction of the rapidly moving vehicle (Boskovic 2001). Land Rover apologized and agreed to pay for advertisements that retracted and replaced the previous message meant to be funny at the expense of a non-Western standard of aesthetics.

See also: Breasts; Exoticize; Jewelry; Mannequin; The "Other."

Further Reading

Bollig, Michael, and Heike Heinemann. 2002. "Nomadic Savages, Ochre People and Heroic Herders: Visual Presentation of the Himba of Namibia's Kaokoland." *Visual Anthropology* 15: 267–312.

Boskovic, Aleksander. 2001. "Out of Africa: Images of Women in Anthropology and Popular Culture." *Etnolog* 11: 177–83.

Cole, Jill. 2013. "Himba in the Mix: The 'Catwalk' Politics of Culture in Namibia. *Women's Studies Quarterly* 41, no. 1 & 2: 150–61.

Van Wolputte, Steven. 1998. *Of Bones and Flesh and Milk. Moving Bodies and Self among the Ovahimba.* Leiden, Netherlands: Katholieke Universiteit Leiden.

Van Wolputte, Steven. 2004. "Hang on to Your Self: Of Bodies, Embodiment and Selves. *Annual Review of Anthropology* 33: 251–69.

HOURGLASS SHAPE

During the 18th century, European women of means wore **corsets** designed to cinch the waist to create an hourglass shape. Waists were routinely reduced during that era to measure 18 or 19 inches around and to create a "handspan" back. Originally constructed of whalebone, corsets also featured tight lacing to minimize the waist, sometimes to such small diameters that they created damage to the inner organs of the wearer. Later, the Spirella corset of the 1900s was made of rust-free spiral steel stays, which was the same wire used in high-grade pianos, and created a very architectural hourglass for the wearer.

According to somewhat controversial theories advanced by the biologically based "mate selection theory," males are more attracted to a female body with a particular ratio of waist to hip fat distribution. This measure is often abbreviated as WHR (waist-to-hip ratio). Sociobiologists argue that fat distribution in women's bodies is a strong indicator of health and fertility, indicating to the male that the female has an idealized hormone profile, greater success for potential pregnancy, and less risk for major diseases. Before puberty, males and females have similar WHRs. However, the WHR in women decreases during adolescence and begins to increase again during menopause, suggesting that women's reproductive capacity can be measured with a degree of certainty by looking at the ratio of the waist to the hips. Whereas evolutionary theory underscores the importance of mate selection in reproductive success (Singh 1993), many anthropologists are uncomfortable with extending purely biological impulses to the complex set of factors that create attraction and the formation of families in human cultures. Beauty and sexual desire are complicated social phenomena that take into account many factors which vary widely by time and place. Critics argue that it's easy to take any feature of "modern" life—such as the **Barbie**-style hourglass figure—and argue that it was genetically predisposed. The search for a single biology of beauty may mask a political agenda that reveals more about the fantasy desires of the group in power than it does about the reality of our DNA (Newsweek 1996).

> "People often say that 'beauty is in the eye of the beholder,' and I say that the most liberating thing about beauty is realizing that you are the beholder. This empowers us to find beauty in places where others have not dared to look, including inside ourselves."
>
> —Salma Hayek

A study conducted by Singh et al. (2010) compared female attractiveness with sample groups composed of both men and women participants from Cameroon (Africa), Komodo Island (Indonesia), Samoa, and New Zealand. The researchers showed line drawing outlines of twelve silhouettes with a range of WHRs and asked participants to pick the most attractive woman. Their findings suggested that the most attractive female profile cross-culturally was the normal-**weight** woman with a 0.7 ratio of waist to hips. (This means that the measurement of the waist at its smallest part is about 70 percent of the measurement of the hips at its widest part, taking into account measurement of the buttocks.) These findings reproduce the findings of other studies conducted in Germany, the United Kingdom, and the United States, where ideal WHR is judged to be 0.67 to 0.80, which suggests that a low WHR is the most attractive body shape. Other studies conducted in Indonesia, the Azore Islands, Guinea Bissau, China, and the Shiwiar tribe of Ecuador suggested that men in these groups prefer women with a higher waist-to-hip ratio, which would mean that in those cultures, women are expected to be "thicker." In Uganda, a study showed that the most attractive women were those who weighed the most, but also had the lowest WHR (Furnham, Moutafi, and Baguma 2002). Yu and Shepard (1998) also demonstrated that among the Matsigenka Indians, an indigenous group living in an isolated part of Peru, men preferred heavier women with high WHR ratios and considered them to be more fertile, suggesting that male preference for particular kinds of women's bodies is not necessarily cultural universally, but rather, varies by culture.

In seeking the ideal hourglass shape, celebrities like Kim Kardashian, Chrissy Teigan, and Amber Rose promote the use of waist trainers made of tight spandex which can be worn during exercise and also clothing to emphasize a tiny waist. Despite the high number of users sharing their best waist trainer photos on social media, some users report nausea or shortness of breath when wearing waist trainers for too long.

See also: Barbie; Corsets, Shapewear, and Weight Trainers; Weight.

Further Reading

Furnham, A., J. Moutafi, and B. Baguma. 2002. "A Cross-Cultural Study of the Role of Weight and Waist-to-Hip Ratio on Female Attractiveness." *Personality and Individual Differences* 32: 729–45.

Newsweek. 1996. "Biology of Beauty." Accessed October 24, 2016. http://www.newsweek.com/biology-beauty-178836.

Singh, Devendra. 1993. "Adaptive Significance of Female Attractiveness: Role of Waist-to-Hip Ratio." *Journal of Personality and Social Psychology* 65, no. 2: 293–307.

Singh, Devendra, B. J. Dixson, T. S. Jessop, B. Morgan, and A. F. Dixon. 2010. "Cross-Cultural Consensus for Waist-Hip Ratio and Women's Attractiveness." *Evolution and Human Behavior* 31: 176–81.

Yu, Douglas W., and Glenn H. Shepard, Jr. 1998. "Is Beauty in the Eye of the Beholder?" *Nature* 396: 321–22.

INDIA

India is a vast country with an ancient history and enormous cultural diversity. The beauty work and beauty practices in India serve to identify and celebrate the distinctiveness of different tribes and regions within the modern nation, while also allowing Indians to creatively explore the intersections of different tribal and local identities. In modern India, beauty practices are one way in which Indians negotiate those multiple identities.

Several ethnic and tribal minorities, as well as regional groups, differ significantly from each other and practice their own distinctly striking forms of beauty. The women of the **Apatani tribe** of northeastern India, for example, employ both wooden nose plugs and elaborate facial tattoos as part of their traditional beauty work. People in the Indian state of Chhattisgarh, however, are known for their use and production of a particular type of silk, kosa silk, for the production of traditional clothing, known as sari (or saree), a type of women's clothing that consists of a long length of silk wrapped around the body (Kalaiyarasi 2014).

Regional and ethnic practices dictate a diversity of beauty work in India. Ancient India practiced Hinduism. Directions for making cosmetics appear in the *Kama Sutra*. Another widely retold story is the *Ramayana*, which recounts the tragic love story of Sita and the Hindu god Ram. Sita becomes obsessed with possessing the alluring *maya mrg* (magical animal), a golden-skinned, silver-speckled deer. Ram, who is himself enchanted by the beauty of Sita, sets off to capture the beautiful animal for his beloved and becomes separated from Sita, exposing her to danger. Scholars have interpreted this text as a powerful metaphor for the ways in which the power of beauty can seduce serious people into becoming vulnerable to an impermanent, sensual world (Zacharias 1994). Beauty has the power to bewitch and to destabilize; nevertheless, it is sought and prized.

Thick, shiny hair was highly prized by Indian women during ancient times and remains a desirable feature today. Historically, Indian women applied coconut oil to their hair and rubbed it into their scalps to achieve a smooth, glossy appearance. Many women still swear by the nourishing effects of coconut oil on the hair. Body hair is frequently removed, especially through an age-old process known as threading, which requires some practice to pull off and uses a long, cotton string to "pinch" unwanted hairs out by the root.

Throughout India, elaborate and dramatic beauty work has traditionally been a significant part of the marriage ceremony for both men and women. Wedding ceremonies are frequently held according to the economic status of the families involved in the union, and little expense is spared, particularly in the preparations of the bride.

Marriages were a time for Indian women to enhance their physical beauty with all means available to them in order to bring honor upon their families of origin. Ancient texts indicate that the morning of the wedding, a bride was to be massaged thoroughly with scented oils. Brides were expected to wear sixteen prescribed pieces of jewelry on the day of her wedding. Her ability to do so in style reflected the status of her family and represented her own personal wealth going into her marriage, known as dowry. Additionally, marital status reflected an important identifier to society. All respectable adult women were expected to marry and have families.

Not all beauty practices in India, however, are limited to use by women. Perfume, for example, has also been traditionally essential to the well-appointed ancient Indian woman and man. Perfumes were part of a global trade network, but many of the best perfumed ointments were locally sourced in India from the profusion of flowers, resins, and woods available. Lemon blossoms, orange blossoms, gardenias, and honeysuckle are used to fragrance the home and are tucked into clothing for additional scent. Sandalwood, in particular, is used by both men and women to this day.

Jewelry is also important. Traditionally, earrings have been worn by both men and women. Married women frequently pierced their noses to wear flat studs or rings (called *nath*), occasionally connected with a gold chain to the ear, especially as part of a bridal costume. Today, many women choose to pierce their noses to enhance their beauty with gems, rings, or semiprecious stones. A *maangtika* is a kind of jewelry that is worn by a woman over the middle part of the hair and rests against the forehead to draw attention to the face. A significant facial marker worn exclusively on the forehead is known as the **bindi**. Today, bindis can be made of stickers or small bits of plastic, but historically, the bindi was applied with red powder to indicate a woman was married. Widowed women either abstained from bindis or wore dark black bindis. Young unmarried women wore bindis in a variety of colors.

A more controversial form of beauty work that is practiced by both men and women in India is the use of skin-lightening creams and treatments. Light skin is, in general, highly prized in India as a signal of high class status, beauty, success, choice, and empowerment (Nadeem 2014). Although the exact origins of colorism, or a prejudice for light skin, are unknown, many scholars suggest that the preference is the product of a combination of both the ancient Hindu class system of caste that existed before the arrival of British colonizers and the reinforcement of that system by the British colonial rulers in the 20th century (Jah 2016). Whatever the origins of the preference for lighter skin, the reality of the 21st century is a modern-day India that prizes light skin as a beauty ideal. The national Miss India beauty pageant, for example, presents a national standard of feminine Indian beauty that is fair, slim, youthful, and light skinned (Jah 2016).

Because of the idealized nature of lighter skin, one trend in 21st-century India is toward the use of skin-bleaching or skin-lightening creams. The market for such skin treatments in India by 2007 had grown to a $200 million a year business, with both men and women purchasing and using the products in the pursuit of lighter skin (Nadeem 2014). Indeed, skin-lightening products specifically targeted at the "delicate" skin of women and the "rough and tough" skin of men, target both genders equally (Nadeem 2014, 227). In the case of both men and women, the message is that lighter skin is necessary to find and marry a desirable partner, succeed in business, and achieve personal and professional success. Although some worry at the toxic levels of chemicals found in the lightening creams, and others object to the repeated message that those with darker skin are worth less, skin-lightening continues to be a widespread, and widely accepted, beauty practice in India (Jah 2016).

Bollywood Style

The Indian city of Mumbai has a film industry popularly called "Bollywood." The multibillion-dollar industry is one of the largest producers of films in the world and is responsible for creating a genre of beautifully set and costumed movies along with a series of world-famous actors and actresses loved for their beauty and style. Although Bollywood has produced documentaries and serious historical films, it is most famous worldwide for romantic musicals that feature beautiful people in elaborate, color-drenched song and dance numbers. The music of a Bollywood film is as important as the jewelry and clothing, and the actors and actresses often transition into music careers. Bollywood is a major driver of fashion in India, and Bollywood style has influenced the look of films and designs in Europe, North America, and Asia.

India is well known today in the West as the origin of yoga, which in recent years has become highly prized for assisting to sculpt a lean, fit body that corresponds to Western standards of beauty for men and women. The principles of Ayurvedic medicine relate well with the basic yogic principles and have been practiced for centuries. The principles advise that beauty is much more than skin deep, but reflects the inner health and well-being of a person. All wellness and beauty are managed through the balance of five elements: air, earth, water, fire, and ether (Sachs 2002). This view sees the appearance of people, their health, and the universe as connected. In the Ayurvedic worldview, human bodies are divided into three distinct categories, or *dosha*. Each of these *dosha* types has distinct health concerns, as well as a distinctive "look." Those who have a *Vata* (wind) characteristic tend to be thin, light, enthusiastic, energetic, and open to change. When there is too much change or movement, however, the Vata person tends to experience anxiety, insomnia, dry skin, and constipation. The *Pitta* (fire) nature creates individuals who are intense, intelligent, and goal oriented; however, when out of balance, these people tend to be irritable and compulsive, and may suffer from indigestion or inflammation of the skin. Those who display *Kapha* tendencies are recognizable for their easy-going, methodical, and nurturing personalities. However, when stressed, the sweet and stable Kapha may experience sluggishness, weight gain, and sinus infections. Each body type requires a unique set of behavioral practices that can assist in achieving and maintaining wellness.

See also: Apatani Tribe, India; Class; Hair Removal; Skin Tone; Skin Whitening.

Further Reading

Guha, Sumit. 2013. *Beyond Caste: Identity and Power in South Asia, Past and Present.* Brill's Leiden, Netherlands: Brill Publishing.

India.gov. 2015. "People and Lifestyle." Accessed November 5, 2015. http://www.archive .india.gov.in/knowindia/culture_heritage.php?id=70.

Jah, Meeta Rani. 2016. *The Global Beauty Industry: Colorism, Racism and the National Body.* New York: Routledge.

Kalaiyarasi, S. 2014. "An Empirical Study of the Preferences and Buying Behavior of Silk: Sarees Among Women Consumers in Vellore Town." *International Journal of Business and Administration Research Review* 1, no. 5: 12–20.

Mohapatra, Ramesh Prasad. 1992. *Fashion Styles of Ancient India.* Delhi, India: BR Publishing.

Nadeem, Shehzad. 2014. "Fair and Anxious: On Mimicry and Skin Lightening in India." *Social Identities* 20, no. 2-3: 224–38.

Sachs, Melanie. 2002. *Ayurvedic Beauty Care: Ageless Techniques to Invoke Natural Beauty.* Delhi, India: Motilal Banarsidass Publishers.

Wallace, Doug. 2013. "Girl Talk: Ayurvedic Skin Care." The Gaia Health Blog. Accessed November 24, 2015. http://www.gaiahealthblog.com/2013/02/19/girl-talk-ayurvedic -skin-care-beauty-is-not-skin-deep-it-goes-much-deeper/.

Zacharias, Usha. 1994. "The Sita Myth and Hindu Fundamentalism: Masculine Signs of Feminine Beauty." In: *Ideals of Feminine Beauty: Philosophical, Social, and Cultural Dimensions*, edited by Karen A. Callaghan, 37–52. Westport, CT: Greenwood Press.

INDONESIA

Indonesia is a nation that covers an archipelago of 6,000 different islands. These islands, before the arrival of European colonizers, were not united as a single nation but rather were home to hundreds of different kingdoms, cultures, languages, and religious traditions. It was not until the arrival of the Dutch, followed by the French and the British, that external colonial control molded the diverse island group into one country (Vltchek 2012).

Today, Indonesia is still a nation of many different languages and cultures and a wide diversity of racial and cultural backgrounds. It was not until the late 19th century that the island group gained its independence and began looking for a way to express a unified Indonesian identity. Over time, one factor that emerged as a commonality was religion: Islam became embraced as the common faith. In 1928, a text proposing a single nation under a single religion, language, and government was published, the first step in the diverse island group coming together as a modern country. Indonesia as a free and independent state, however, would not become a reality until the last colonial power, the Japanese, were expelled in 1945 at the end of the second world war (Vltchek 2012).

> "The more people explore the world, the more they realize in every country there's a different aesthetic. Beauty really is in the eye of the beholder."
>
> —HELENA CHRISTENSEN

This particular history means that there continues to be a diversity of cultural practices, alongside some generally shared ideas and notions across Indonesia in the 21st century. The mix of a variety of native Indonesian cultures, along with the influences of the European and Asian colonizers, created a contemporary Indonesian hybrid culture (World Trade 2011). Traditional clothing and style, such as the fabric known as batik, combines with kimonos from the Japanese tradition and European suits.

One of the longest-standing elements of beauty for women in Indonesia is light skin. Classic texts from BCE 300 describe beautiful women as having faces that are "white like moons." Because of the continuing preference for whiter, lighter skin, Indonesia is a major consumer of skin-lightening products and treatments. International cosmetics companies spend millions in advertising the skin treatments, and skin bleaching products are the number-one seller among all cosmetics in the nation (Saraswati and Muse Project 2013). Studies report that more than one-third of Indonesian women use skin lightening creams (Gold Coast 2004).

The integration of the Islamic faith into the governmental structure means that clothing, especially for women in Indonesia, is typically very modest. Since the 1980s, when modest dress started to become more common in public and in the workplace, women typically cover their legs and arms at all times with long dresses or skirts with long-sleeved blouses. Wearing headscarves or *hijab* is also a widespread practice, and in some areas, headscarves are compulsory for Muslim women (World Press 2011).

It is important to note that the modest clothing for women in Indonesia still follows fashion trends. In this, it is another indication of the diversity of cultural practice, combining the traditional symbolic system of veiling with ever-changing and globally influenced style. This specific practice is sometimes called "fashion-veiling" (Bucar 2016).

The practice of wearing modest clothing, which began in Indonesia in the 1980s as a political and religious response to the corruption of the dictator Suhartho's government, underwent drastic changes in the 1990s. The modest fashions, which were originally solid, pastel-colored, loose fitting gowns and veils (called *jiljab*) in the late 1990s changed to become more elaborate and vibrantly colored (Bucar 2016).

Twenty-first-century *jiljab* in Indonesia gives a wide range of modest, yet stylish, choices. Women can choose from long, flowing skirts or tunics that are worn over leggings. The long-sleeved tunic can also be worn over jeans, and a recent style trend is the wearing of tightly fitted long-sleeved shirts and leggings under a spaghetti-strap dress. All of these clothing choices come in tie-dye, flowered print, and sequined versions (Bucar 2016).

The headscarf is also a way in which women express both adherence to religious ideas of modesty and fashion. The scarf may be worn over an elaborately beaded skullcap, and is often layered with other scarves in contrasting colors. Headscarves may be beaded or embellished with silk flowers, and are often tied in elaborate, decorative knots (Bucar 2016).

Due to the increased popularity of modest dress in Indonesia, the world's most populous Islamic nation, the Islamic fashion industry is booming. According to data from the Indonesian Ministry of Industry, the Islamic fashion industry in Indonesia generates one hundred million dollars a year and is only expected to increase over time (AP 2011).

See also: Makeup and Cosmetics; Skin tone; Skin whitening.

Further Reading

AP. 2011. *Islamic Fashion Boom in Indonesia*. Associated Press Video Collection. Accessed August 1, 2016. https://www.youtube.com/watch?v=IlxvU7NeIc8

Bucar, Elizabeth M. 2016. "Secular Fashion, Religious Dress, and Modest Ambiguity: The Visual Ethics of Indonesian Fashion-Veiling." *Journal of Religious Ethics* 44, no. 1: 68–91.

Gold Coast Bulletin, The . 2004. "Asians Embracing Lightening Lotions." March 27: *Newspaper Source*. Accessed August 2, 2016.

Saraswati, L. Ayu, and Muse Project. 2013. *Seeing Beauty, Sensing Race in Transnational Indonesia*. Honolulu: University of Hawaii Press.

Tedjasukmana, Jason. 2007. *Time International (South Pacific Edition)*, October 1, no. 38: 21.

Vltchek, Andre. 2012. *Indonesia: Archipelago of Fear*. London: Pluto Press.

World Trade Press. 2011. *Indonesia: Society & Culture*. Petaluma, CA: World Trade Press.

INJECTIONS

The American Society of Plastic Surgeons defines "cosmetic" plastic surgery as "surgical and nonsurgical procedures that reshape normal structures of the body in order to improve appearance and self-esteem" (ASPS 2015). When the society refers to "nonsurgical procedures," one of the techniques to which they refer is the injections of substances into the body. Worldwide, both certified plastic surgeons and unlicensed practitioners inject botulism toxin, collagen, estrogen, fat, silicone, and other liquids into patients' faces, muscles, breasts, and buttocks in order to effect a change in appearance.

Historically, some of the first cosmetic surgery procedures involved injectable substances. In the first decade of the 20th century, paraffin was injected into women's breasts both in the United States and Europe in order to increase breast size. German physicians later experimented with the injection of Vaseline, either alone or mixed with olive oil, wax, or glycerin, into women's breasts (Haiken 1999). By the mid-1900s, liquid silicone had gained popularity as a way to increase the size of breasts and shape other parts of the female body, a practice that was particularly popular in Asian nations such as Vietnam (Haiken 1999).

The injection of these substances has not been limited solely to women, however. Researchers find that men seeking to "bulk up" or augment their muscles and their general body image have regularly injected anabolic steroids, plant oils, silicon, Vaseline, and paraffin into their muscles (Abdul Gaffar 2014). Anabolic steroids in particular, used in World War II by Hitler to increase the bulk of his soldiers, then gained widespread use and popularity in the 1950s in the United States as body builders and athletes began using testosterone and other androgens to increase muscle mass and improve appearance (Walker 2008).

These earlier experiments in the injections of liquids, however, have often led to disastrous results. The direct injection of liquid substances into male and female bodies can lead to a host of negative consequences, including the development of cysts, abscesses, and tumors (Abdul Gaffar 2014). In other cases, the injection of liquid silicone as a filler has been directly linked to kidney failure and death, and the injection of anabolic steroids to kidney and liver failure, heart failure, and psychological disorders (Branton, Bivens, and Terrado et al. 2008, NIH 2012).

Although most of the injections listed here have been discredited and warned against by medical professionals, patients in the 21st century still continue to seek unlicensed practitioners for the injection of silicone and often resort to self-injection for substances such as anabolic steroids. In the male bodybuilding community, for example, researchers were forced to conclude that "the practice of unsupervised injection is probably common in the sports community" with as many as 15 percent of high school and college athletes in the United States self-injecting steroids in their lifetime (Abdul Gaffar 2014, 1; Lyman 2009, 15).

Illicit injections continue to be applied to men and women; however, in the 21st century, licensed medical practitioners also carry on providing a range of injectable beauty treatments, including botulism injections (commonly known as "Botox") and collagen and fat transfer (from a patient's own body). These substances and a variety of other permanent and nonpermanent substances are collectively known as "fillers" (ISAPS 2015a). These procedures and injections are most commonly used on the face to smooth and fill in lines. Injections are also common, however, in areas such as the breasts and buttocks to increase size.

In general, nonpermanent fillers, such as a transfer of fat from one area to another of a patient's own body, is much safer, but the results are not long lasting and can vary, as the patient's body will often reabsorb most, or all, of the transferred fat (ISAPS 2015a). Permanent fillers, however, carry many more potential health consequences, including lumps, infections, and other risks that often require surgery (ISAPS 2015b).

Although many injection procedures are available from properly trained professionals, in the 21st century, international experts from the United Kingdom to South Korea express fear and caution, particularly about the use of fillers (Schlesinger, Smyth, and Magill 2012). The International Society of Aesthetic and Plastic Surgery (ISAPS) cautions potential patients to always "demand fillers that are generally accepted, or FDA approved" and to always be sure to check out the filler that a practitioner will be using. The ISAPS further warns that "[f]or all fillers, risks include irregularities or lumpiness, over- or under-correction, asymmetry and infection. Permanently visible lumps or late reactions with some permanent fillers can result" (ISAPS 2015a). In 2008 the American Society of Plastic Surgeons additionally cautioned patients against seeking permanent fillers, naming the procedure one of the top ten cosmetic procedures to avoid (Childs 2008).

See also: Bodybuilding; Breast Augmentation and Reduction Surgeries; Buttocks Lifts and Implants; Plastic Surgery.

Further Reading

Abdul Gaffar, Badr. 2014. "Illicit Injections in Body builders: A Clinicopathological Study of 11."
ASPS. 2015. "Cosmetic Procedures." Accessed September 8, 2015. http://www.plasticsurgery.org/cosmetic-procedures.html.

Branton, M., A.D. Bivens, L. T. R. Terrado, et al. 2008. "Acute Renal Failure Associated with Cosmetic Soft-Tissue Filler Injections—North Carolina, 2007 (cover story)." *MMWR: Morbidity & Mortality Weekly Report* 57, no. 17: 453–56.

Cases in 9 Patients with a Spectrum of Histological Reaction Patterns." *International Journal of Surgical Pathology* 22, no. 8: 688–94.

Childs, Dan. 2008. "10 Cosmetic Procedures that You Should Avoid." April 7. Accessed November 24, 2015. http://abcnews.go.com/Health/PainManagement/story?id=4585277&page=1.

Haiken, Elizabeth. 1999. *Venus Envy: A History of Cosmetic Surgery*. Baltimore: Johns Hopkins University Press.

ISAPS. 2015a. "Fat Transfer." Accessed September 10, 2015. http://www.isaps.org/procedures/fat-transfer-facial.

ISAPS. 2015b. "Fillers." Accessed September 10, 2015. http://www.isaps.org/procedures/dermal-fillers.

Lyman, Kaitlin J. 2009. *Men and Addictions: New Research*. New York: Nova Science Publishers, Inc.

NIH. 2012. "DrugFacts: Anabolic Steroids." Accessed September 10, 2015. http://www.drugabuse.gov/publications/drugfacts/anabolic-steroids.

Schlesinger, Fay, Chris Smyth, and Sasha, Magill. 2012. "Alert Over Dangers of Cosmetic Injections." *The Times (United Kingdom)* p. 1.

Walker, Ida. 2008. *Steroids: Pumped Up and Dangerous*. Broomall, PA: Mason Crest Publishers.

IRAN

The issue of beauty, especially for women in 21st-century Iran, is problematic. Iran is a conservative Muslim nation with strict legal dress codes for women in public, and women negotiate complex issues of morality, religion, and freedom of expression (Homa 2015). This has not always been true, however. Iran is also an ancient nation, and ideas governing beauty for men and women have changed much over the course of centuries.

Iran, also known as Persia, has a much longer history than most nations and stands as one of the world's oldest civilizations. What is now known as Iran began as a civilization of a people called Pars in the time period of the Ancient Greeks, in BCE 600. The Greeks called the empire of the Pars "Persian" over time, using that name to describe the civilization and its member states (Axworthy 2010). Through the 19th century, much of the world called the area and its states "Persia," whereas the people in those states called themselves "Iran." However, the names can be used to understand the same group of people and their culture.

In the Qajar period of Iran, which ran from the late 1700s to the early 20th century, beauty standards and norms were strikingly similar for men and women. In both literature and art, men and women are described with the same adjectives to express their beauty. During this time, the preference was for black hair, full and rosy lips, crescent-shaped eyebrows, narrow waists, and pale and rosy faces (Najmabadi 2001). These descriptors applied equally to men and women, and at times the difference between the genders in paintings is only noticeable from the depictions of what they wear on their heads, from scarves to hats (Najmabadi 2001).

Through the 19th and early 20th centuries, Iran was governed by a monarch, called the Shah, a secular leader. In the 1930s, Reza Shah followed a plan of modernization and secularization that called for women to receive more education and participate more in the workforce. As part of this plan of modernization, Reza Shah actually banned the wearing of the headscarf and veil in Iran. Reza Shah's desire was for both men and women to dress in the Western fashion and forgo traditional dress (Axworthy 2010). It was not until the Islamic revolution in 1979 that the veil and the dress codes seen today became law.

Since the late 1970s, by law Iranian women must be fully covered in public except for their hands and faces. Women are required to wear a headscarf, or *hijab*, over their hair, and a long overcoat known as a manteaux while in public. To break or bend the dress code is not only to break the law, but also to risk punishment at the hands of vigilantes, who attack women who they believe are in violation. Acid attacks, where acid is thrown in the face of women who these informal police believe are in violation, are not common, but also not unknown and in 2014, the Iranian parliament passed a law protecting assailants who attack women, "enjoining good and forbidding wrong" (Homa 2015).

Despite these laws, Iran is a society that also recognizes a woman's beauty as essential to her personal worth. Women in modern Iran are judged by beauty norms that seek a small and pointed nose, full lips, and an hourglass figure with large breasts and buttocks. It is by these standards that women are deemed marriageable or unmarriageable (Homa 2015). Because the conservative nature of Iranian society expects women to be financially dependent on a husband, the status of a woman as attractive or not to potential husbands is of utmost importance. It is perhaps for this reason that women continue to challenge and flout morality laws and dress codes seeking to appear more beautiful.

Women seeking to skirt the dress codes in search of beautiful appearances experiment with fashion, cosmetics, and plastic surgery. Because the face is one of the only areas visible on a woman in public, plastic surgery, especially for the nose, is widely practiced. The nose is of particular importance in beauty norms in Iran, where citizens will openly make fun of strangers on the street if they believe their nose is too big (Peterson 2000). The nose is a woman's most visible asset, and rhinoplasty to create the ideal nose is increasingly common. In 2014, despite its small size, surgeons in Iran performed the fourth most nose jobs in the world, only behind Brazil, Mexico, and the United States (AFP 2016).

Cosmetics for the face, although technically forbidden, are another way in which women seek the facial appearance that is so essential in the marriage market. The centuries-old preference for ruby or rosy lips can be achieved more readily through lipstick, as can the preference for a pale and delicate face. Under the letter of the dress code, the face is one of only two areas of skin visible for women in public. As a result, a 2010 study found that Iran had become the world's seventh largest consumer of cosmetics, spending 2.6 billion annually (Iranian 2010). Women also use fingernail polish on the hands, another visible body part, as a way of seeking to portray beauty.

This use of cosmetics is one way to work within the dress codes to find a way to adhere to beauty norms. Clothing is another. Although the law requires women to be fully covered except for the face and hands, some women push the boundaries by wearing form-fitting jumpsuits or tight trousers to display their hourglass figures (Homa 2015). Given the 21st-century laws regarding clothing for women, the fashion industry in Iran is both clandestine and illegal. Fashion shows happen in secluded basements and back rooms. Designers push the boundaries of what is acceptable to enforcers, and women choose more expressive colors and styles with the risk of being arrested and attacked (Sewn 2009.

See also: *Hijab*; Makeup and Cosmetics; Nose Jobs.

Further Reading

AFP. 2016. "Iran Leaps into World's Top 10 Countries Performing Plastic Surgery." January 4. Accessed July 29, 2016. http://www.thenational.ae/arts-life/beauty/iran-leaps-into -worlds-top-10-countries-performing-plastic-surgery.
Axworthy, Michael. 2010. *A History of Iran: Empire of the Mind*. New York: Basic Books.
Homa, Ava. 2015 "Beauty Is Mandatory Yet Illegal in Iran." *Herizons* 29, no. 1: 31.
"Iranian Beauties." 2010. *Gold Coast Bulletin,* April 12. Accessed July 29, 2016.
Najmabadi, Afsaneh. 2001. "Gendered Transformations: Beauty, Love, and Sexuality in Qajar Iran." *Iranian Studies* 34, no. 1/4: 89–102.
Peterson, Scott. 2000. "In Iran, Search for Beauty Leads to the Nose Job." *Christian Science Monitor*, March 9. Accessed February 7, 2017. http://www.csmonitor.com/2000/0309 /p7s2.html
"Sewn in Secret." 2009. *Newsweek (Pacific Edition)* 154, no. 13 (September 28): 54.

ITALY

In ancient Rome, citizens concerned themselves with issues of health, hygiene, cleanliness, and beauty. Despite their Mediterranean climate, early Romans wore woolen dresses and shirts. These clothes were cleaned by *fullones*, who treated the clothing with an alkaline cleaning solution of men's urine and water and then stomped them clean. Urine was collected in large vats made available in public places (Sandbeck 2010). *Fullones* also added fuller's earth, a light, fine clay that absorbs grease, to the clothing.

A number of intriguing recipes for ancient Roman beauty treatments have been turned up by historians. One version of a lash-lengthening mascara used by ancient Romans called for the beating of baby mice into old wine until it formed a creamy salve. The poet Ovid described several exotic skin-beautifying products made from a variety of surprising ingredients, including a wrinkle cream to combat the effects of **aging** made by soaking the fronds of maidenhair fern in the urine of a young boy and a skin cream that started with a base of goose grease, honey, and vinegar and added a combination of kingfisher, mouse, or crocodile dung; deer antlers; placenta; bone marrow; genitalia; bile; and calf, cow, bull or mule urine (Sandbeck 2010). Pliny the Elder recorded a recipe for restoring the color and texture of damaged skin with a salve containing the lungs of sheep, the ash of an immolated green lizard, a snake's skin boiled in wine, pigeons' dung in honey, the white part of a hen's dung kept in oil, bat's blood, or a hedgehog's gall in water.

During the Middle Ages, women across Europe were discouraged from drawing attention to their external beauty, which could lead men to sin (Lowe 1994). Early Christian writers, like the theologian Jerome, born in what is now northeastern Italy in 347, believed that women were inferior and incapable of self-control. Jerome warned women that the only way they could live a moral life was through renunciation of their beauty. He advised "let paleness and squalor be henceforce your jewels" (Lowe 1994, 24). Control over the body was believed to be a fundamental means for enacting social power and for unlocking the keys to a religious afterlife. True beauty was imagined to be spiritual, and women and men likely felt a great deal of ambivalence over the value and nature of physical beauty that was so thoroughly denigrated by the strict clerics of the era.

Italian women during the Renaissance period were among the most literate in the world, and a relatively large number of women came to be noted for their accomplishments, including Christine de Pizan, Catherine de'Medici, and Lucrezia Borgia. In addition to the nation's reputation for food and wine, Italian women have captured an international reputation for being among the most beautiful in the world. Many attribute this natural beauty to the prevalence of sensible eating habits central to the Mediterranean diet, which features fresh, locally sourced, high-quality fruits, vegetables, beans, fish, poultry, olive oil, tomatoes, whole grains, dairy, and red wine. Traditionally, Italians ate very little red meat, and they created leisurely, social experiences around dining on several courses of small portions over several hours that allowed them to savor a balanced plate of healthy foods at every meal. The traditional Italian diet avoided sugars, fried foods, and mayonnaise. According to the International Association for the Study of Obesity, only 9 percent of Italians are considered obese (compared with 32 percent in the United States) (Kovacs 2007).

In the rural Italian province of Calabria, "plumpness came to be considered as a symbol of well-being and alimentary happiness, of beauty, wealth, power and dominance" (Teti 1995, 4). Fatness and good food, strength, physical force, erotic capacity, and beauty were ideals to be aspired to and very difficult to achieve for poor, undernourished people. The differences between the worlds of "full stomachs" and "empty ones" are central themes in 19th- and early 20th-century literature, poetry, songs, proverbs, and prayers, but the most distinct way that the beauty of robust size is noted is in the folk literature of the Christian season of Lent. Nursery rhymes and folk tales reveal a popular rejection of thinness, ugliness, and forced abstinence. Thin bodies were viewed as worrying figures, both threatening and dangerous, possibly even aligned with "witchcraft." The robust man, the man who could afford meat to eat, embodied cheerfulness, the capacity to work, and sexual virility. This **obese** ideal has been called "the carnival body" (Bakhtin cited in Teti 1995, 15) to reflect a celebration of abundance, good foods, and the popular longing to die from overeating.

Today, Italy is synonymous with glamour and noted as one of the fashion capitals of the world. Perhaps the most famous Italian beauty, known for her effortless luminosity, sensuality, and serene composure, is Sophia Loren. Born in the 1930s, former **pageant** contestant Loren captured the attention of the world when she signed a five-film contract with Paramount in 1956. She once famously credited the secret to her beauty to pasta.

The term "*sprezzatura*" refers to the art of dressing and looking good, usually for men, without appearing to try very hard (McKay 2009). The overall principle relies on an appearance that maintains an unstudied trend of nonchalance and carefree self-presentation, such as a scarf tossed casually around the shoulders or an unusual color combination, even if the look itself is quite expensive or time consuming to put together.

See also: Obesity; Pageants—International, National, and Local Contests.

Further Reading

Kovacs, Jenny Stamos. 2007. "Popular Diets of the World: The Italian Way with Food." *WebMD*. January 1. Accessed July 17, 2016. http://www.webmd.com/food-recipes/the-italian-diet.

Lowe, Ben. 1994. "Body Images and the Politics of Beauty: Formation of the Feminine Ideal in Medieval and Early Modern Europe." In: *Ideals of Feminine Beauty: Philosophical, Social, and Cultural Dimensions*, edited by Karen Callaghan, 21–36. Westport, CT: Greenwood Press.

McKay, Brett, and Kate McKay. 2009. "In Praise of Sprezzatura." Art of Manliness. July 14. Accessed March 15, 2016. http://www.artofmanliness.com/2009/07/14/in-praise-of-sprezzatura-the-compleat-gentleman-giveaway.

Sandbeck, Ellen. 2010. *Green Barbarians: How to Live Bravely on Your Home Planet*. New York: Scribner.

Teti, Vito. 1995. "Food and Fatness in Calabria," translated by Nicollete S. James. In: *Social Aspects of Obesity*, edited by Igor de Garine and Nancy J. Pollock, 3–31. Amsterdam: Gordon and Breach Publishers.

JAPAN

Influenced by the action-based religious worldview known as Shintoism, traditional Japanese culture embraced an extremely rich ritual tradition intent upon establishing and maintaining a connection between the contemporary world and the ancient past. Often referencing the grace and serenity of the natural world, attention to harmony, balance, and elegance in daily practice carries through to Japanese standards of beauty. Bathing and personal hygiene set the foundation for a beautiful body. Traditional Japanese culture devoted a great deal of time to the bathing of the body and the removal of body hair for both aesthetic and religious reasons. Shinto shrines were attended by female priestesses, called *miko*, who were trained to perform sacred cleansings and ritual ceremonies. Traditionally, a *miko* wore loose red trousers (called *hakama*) and a white *haori* (kimono jacket), symbolizing purity. The hair was dressed with white or red ribbons.

The highly stylized art of Japanese tattooing, called *irezumi*, dates to the Edo period (1600–1860) and imitates the effect of wood-block prints. Japanese decorative tattoos are distinctive in the world of tattooing, comprising eye-catching displays of color and design that span the entire body. The technique is very time consuming as the ink is inserted into the skin entirely by hand. Though beautiful, *irezumi* tattoos were frequently considered shameful and hidden in classic times because of a stigma associated with the tattooing of criminals. *Irezumi* tattoo artists were often secretive about their craft and difficult to find. The revival of this colorful art form in recent years has occurred due in large part to interest in Japanese techniques from the outside world. The range of naturalistic motifs (including koi fish, tigers, snakes, waves, clouds, lotuses, chrysanthemums, and cherry blossoms), as well as mythological beasts like dragons, have inspired a generation of American tattoo artists, including Ed Hardy.

Along with the tea ceremony (*sado*) and the art of flower arranging (*kado* or *ikebana*), perfumery (called *kodo*, or literally "the way of the fragrance") represented one of the three key classical feminine arts that Japanese women of refinement were expected to master. Instead of applying the fragrances directly to the body, it is probably best to think about *kodo* as a kind of aromatherapy: the goal was to create pleasant-smelling spaces that enhanced the beauty of all within the space.

Hair is another important consideration for Japanese beauty, including the sheen, thickness, and style of the hair. Historically, washing hair and applying oils to it could be a time-consuming process, and hair salons employed specialists with many years of training to engineer the elaborate hairstyles favored by maiko, geisha, and other women of means. The basic traditional hairstyle involves dividing the hair into six sections, roughly corresponding to the front, sides, back, center, and a chignon, located close to the neck. Styles varied widely depending upon one's profession and social status, but using combs, pads, and frames, hairstyles usually intertwined and piled each of the sections in such a way that they eventually created the desired height and met at the center.

Special hair jewelry, known as *kanzashi*, is frequently associated with the elaborate hairstyles of well-dressed Japanese women. These long hair sticks or hair pin ornaments usually have some item of interest at the end, which is inserted into the coiffure to secure the hair, but also to add color, movement, or visual interest to the outfit. Some ornaments are of the fluttering or dangling style, composed of metal strips attached by rings to the stick of the ornaments so that they may move independently and even create a pleasant tinkling sound. Other forms may be heavily jeweled or include designs of flowers, butterflies, or other motifs that sit closer to the scalp. There are ceremonial versions of the hair ornament more suited to geisha or brides, including a *kanzashi* design shaped like a fan with aluminum streamers attached to the sides allowing for movement. Hair ornaments are highly sensitive to the season, and so it was not uncommon to see well-dressed women of previous eras match the jewelry of their hairstyle to a preferred color scheme or naturalistic motif according to the month of the year. The famous Japanese cherry blossom (*sakura*), for example, was celebrated in April with a mixture of butterfly and lantern motifs on hair ornaments. November designs featured trailing autumnal leaves of the popular Japanese maple. *Kanzashi* are made of a wide variety of materials, including precious metals, tortoiseshell, coral, jade, small pieces of elaborately tucked silk made to resemble flowers, and even plastic. In some dramatic film moments, the sharp end of a strategically placed *kanzashi* hair stick can also be used as handy weapons in self-defense.

Even outside of Japan, many are familiar with the beautiful femininity of the geisha, a woman accomplished in the art of entertaining men. Geisha means "one who lives by art," and women in this profession were trained to speak, move, sing, write, dance, and serve food and drinks in ways that were considered graceful and beautiful.

Noh theater features large, expressive masks worn exclusively by male performers. Through the mask and their costuming, men are expected to enact the qualities of ideal femininity at different stages of a woman's life. Noh masks are made from a honey-colored, close-grained wood of medium weight crafted from (endangered) Kiso cypress wood. When portraying a woman, the costume should also include the richest, most spectacular kimono possible; a fan; and a profusion of thick, jet-black hair. The mask itself should have a splash of red, often with blackened teeth and a protruding lower lip to accentuate the vibrant red color of the lipstick. These masks also feature very high eyebrows, because aristocrats of both sexes historically depilated themselves and painted dramatically high arches on their faces. The essence of beauty in Noh comes from restraint and a curtailing of movement: performers report that the wig and the mask are actually painful, but the movements seen by the audience should appear dreamy and effortless. This requires the male performer to endure discomfort as part of the illusion of beauty.

The aesthetics of Japanese anime represent an important contribution to contemporary standards of beauty. Contemporary youth culture in Japan often borrows elements from Western cultures, but with very distinct ways of marking it as distinctly Japanese. The popular *ganguro* style (which is itself a subculture of the urban, hip-hop–inspired Kogal style) refers to dyeing very dark hair either blonde or some shade of red.

See also: Geisha; Hair; Makeup and Cosmetics; Perfume and Scented Oils; Yaeba; Youth.

Further Reading

Allison, Anne. 1994. *Nightwork: Sexuality, Pleasure, and Corporate Masculinity in a Tokyo Hostess Club*. Chicago: University of Chicago Press.
Golden, Arthur. 1999. *Memoirs of a Geisha: A Novel*. New York: Vintage.
Miller, Laura. 2006. *Beauty Up: Exploring Contemporary Japanese Body Aesthetics*. Berkeley, CA: University of California Press.
Morris, Ivan. 1964. *The World of the Shining Prince: Court Life in Ancient Japan*. Tokyo, Kodanasha International.
Nakato, Hiroko. 2002. "Craftsmen Keep Alive Hair Ornaments that Were All the Rage in the Edo Period." Japan Times. April 27, 2002. Accessed July 27, 2016. http://www.japantimes.co.jp/news/2002/04/27/news/craftsmen-keep-alive-hair-ornaments-that-were-all-the-rage-in-edo-period.
Vollmann, William T. 2010. *Kissing the Mask: Beauty, Understatement and Femininity in Japanese Noh Theater*. New York: HarperCollins.

JEWELRY

Nearly any part of the face or body can be adorned with jewelry. Body ornamentation not only beautifies the self, but it may also render the boundaries of the individual or group identity into physical form. Evidence of jewelry is found in every known culture and worn on appropriate occasions by some combination of women, men, children, and even animals. A wide range of materials can be used to create jewelry, presented alone, strung together, or set into metals, including pearls, coral, bones, teeth, or amber. Other materials can also be used to make jewelry, including plastic or found objects of any type.

According to archaeologists, early humans made and wore jewelry as long as 135,000 years ago. Perforated beads made from the shells of sea snails were discovered at a Stone Age site in Skhul, Israel, and necklaces of shell ornaments stained with hematite or ochre are commonly found in burials associated with Neanderthal burial, dating to about 50,000 years ago (Zilhao). The oldest stone bracelet, found in the Altai region of Siberia, dates to Denisovan occupation of a cave complex and was made by carefully drilling chlorite, probably with an antler or bone boring tool. Chlorite does not occur naturally in the vicinity of the cave, leading archaeologists to believe that the precious stone, which was polished to reflect the light, was traded as a luxury or prestige item, and the resulting bracelet was worn by someone of high social status.

The invention of metallurgy allowed metals, especially bronze, gold, and silver, to be fashioned into ornaments. The oldest gold jewelry, a 24-karat, two-gram pendant, was unearthed in the Varna region of Bulgaria and dates to 6,600 years ago. The gold was soft enough to have been hammered into shape, and it is unknown whether it was worn by a man or a woman. Because jewelry tends to be relatively small, the skill of the metal worker is tested to render exquisite detail. Two gold earrings were found in the tomb of a 1,500-year-old woman named Farong buried in Datong City, China. The earrings are extraordinary in their tiny, detailed representation of two dragons and a human figure, with a cascading trail of jade, turquoise, and amethyst, held aloft by tiny chips of precious stones in an elaborate teardrop-shaped setting that decorates the sides of the earrings (Jarus 2016). Today, platinum and titanium are also used extensively in jewelry.

The female Sumerian dignitary buried in the Royal Tomb of Ur, nicknamed Queen Pu-abi during the excavation, wore an estimated 14 pounds of jewelry composed of an elaborate gold leaf headdress and hair ornaments, two sets of large gold lunate (hoop) earrings, a wide, choker-style necklace, and a "cape" and "belt," each made of semiprecious stone beads and gold and silver rings. She also wore a wrist cuff and ten rings. Elaborate jewelry is found in burials across Mesopotamia. Jewelry was used as a wedding gift, as well as a convenient way to store wealth used in dowries and inheritances. Mesopotamian men also wore earrings, necklaces, armlets, bracelets, pectoral ornaments, and headbands. Elite women also wore diadems (crowns or headbands) made of semiprecious stone beads and gold. Many of the materials used in the jewelry were imported from very far distances, adding to their value. Jewelry found in Mesopotamian burials serves as markers of individual and family wealth, and underscores the differentiation of the people of this era into social **classes**.

Labrets, disc-shaped jewelry worn as piercings in the skin below the lower lip, are also found around the world dating to the prehistoric period. In ancient Chile of the El Molle period (1–700 CE), labret jewelry functioned to denote and perhaps even create identities through the social processes necessary to acquire the ornamentation Archaeologists have identified a relationship between heavily labretted men and warriors of the society who were at risk for high rates of traumatic injury through warfare, suggesting the right to display jewelry was connected to **masculinity** in that culture (Torres-Rouff 2011).

Stiff neck rings called torques (also called "torc") are most commonly associated with the European Iron Age (from BCE 8th century to the 3rd century CE) era. They were usually made either as a single piece of metal or with metal strands twisted or braided together with an opening at the front. Torques would have been difficult to remove and became permanent daily wear after they were originally placed on the wearer. Archaeologists have found torques made of bronze, silver, and gold (often mixed with other metals to improve strength and durability) in the Scythian, Thracian, Illyrian, and Celtic cultures. Similar bracelets, anklets, and armlets worn around the bicep have also been found. Celtic torques became quite elaborate, depicting images of animals, gods, and cultic symbols. They would have been very valuable, and appear as grave goods associated with the burials of both male and female high-status Celts.

In addition to being pleasing to the eye or used to reinforce messages about femininity or masculinity, jewelry often has a functional spiritual or religious significance, or may be designed as a talisman to protect the wearer from harm. Amulets, objects with the power to ward off evil, are sometimes used as pendants and hung from necklaces, bracelets, rings, or other forms of jewelry. Amulets can be quite beautiful and fashioned from precious stones, gems, plants, bones, or other objects. "Sacred eye" agate beads (called "*dzi*") are used widely in Tibet to ward off evil (Childers 2011). In Asian countries, amber beads are also commonly thought both to be beautiful and to offer protection from ill-wishers. The hand-shaped hamsa design (sometimes called the "Hand of Fatima") is an ancient symbol in the Middle Eastern world dating back to Mesopotamia as a universal sign of protection, blessings, power, and strength associated with the goddess Ishtar.

To increase the dramatic effect of jewelry, stones—referred to as "jewels"—were set into worked metals. The most valuable gems include diamonds, rubies, emeralds, and sapphires, prized for the way they are cut to reflect the light. There are also many semiprecious stones, typically chosen for their bright colors, including the regal purple of amethyst; the various shades of blue in aquamarine, lapis lazuli, and turquoise; and the bright orangey-pink of carnelian (a form of agate). Of course, many other semiprecious stones exist, including tourmaline, chrysoberyl, alexandrite, peridot, garnets, and tanzanite.

Egyptian tombs are famous for the discovery of "scarabs," elaborately jeweled beetle designs. The beetle hieroglyphic is usually translated as "to come into being," and so it is likely that in addition to being attractive, the design carried a spiritual symbolism. These ornamental scarabs were central to a wide variety of jeweled designs that included brooches, earrings, and diadems meant to be worn on the head much like a crown or a tiara. Upper arm bracelets were also commonly worn

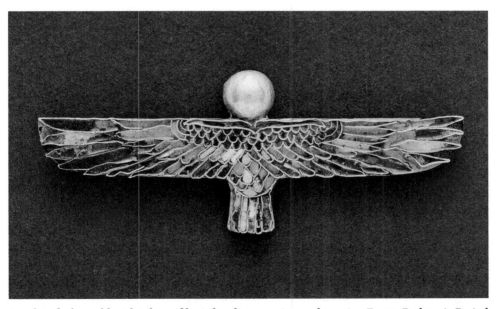

Amulet of a *ba*, gold with inlays of lapis lazuli, turquoise, and steatite, Egypt, Ptolemaic Period (332–30 BCE). In ancient Egyptian mythology, the ba was represented as a bird with a human head, arms, and hands. The ba may come closest to Western notions of a "soul." (Los Angeles County Museum of Art)

by ancient Egyptians, sometimes fashioned into the shape of a serpent. Possibly the most distinct form of ancient Egyptian jewelry is known as the "pectoral," a large collar necklace worn by pharaohs and other elites for aesthetic purposes and to display wealth. Pectorals were usually made of gold with gem inlays. Ancient Egyptians also wore a variety of amulets, frequently elaborated with gems or precious metals.

Classical Greek jewelry featured a number of animals fashioned into hoop earrings, bracelets, necklaces, and brooches, including motifs of the ram, owl, bull, stags, and lions. These were fashioned into jewelry from eighteen-carat gold by heat treatment and skilled hammering.

Gradually, fine jewelry became democratized and more affordable for those who were not royalty. The growing middle class developed a taste for elegant jewelry in their pursuit for conspicuous consumption. In the post–World War II reconstruction period, Rome became the worldwide center of glamour as the budding young celebrities of Hollywood flocked there to make high-profile films. Many of the starlets of the age frequented European jewelers, adding to the "material girl" reputations of famous women of the age like **Marilyn Monroe**, Elizabeth Taylor, and Sophia Loren.

Fine jewelers also view the current trend in body jewelry as a new opportunity for experimentation and aesthetic impact, including body chains, multiple ear piercings, navel rings, anklets, and labrets. One of the "youngest forms of fine jewelry" (Childers 2014) is the wristwatch.

See also: Class; Egypt; Greece; Lips; Masculinity; Monroe, Marilyn.

Further Reading

Balter, Michael. 2006. "First Jewelry? Old Shell Beads Suggest Early Use of Symbols." *Science* 312, no. 5781: 1731.

Chapman, Martin, and Amanda Triossi. 2014. *The Art of Bvlgari: La Dolce Vita and Beyond, 1950–1990*. New York: Fine Arts Museums of San Francisco/Delmonico Books.

Childers, Christine. 2011. *Jewelry International: The World's Finest Jewelry Book*, Volume 3. New York: Rizzoli Publications.

Childers, Christine. 2014. *Jewelry International: The World's Finest Jewelry Book*, Volume 5. New York: Rizzoli Publications.

Jarus, Owen. 2016. "1500 Year Old Tomb of a Chinese Woman Named Farong." Live Science August 17. Accessed August 29, 2016. http://www.livescience.com/55789-photos -ancient-tomb-of-chinese-woman.html.

Liesowska, Liona. 2015. "Stone Bracelet Is Oldest Ever Found in the World." *Siberian Times*. May 7. Accessed August 29, 2016. http://siberiantimes.com/science/casestudy/features /f0100-stone-bracelet-is-oldest-ever-found-in-the-world.

Torres-Rouff, Christina. 2011. "Piercing the Body: Labret Use, Identity, and Masculinity in Prehistoric Chile." In: *Breathing New Life into the Evidence of Death: Contemporary Approaches to Bioarchaeology*, edited by Aubrey Baadsgaard, Alexis T. Boutin, and Jane E. Buikstra, 153–78. Santa Fe, NM: SAR Press.

Volpicelli, Gian. 2015. "Is This the World's First Bling?" *Daily Mail*. November 20. Accessed August 29, 2016. http://www.dailymail.co.uk/sciencetech/article-3327210/Is-world-s -oldest-BLING-6-600-year-old-golden-pendant-prehistoric-Bulgarian-settlement.html.

Winkel, Bertie, and Dos Winkel. 2006. *Vanishing Beauty: Indigenous Body Art and Decoration*. Munich, Germany: Prestel.

Zilhao, Joao. 2007. "The Emergence of Ornaments and Art: An Archaeological Perspective on the Origins of Behavioral Modernity." *Journal of Archaeological Research* 15, no. 1: 1–54.

KAYAN (KAREN) NECK RINGS ("PADAUNG NECK RINGS")

Gradual stacking of brass or bronze coils, often called "rings," around the neck is practiced among the indigenous, Karenic-speaking people of the hills of northern Thailand and Myanmar, a region often referred to as the Golden Triangle. These women are sometimes known as the "giraffe women" and are highly photographed by curiosity seekers. Long necks are associated with wealth and beauty, and are said to give young women more options in attracting a successful husband.

Padaung women are fitted with these metal coils gradually from childhood, usually at the age of 5 or 6, to give the illusion of a longer, more slender neck. Each year, women are able to add more rings according to their ability to afford them. Adult women can wear about 20 of the rings, although there are examples of women with up to 25 rings, each ring weighing about 4 to 5 pounds. The look is so striking some outsiders worry that "stretching" the neck in this way can cause orthopedic damage. In fact, the rings do not actually lengthen the neck, but instead, the heavy weight associated with the coils forcibly push down the collarbone to create the visual appearance of a longer, more pleasing neck. The ligaments and cartilage attaching the clavicle to the sternum also can be slowly stretched to accommodate more and more rings. Over time, this process begins to press on the upper ribs, further opening the space for the rings to be stacked.

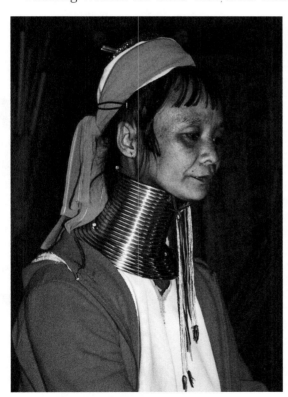

A Kayan woman wears a stack of neck rings, Chiang Mai, northern Thailand. Neck rings may be added gradually over the course of a woman's life, according to her social status. (J. J. Spring/Dreamstime.com)

Tribal women of the region are noted for their jewelry, which may also include silver chains, an assortment of glass beads, buckles, earrings, and finger rings. Women also favor decorative additions in the form of tassels, seeds, shells, and other natural products that may be attached to clothing or worn in an ornamental way. The value of a woman's jewelry represents the wealth of her family and may attract suitors to the young woman. Within the region, marriage negotiations are often made using silver as the standard for exchange, though brass and copper are also used widely. The Padaung observe matrilineal descent patterns, which means that ornaments and jewelry may pass from mother to daughter, although they are also bought independently whenever possible. The coils are carefully wrapped, usually by a local spiritual leader, who also anoints the neck with protective ointments and cushioning.

Less dramatic, but still notable in Karenic women's appearance, is the presence of large, "gauge-style" earrings, originally made from the ivory of elephant tusk. Until recently, men also wore these distinctive ear plugs with projections of varying lengths. Like the neck rings, these gauges are fitted into the earlobes of young girls, and the lobe is stretched progressively to achieve a pleasing size. The women also wear brass rings around their calves.

According to the legends of the people, the neck rings were originally designed to give women the striking appearance of a dragon or possibly to prevent tigers from fatally attacking women. Another explanatory story suggests that women were fitted with the neck rings to discourage being kidnapped by neighboring tribes, who might find the longer necks unappealing.

Once attached, the rings are rarely removed, and women wear them for the duration of their lives. The region is also noted for the high-quality looms which allow the locals to spin thread from their own cotton and create intricate textile patterns of bright colors from locally sourced dyes. Women also traditionally wear their hair long and tied into a knot at the top of the head, covered by a turban-like head covering with a long fringe. Young women often add brightly colored pompoms around the head covering, which may hang down and swing attractively close to their neck rings.

In the last few decades, political unrest in the region has pushed increasing numbers of Karenic people from Burma into Thailand.

Ndebele Rings

Historically, Ndebele women of South Africa wore copper and brass rings around their necks, arms, and legs called *idzila* following marriage to indicate marital fidelity. The more rings a woman's financial and social situation allowed her to wear, the greater the prestige of her husband. Unlike the Padaung neck rings of southeast Asia (featured on the cover), which are really more like coils, the neck and limb rings worn by these southern African people were typically left open in the back to allow flexibility for opening the ring to place around arms, ankles, or the neck. The rings were often believed to be imbued with ritualistic power and were typically only removed by a woman after the death of her husband. Ndembele women also adorned themselves with brightly colored beaded jewelry, including handmade, beaded neck coils (called *izigolwa*), aprons, and belts.

Today, the government of Myanmar (formerly Burma) actively discourages the practice of adding neck rings to young girls' growing bodies. However, many Thai tour companies offer treks with the explicit promise of viewing the extraordinarily long necks of these "hill-women," leading to serious consideration about whether or not the desires of outsiders to pay to see "exotic" women in their native habitat is not a form of exploitation (Waddington 2002).

See also: Body Modification; Jewelry.

Further Reading

Lewis, Paul, and Ellen Lewis. 1998. *Peoples of the Golden Triangle: Six Tribes in Thailand*. London: Thames & Hudson.
Waddington, Ray. 2002. "The Karen People." The Peoples of the World Foundation. Accessed September 13, 2015. http://www.peoplesoftheworld.org/text?people=Karen.

KAYAPO

The anthropologist Terence Turner argues, "Man is born naked but is everywhere in clothes or their symbolic equivalents" (1980, 112). The act of decorating, covering, uncovering, or modifying the human form, however inconsequential or frivolous that act may seem, conveys accordance with the social notions of propriety, morality, the sacred, status, changes in status, and beauty for every society.

The Kayapo are an indigenous people of the southern Amazonian rainforest who have garnered a great deal of world attention in recent years due to the highly publicized protests of the Belo Monte hydroelectric dam on the Xingu River of Brazil. Though they seem to wear very little "clothing," the body paintings, hairstyles, and **body modifications** of individual Kayapo people convey an extraordinary amount of meaning to those who know how to "read" the symbolic trappings of their self-presentation.

For the Kayapo, beauty includes a distinct importance on a high standard of cleanliness. All Kayapo **bathe** at least one time a day in a river or with a quantity of water drawn from the abundant water sources in their rainforest environment. Being clean is the minimal standard for beauty: it also conveys a dimension of being human, as animals are not considered clean. To be "clean" for the Kayapo also includes the removal of all **hair** from the body except that of the head. Though hair on the head is most commonly kept short, certain categories of people in Kayapo culture are allowed to wear their hair long. Nursing infants, women who have borne children, and men who have been through the initiation to adulthood are allowed to wear long hair.

There are two main aspects to Kayapo body painting: the colors (black and red) and emphasis of different regions of the body, which indicate Kayapo ideas about the social nature of the person. The color black is associated with the domain of nature and the world of death. Black paint is applied to those parts of the body that are thought of as the source of "natural" powers and energies, like the trunk, internal and reproductive organs, and major muscles, such as the upper arms and thighs. Red paint is associated with vitality, energy, and intensification, especially

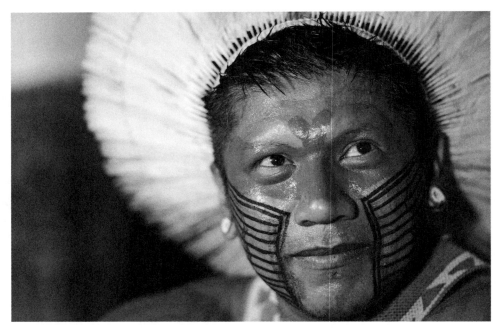

A Kayapo man attends the cultural festival of the World Indigenous Games in Palmas, Brazil, October 21, 2015. (AP Photo/Eraldo Peres)

as may be demonstrated by remarkable achievements or powerful personal qualities. Red is usually the color applied to the eyes, especially of children, who are deep in the process of active learning through observation, and also the mouth, which is the source of speech, ideas, and dreams. The bodies of children are much more elaborately decorated than those of adults. Children are painted by their mothers or grandmothers with intricate, black geometrical designs composed of lines and dots, which trace the major organs from the neck to the knees. Though there are similarities between the patterns by family or lineage, there are also significant differences depending on the qualities and health of the individual person. No two sets of patterns are exactly alike. Older girls and women continue to paint each other in fairly elaborate patterns, but in general, as one ages, one comes to be painted with more standardized designs, many of which have names to indicate the animal that the pattern resembles or represents. Men also paint other men with standardized patterns, but typically only for rituals. The social context of application of body paint is collective and reinforces the unity and ideology of the group in an intimate, personalized way.

Similar to **lip plates**, Kayapo men may also wear lip plugs. Only men have their lips pierced, and lip plugs may reach a large size among older men. The piercing is given soon after birth, but at first, only a string of beads and bit of mussel shell is used to keep the hole open. After initiation into manhood, young men begin to use progressively larger wooden pins to stretch the lip hole. Wooden lip plugs are common, but men who earn prestige may also wear cylindrical lip plugs of ground or polished rock crystal, which may reach six inches in length and one inch in diameter. To keep the plug from slipping, it may have two small flanges at the upper end. These plugs are hard to make and are highly valued for their beauty. They may be passed down as family heirlooms. The larger lip plug of the senior male is viewed as a physical expression of a man's oral assertiveness and skill as an orator, symbolizing both his social dominance and the expressive beauty of elder men. Both men and women may wear ear plugs. Again, the first piercing in the lobes of infants is made shortly after birth. At weaning, the ear plugs are removed and little strings of beads are tied through the holes to keep them open. Both Kayapo men and women wear these bead earrings into adulthood. Adult men also wear penis sheaths after their initiation into manhood. The purpose of the sheath is understood as a way to restrain the spontaneous, "natural" form of socially unrestrained male libidinal energy, the erection. The sheath is made into a cone shape from a small palm leaf, woven at both the wide and narrow ends to fit over the tip of the penis. The penis is then drawn through the sheath and secured by tucking the foreskin through the narrow end of the sheath.

At more elaborate communal ceremonies, adult men of the village also augment their appearance with elaborate coiffures, many of which include feather headdresses and ritual regalia. The headdresses of the most important men may include the breast plumage of the red macaw, highly prized for its color and rareness. All members of the group also wear symbolic **jewelry** appropriate to their rank and earned through various life course trials, including bracelets, ear and lip plugs, and belts and leg bands made with beads, bones, freshwater mussel shells, and hooves from forest animals. Each individual earns and receives different types of adornment to denote an aspect of social identity of the wearer. Body adornment is serious business for the Kayapo, who also bestow "beautiful" names at ceremonies, which may be passed down by kinsmen. The beautiful, symbolic jewelry pieces made for these ritual occasions comprise the only goods for which the Kayapo language contains the terms for "wealth," "valuables," or "riches." The connection between "beauty" and "wealth" is articulated in songs and stories. It is important to note that though individuals may be deemed "beautiful," the true measure of beauty of the Kayapo is the capacity of the individual to be connected to others in meaningful and symbolic ways that may be reflected in elaborate costumes. Turner says, "Beauty is an ideal expression of society itself in its holistic capacity. It is, as such, one of the primary values of Kayapo life" (1980, 137–38). For the Kayapo, to be properly socialized is to be "beautiful."

See also: Bathing and Showering; Body Modification; Hair; Jewelry; Lip Plates.

Further Reading

Turner, Terence. 1980. "The Social Skin." In: *Not Work Alone: A Cross-Cultural View of the Activities Superfluous to Survival*, edited by Jeremy Cherfas and Roger Lewin, 112–40. London: Temple Smith.

LABIAPLASTY

Labiaplasty is a relatively new form of surgical **body modification** designed to minimize, augment, or change the appearance of the labia and vagina. Sometimes called "cosmetic gynecology" or "sexual enhancement surgery" (Loy 2000), labiaplasty procedures can include vaginal tightening (sometimes called "vaginal rejuvenation"); liposuction and lifting of the labia to appear more aesthetically pleasing or more youthful; "repair" of the hymen; clipping and re-sculpting of labia to appear more symmetrical; "unhooding" the clitoris to improve friction during sexual activity; and injecting fat, usually taken from the inner thigh, into labia to make them appear plumper.

Despite other cultures that practice labial stretching to create **elongated labia** designed to enhance sexual pleasure, in the West, long labia are believed to inhibit sexual pleasure and to be an embarrassment (Jeffreys 2014, 34).

The ubiquity of pornography and pornographic images of genitalia have created a "pornographication" of Western culture (Jeffreys 2014, 67). Some commentators note that the rise of Playboy magazine in the 1960s and 1970s gave rise to an increased demand for breast augmentation, while the increasing tolerance for "crotch shots" in *Penthouse* and mass-produced pornographic videos has contributed to the rise in desire for labiaplasties (Jeffreys 2014, 82). The aesthetic values of pornographic practices have been increasingly over-represented in Western standards of beauty since the 1980s, as clearly demonstrated by the increasing frequency of shaved and waxed women's genitals and the widespread acceptance of "the Brazilian" as the standard of acceptable bodies promoted by men's magazines and Web sites. One woman interviewed for a popular woman's magazine explained that after receiving a Brazilian wax, she became more aware of the shape of her inner labia and the consequent "need" to seek surgical grooming of her vagina's inner lips (Jeffreys 2014, 84).

Additionally, labiaplasty appears to promise that the procedure will make women more sexually acceptable to men. One way to increase sexual desirability can be achieved either through "tightening" vaginal muscles that may have been "enlarged" during childbearing in order to satisfy a male sexual partner more intensely. Alternatively, labiaplasty offers the possibility of "repairing," or surgically reconstructing, a hymen, especially for women from cultures subject to more traditional patriarchal codes of gendered and sexual morality, where virginity may still be necessary at the time of marriage to avoid dishonor upon the family or the individual woman.

In her passionate 2008 documentary about British women seeking labiaplasty, Lisa Rogers reveals that girls as young as 14 are seeking vaginal surgery, concerned that their genitalia are somehow disfigured or malformed. Women who seek the surgery confess to feeling anxiety and self-consciousness about the supposed ugliness of their labia, but there is also evidence to suggest that most women do not actually know what other women's "normal," nonpornified genitals look like (Jeffreys 2014, 83).

A special report prepared in 2002 for the United Nations High Commission on Human Rights drew special attention to practices that "do not respect the integrity of the female body" (Coomaraswamy 2002, 8) and paid particular attention to "cultural practice that brutalizes the female body." The report refers almost exclusively to non-Western practices of female genital modification, but does not directly address the issue of labiaplasty. However, it can be hard not to see parallels with the intimate tyrannies demanded of women's body parts to conform to arbitrary and impossible standards of beauty (Jafar 2012), despite the cost or pain that may be involved.

See also: Body Modification; Elongated Labia.

Further Reading

Coomaraswamy, Radhika. 2002. "Cultural Practices in the Family that Are Violent Towards Women." United Nations High Commission on Human Rights Report of the Special Rapporteur on Violence Against Women." Accessed March 3, 2016. http://www.awf.or.jp /pdf/h0016.pdf.

Holloway, Kali. 2015. "The Labiaplasty Boom: Why Are Women Desperate for the Perfect Vagina?" *Alternet*. February 13. Accessed March 3, 2016. http://www.alternet.org/news -amp-poliRtics/labiaplasty-boom-why-are-women-desperate-perfect-vagina.

Jafar, Afshan. 2012. "Progress and Women's Bodies." *TEDxConnecticut College*. Accessed March 3, 2016. https://www.youtube.com/watch?v=BaxnvwffWbE.

Jeffreys, Sheila. 2014. *Beauty and Misogyny: Harmful Cultural Practices in the West*. New York: Routledge.

Loy, Jen. 2000. "A Look at Labiaplasty." *Alternet*. May 28. Accessed March 3, 2016. http:// www.alternet.org/story/9217/a_look_at_labiaplasty.

Rogers, Lisa. 2008. "The Quest for the Perfect Vagina." *The Guardian*. August 15. Accessed March 3, 2016. https://www.theguardian.com/culture/tvandradioblog/2008/aug/15/the questfortheperfectvagi.

Rogers, Lisa. 2008. *The Perfect Vagina*. Film. Directed by Lisa Rogers. Channel 4 Television.

LEG LENGTHENING SURGERY

In the venue of cosmetic plastic surgery, there are many different procedures designed to provide patients with a desired change in appearance. Facelifts, eyelid opening surgery, and breast augmentation are among the most popular cosmetic surgeries performed worldwide, with tens of thousands of procedures being performed every year, making then relatively commonplace (ISAPS 2015). There are, however, less common and more radical surgeries that take place around the globe, including a procedure designed to lengthen the patient's legs.

Leg lengthening was originally pioneered in Russia in 1951 as a remedy for people with stunted growth, mismatched leg length, or certain genetic conditions (Kirit

2013). In the 21st century, the procedure is now being used by patients seeking to simply be taller. This procedure is especially common in China, where height is of great importance to citizens and considered a key element of beauty and the procedure is known as "*duango zenggao*" [breaking legs and getting taller] (Hua 2013). Some clinics in China in the early 21st century reported performing as many as 600 leg-lengthening procedures per year (Marie Claire 2003).

Lengthening a patient's legs is a long and painful three-step process. First, the tibiae (or shin bones) in the patient's legs are broken completely through, and screws are placed in the bones, penetrating the skin. These screws are then attached to an external frame built around the patient's legs. The frame around the patient's legs is then progressively opened over the course of several months, stretching the lower part of the shin bone away from the upper part, lengthening and creating space in the soft tissues surrounding the bone. During this time, the bone regenerates to fill the gap between the broken ends, effectively creating a longer shin bone. When the procedure is complete, steel pins are inserted to provide extra support for the newly grown bone. The end result of the surgery can add up to ten centimeters (about four inches) to a patient's height (Watts 2004).

This process is exceedingly painful and requires the patient to remain on bed rest for the entire procedure. The procedure is also dangerous and filled with potential side effects and risks. Legs stretched too quickly will not develop new bone that is hard enough to support the weight of the patient and may remain so brittle that even slight blows will break them. If sufficient care is not taken to lengthen the legs at equal speeds, nerve damage and mismatched misshapen legs may result. Other potential risks include loss of a full range of motion in the legs and the splaying out of the feet or dangerous infections from the frame (Watts 2004). Because of these dangers, the surgery is banned in some nations and nearly unavailable in other nations, such as the United States, where the procedure is still only regularly performed for patients with reconstructive needs, not cosmetic ones (Kirit 2013).

The pain and danger involved in the procedure highlight the significance of height as a desirable element of appearance, especially in Asian nations. In China, many professions have height minimums for potential applicants clearly listed in job descriptions. Male members of China's foreign ministry, for example, must be at least five feet, seven inches tall, and women must be at least five feet three inches tall. Chinese stewardesses must be more than five feet five inches tall, and to get into law school, male students must be more than five feet five inches tall (Watts 2004).

Chinese patients are not the only ones continuing to seek the surgery, however. Some residents of nations such as Australia, Great Britain, or the United States also undergo the procedure. In those nations, however, it can be difficult to find access to a doctor or afford the procedure. In the United States, for example, only a few doctors perform the surgery, and in 2012, the average cost topped $85,000 (The Week 2012). The most popular locations to undergo the process, then, continue to be Russia and China, where medical tourists from around the world have the surgery performed (Kirit 2013). Travelers and locals alike seeking the procedure are still urged to take care in these nations, where many of the surgeries are performed in hospitals and clinics that are not licensed or regulated by the Russian or Chinese governments (Hua 2013).

Leg-lengthening surgery is risky, invasive, and dangerous enough that plastic surgery's main international governing body, the International Society of Aesthetic and Plastic Surgeons, does not recognize or offer advice on the procedure. The American Society of Plastic Surgeons, for their part, has named leg lengthening as one of the "top ten cosmetic procedures to avoid," a list that is designed to demonstrate procedures that are least likely to offer results that are worth the risks associated with the procedures (Childs 2008).

See also: China; Height; Plastic Surgery.

Further Reading

Childs, Dan. 2008. "10 Cosmetic Procedures that You Should Avoid." April 7. Accessed November 24, 2015. http://abcnews.go.com/Health/PainManagement/story?id=4585277 &page=1.

Hua, Wen. 2013. *Buying Beauty: Cosmetic Surgery in China.* Hong Kong: Hong Kong University Press.

ISAPS. 2015. "ISAPS International Survey on Aesthetic/Cosmetic Procedures Performed in 2014." Accessed August 20, 2015. http://www.isaps.org/Media/Default/globalstatistics /2015%20ISAPS%20Results.pdf.

Kirit, Radia. 2013. "Leg Lengthening Patient Hopes to Grow By 3.3 Inches With Painful Procedure." Accessed September 15, 2015. http://abcnews.go.com/Health/leg-lengthening -patient-hopes-grow-33-inches-painful/story?id=19451057.

Marie Claire. 2003. "The Height of Vanity." *Marie Claire (US Edition)* 10, no. 4 (April 2003): 92.

Watts, Jonathan. 2004. "China's Cosmetic Surgery Craze. Leg-Lengthening Operations to Fight Height Prejudice Can Leave Patients Crippled." *Lancet (London, England)* 363, no. 9413: 958.

The Week Staff. 2012. "Limb-lengthening: The 'Radical' New Plastic Surgery Craze." February 27. Accessed September 15, 2015. http://theweek.com/articles/477795/limbleng thening-radical-new-plastic-surgery-craze.

LIPOSUCTION

Sometimes known simply as "lipo," liposuction is a cosmetic surgery procedure that removed unwanted fat from the body and face. The International Society of Aesthetic Plastic Surgeons (ISAPS) explains that liposuction surgery is a procedure normally carried out with a tube and suction device, allowing the doctor to target specific areas of concern for the patient (ISAPS 2015b).

While the allure of simply removing unwanted fat had been around in various stages and experimentation processes since the 1920s, modern-day liposuction techniques date from a blunt tunneling technique developed by surgeons in Italy in the 1970s. To that tunneling technique, the French surgeon Dr. Yves-Gerard Illouz added the concept of a suction device to remove the fat cells, and the practice of liposuction was born (Mandal 2015).

With the arrival of the procedure in the United States, surgeons began experimenting with different forms of anesthetic in the 1980s, and eventually also introduced the practice of using ultrasound to liquefy the fat prior to extraction. By the 1990s, complications of the procedure were rarer, and the practice began to be widely used in the United States and abroad. In 1993, liposuction was the top cosmetic surgery procedure chosen by women in the United States, and the notorious Venezuelan terrorist Carlos the Jackal was apprehended in Africa in 1994 when the plastic surgeons he had contacted about performing liposuction on his belly turned him in once he was under the anesthesia (Haiken 1999).

Although liposuction is often associated with belly fat, the abdomen is far from the only place that the practice is used. Patients have the procedure performed to reduce under-eye bags, to eliminate the "wattle" below the neck, and to slim calves and ankles. The ISAPS reports that the most common places where the procedure is performed are the chin, cheeks, neck, and upper arms; the area above the breasts; abdomen; buttocks; hips; thighs; knees; calves; and ankles (ISAPS 2015b).

In the 20th and 21st centuries, the practice of liposuction has also led to the creation and practice of analogous fat transfer, or "lipofilling," a procedure in which "a person's own fat is used to fill in irregularities and grooves." Although this process can be used to fill in such areas as deep grooves that run from the cheekbone to the mouth, lipofilling is most commonly used as a way to plump up lips (ISAPS 2015a).

In 2014, worldwide, liposuction was the second most popular form of cosmetic surgery (behind blepharoplasty), with the United States, Brazil, Mexico, and Germany performing the most liposuction procedures. Fat grafting was the fourth most popular cosmetic surgery procedure internationally, with the United States, Brazil, South Korea, and Mexico performing the most lipofilling procedures (ISAPS 2015b).

Liposuction is an outpatient procedure that lasts one or two hours and only requires general anesthesia in some cases. Liposuction can leave patients bruised and sore in the short term, and has some long-term risks, including serious infection, a permanently asymmetrical appearance of the treated area, rippling of the skin, changes in skin tone, or other injuries to the skin (ISAPS 2015c).

See also: Eyelid Surgery; Injections; Plastic Surgery.

Further Reading

Haiken, Elizabeth. 1999. *Venus Envy: A History of Cosmetic Surgery*. Baltimore: Johns Hopkins University Press.

ISAPS. 2015a. "Fat Transfer." Accessed January 29, 2017. http://www.isaps.org/procedures/fat-transfer-body.

ISAPS. 2015b. "Global Statistics." Accessed January 29, 2017. http://www.isaps.org/Media/Default/global-statistics/2015%20ISAPS%20Results.pdf.

ISAPS. 2015c. "Liposuction." Accessed January 29, 2017. http://www.isaps.org/procedures/liposuction.

Mandal, Ananya. 2015. "History of Liposuction." January 11. Accessed January 29, 2017. http://www.news-medical.net/health/History-of-Liposuction.aspx.

LIP PLATES

Lip plates, also called labial plates, are a form of body art that emphasize the stretched flesh of the lower lip to accommodate a prominent, flat disc, sometimes decorated. Typically, these plates may only be worn after a period of initiation and dedicated efforts to achieving the desired look. Lips are perhaps a likely facial feature to emphasize due to their extremely malleable nature and their prominent position bordering the mouth, which may be thought of as a key symbolic passageway for language and self-expression and thus marks the contact point between nature and culture (Geoffrey-Schneiter 2006, 65).

Historically, lip plates were worn by **Kayapo** and Suyá men of the Xingu River in Brazil. The wooden plates, which measure from three to eight inches across, were worn by married men. They are not worn anymore. Until recently, the Sara and Lobi women, who live along the Chari River in neighboring Chad, and women of the Makonde of Tanzania and Mozambique, also wore lip plates. Today, the Mursi (sometimes called the Mun) are one of the only groups still practicing the technique (though ritual lip plates may also be seen among a very few, elite Kayapo men in Brazil). The Mursi live between the Omo and Mago rivers in a valley of southwest Ethiopia. They are pastoralists, relying on cattle herding and plant cultivation for their livelihoods.

In form and function, lip plates are exaggerated versions of labrets, which are piercings that puncture the bottom lip, usually directly in the center. This is how the Mursi lip plate placement begins, when the perforation is made as part of a ceremony by a female relative of the girl. Girls and women gradually add larger plates to stretch the piercing that begins as a much smaller hole. Archaeological finds in neighboring Chad place quartz labrets in the region hundreds of years ago. Smaller labrets are still worn by the Bodi, who live close to the Mursi, and aluminum labrets were reportedly worn by the Karamojong people of Uganda. Labrets designed to protect against evil spirits that may enter through the mouth are also worn

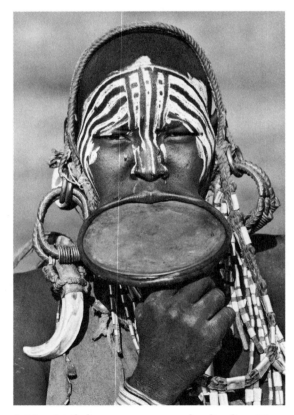

A Mursi tribal woman wears a clay lip disc, Mago National Park, southern Ethiopia. The Mursi women are famous for wearing plates in their lower lips. (Uros Ravbar/iStockphoto.com)

by the Lobi women of Ivory Coast and Ghana and Kirdi women of Cameroon (Pitt Rivers Museum 2011).

The process of stretching soft flesh must be done with some care and sophistication to avoid rips or tears that would ruin the effect. The entire process of stretching, similar to the earlobe stretching known as "gauging," to accommodate a large lip plate for the Mursi takes several months to a year. Though the stretching process begins before marriage, usually only married women wear lip plates, and they are understood as a symbol of female social adulthood. It has been reported that, at least historically, the size of the lip plate correlates to the amount of bridewealth that trades hands at the time of marriage. However, this point has been disputed by anthropologist David Turton (2004) who lived among the Mursi for several years. The women themselves determine how long they will continue to stretch their lips and the ultimate size of their lip plates. Typically, two bottom teeth are extracted to accommodate the size of the lip plate as it gets increasingly larger. Some women remove up to four teeth from their lower jaw. The plates may be removed, but after a certain point in the process, the original shape of the lips can never be restored.

The heavy pottery plates worn by Mursi women are shaped from clay, decorated, and fired individually by each woman herself. The process is deeply spiritual, connecting the woman to the earth. Made of fired clay, the plates are reasonably fragile and must be remade frequently. As with other non-Western people, the Mursi people view their entire bodies as a living canvas that reflects their intimate relationship with the environment. Both women and men also paint their faces and bodies with white chalk from the riverbank for ritual occasions. A BBC television documentary called *Tribe* aired in 2004, highlighting the significance of body painting at the river in a nearby group called the Suri (Surma). The video sensationalized the body paint as part of a stick-fighting ceremony called *donga*.

A reason that is often given for the origin of this "disfiguring" lip plate practice comes from a 1938 report by British explorers who claimed that lip plates were originally worn to discourage slave traders. Given that lip plates have also been worn in other regions around the world and that it continues to the present day, this explanation seems unlikely. However, during the colonial period, the wearing of lip plates by Mursi women was identified as a "harmful cultural practice" on the grounds that piercing and stretching the lips introduced unnecessary health risks. A series of targeted interventions by the government in the last few decades have reduced the number of women wearing lip plates from 95 percent to 50 percent (LaTosky 2015). However, many anthropologists feel that these interventions into cultural practices are condescending and imperialistic. Ethnographic research shows that the Mursi are well aware of the health risks involved with lip stretching and that the women in these groups have traditional ways of preventing and curing infections, repairing torn lips, and avoiding dental problems (LaTosky 2015). The girls and women of the Mursi for whom this practice continues to have significance are largely left out of the debates about what is "best" for them. Some advocates suggest that the decisions about these women's bodies should be left to them.

During the 1930s, female members of the tribe were exhibited in the famous Ringling Brothers and Barnum & Bailey Circus. The sensation around the **exoticizing** of these women resulted in the derogatory term "Ubangi Savages," named for the Ubangi River in central Africa where the women were said to originate (Thomson 1996). In Central Africa, the process of lip stretching reportedly emulated the beaks of graceful water birds in the vicinity (Pitt Rivers Museum 2011).

Like many traditional pastoralist groups around the world, the Mursi have fallen on hard economic times in the last few decades, and the society is changing rapidly. Many young people leave the group to look for wage-based employment in the cities. Due in part to the extreme age differences between young women and their husbands, some young women and their lovers have fled rural life to the city (Simpson-Hebert 2005), where they pose for photographs by curious tourists with their lip plates on prominent display in order to earn much-needed money. Tourists can also book a six-hour round trip from Mago National Park to visit a Mursi village, take photographs (for an additional fee), and purchase chipped lip plates to take home as souvenirs. The various ways that Mursi are now in the unfortunate position of having to **perform** authenticity lends a dimension of concern to the "predatory" (Sontag 1979, cited in Turton) act of taking souvenir photographs.

See also: Exoticize; Kayapo; Performance/Performativity.

Further Reading

Abbink, Jon. 2009. "Suri Images: The Return of Exoticism and the Commodification of an Ethiopian 'Tribe.'" *Cahier d'études africaines* 4, no. 196: 893–924.

Geoffrey-Schneiter, Bérénice. 2006. *Vanishing Beauty: Indigenous Body Art and Decoration*, photography by Bertie and Dos Winkel. Munich, Germany: Prestel.

LaTosky, Shauna. 2004. "Reflections on the Lip-Plates of Mursi Women as a Source of Stigma and Self-esteem." In: *The Perils of Face: Essays on Cultural Contact, Respect and Self-Esteem in Southern Ethiopia*, edited by Ivo Strecker and Jean Lydall, 382–97. Lit Verlag, Germany: Münster.

LaTosky, Shauna L. 2015. "Lip-Plates, 'Harm' Debates, and the Cultural Rights of Mursi (Mun) Women." In: *Interrogating Harmful Cultural Practices: Gender, Culture, and Coercion*, edited by Chia Longman and Tamsin Bradley, 169–91. London: Routledge.

The Pitt Rivers Museum, University of Oxford. 2011. "Body Art: African Lip Plugs" [Web site]. Accessed July 1, 2016. http://web.prm.ox.ac.uk/bodyarts/index.php/permanent -body-arts/reshaping-and-piercing/158-african-lip-plugs.html.

Simpson-Hebert, Mayling. 2005. "Ethiopia's Pastoral Women Speak Out." University of Oxford [Web site]. Accessed July 1, 2016. http://dana.nonuniv.ox.ac.uk/pdf/ethiopian pastoralwomen.pdf.

Sontag, Susan. 1979. *On Photography*. New York: Penguin Books.

TatRing. 2016. "Traditional African Mursi Lip Plates." Accessed January 29, 2017. https:// tatring.com/piercing-   types/Have-Mursi-on-the-Lip-Plate.

Thomson, Rosemarie Garland. 1996. *Freakery: Cultural Spectacles of the Extraordinary Body*. New York: New York University Press.

Turton, David. 2004. "Lip-plates and 'The People Who Take Photographs': Uneasy Encounters between Mursi and Tourists in Southern Ethiopia." *Anthropology Today* 20, no. 3: 3–8.

LIPS

The ratio of lip size to other facial features was a crucial measurement in determining the "golden ratio" of beauty for the Greeks. Plastic surgeon Dr. Stephen Marquardt developed the "Marquardt Beauty Mask" through careful measurement and examination of symmetry in beautiful faces from classical paintings. He discovered that the ratio of phi (1.618) frequently repeats in the proportions of faces considered most beautiful around the world (for example, in ratios of the top of lips to the center of lips to the bottom of lips, and repeated in ratios from the nose flair to the bottom of lips to the bottom of the chin). The formula is used widely by professional aestheticians in order to make recommendations to clients looking for lip augmentations.

Despite Marquardt's evidence that idealized facial ratios are universal, there is some variation in cultures around the world regarding idealized lip size and shape. In some eras and in some cultures, large or fuller lips are preferred. This preference for larger lips can sometimes vary by gender as well. In ancient **Greece**, sculpture attests to the preference for cupid's-bow lips that were full, sleepy, and decadent with gently upturned corners and square bottom lips for both men and women. Large pink lips were the focus of many paintings of aristocratic beauties from the 1700s in France. The 1970s decade of free love and long hair also featured big, pouty lips made famous by Mick Jagger and American fashion models. In the 1990s, Julia Roberts' broad, expressive mouth set the standard for beauty with full-lipped smiles.

However, many cultures are less invested in the size of the lips, but more concerned with the ideal lip shape. In ancient **India**, a beautiful woman's lips were expected to be lush and in the shape of a rosebud as demonstrated in sculptures devoted to Parvati, the Hindi goddess of romance. This shape is still preferred in India, where Bollywood stars Aishwarya Rai and Priyanka Chopra set the standard for contemporary beauty with full lips that don't show a tip in the top curve. In Japan, women's lips were ideally "petal" shaped, slightly larger on the top lip than the bottom. During the 1500s in northern Europe, early Renaissance painters focused on smallish lips for women subjects, emphasizing instead a deep, expressive philtrum (or dip) in the upper lip. This trend continued into the 1600s, with Dutch painters emphasizing the distinction between the two lips, slightly parted.

In general, West African beauty standards align closely with ideals of good behavior, so that the word for "beauty" is often synonymous with the word for "good." However, many African cultures focus on mouths with prominent lips as one indicator of beauty. For example, the Mende of Sierra Leone prefer the mouths and lips (*nda*) of a woman to be smooth and free of blemishes and with breath that is fresh and sweet. Mende people like mouths to be full and well rounded, with a lip line that appears to be "cut" into a sharply defined shape (Boone 1986). They prefer lips that are not overly large or "blubbery" and also not too thin, which is regarded as an animalistic facial characteristic such as may be seen in monkeys. Mouths in general should be smiling. In general, most studies of beauty diversity within the United States find that African American women are less likely to hold uniform ideas of beauty than Latina or "white" women, and they are far more likely to describe beauty in terms of personality traits rather than physical ones (Landrine, Klonoff, and Brown-Collins 1992).

Lipstick, of course, exists to emphasize the prominence of the mouth and to shape the lips into a certain shape, to look larger or more beautiful. Women around the world and deep into history have augmented their lips with naturally occurring substances, as evidenced by archaeological evidence found in Egyptian burials. In the puritanical United States of the 1800s, marketing artificial lip colors to women was initially considered to be controversial because of the frank association between lips and implied sexuality (Peiss 2008). The task of the cosmetic industry was to make lipstick appear to be "natural." The famous Gibson Girl look from the late 1800s emphasized large lips with a high cupid's bow and plump volume of the lips. American "flappers" of the 1920s, the first women of the United States who could cast a vote, continued to exaggerate the "poutiness" of this look with a huge cupid's bow on the top lip and a matching, petulant bottom lip painted bright red. By the 1930s, lipstick had become a daily staple for most Euro-American women's beauty regimens (Peiss 2008). The 1950s Hollywood glamour era emphasized the bottom lip with bright lipstick to accentuate a wide, richly colored smile.

At other times or in other places, the emphasis placed on lips is less important. According to our understanding of art from ancient **Egypt**, ideal beauty standards highlighted strong facial symmetry of large eyes and regal, straight noses, but lips were not necessarily prominent. In ancient Nepal and the Ming Dynasty of **China**, women with dainty, small mouths were celebrated as the great beauties of their day. The illusion of a smaller mouth could be achieved with elaborate makeup that lined the darker shade of the lip with white in order to deemphasize the lip's natural shape. Art from medieval Europe attests to a preference for women with thin, barely visible lips that were not highlighted in any way with color. Following the pouty lips of the 1970s, American preference in the 1980s switched back to an emphasis on large, shiny, toothy smiles, with thinner, well-defined lips.

Kylie Jenner, from the popular reality television program *Keeping Up With the Kardashians*, became a prominent spokesperson for a dramatic "beestung" lip aesthetic in 2015 when she swept social media with the #kyliejennerchallenge. Thousands of fans posted their own versions of Jenner's recommended lip augmentation process, which consisted of creating an airlock around the lips using a shot glass or other glass container in order to swell both upper and lower lips to twice their size.

Female lips are, on average, a little bit fuller than male lips. Overly full male lips can cause facial features to appear "feminized." A number of factors can deflate lip fullness over time, including aging, sun damage, smoking, and hereditary factors. "Atrophic" lips are those that appear very thin, lacking anatomic distinctions, inflection points, and vermilion (the darker, reddish coloration of many lips). A range of **cosmetic** and surgical options exist to enhance lip size and shape. Most commonly, the lips can be surgically enhanced through injections of hyaluronic acid and polyacrylamide, called "fillers." Such options may also be used to treat perioral rhytides (lines that appear around the mouth, especially above the upper lip, which may cause the upper lip to look less prominent) and mentolabial folds (a fold or indentation between the lower lip and the chin, which may make the lower lip look less prominent).

See also: Body Modification; China; Greece; India; Lipstick and Lip Tattoos; Plastic Surgery.

Further Reading

Boone, Sylvia Arden. 1986. *Radiance in the Waters: Ideals of Feminine Beauty in Mende Art.* New Haven, CT: Yale University Press.

Elliott, Annabelle Fenwick. 2015. "Disturbing New Kyle Jenner Challenge Sees Teens Suck Shot Glasses to Blow Lips to Double Their Natural Size." Daily Mail (UK). April 20. Accessed January 29, 2017. http://www.dailymail.co.uk/femail/article-3047484 /Disturbing-new-Kylie-Jenner-challenge-sees-teens-suck-shot-glasses-blow-lips-double-size -disastrous-results.html

Jefferson, Deana L., and Jayne E. Stake. 2009. "Appearance Self-Attitudes of African American and European American Women: Media Comparisons and Internalization of Beauty Ideals." *Psychology of Women Quarterly* 33, no. 4: 396–409.

Landrine, Hope, Elizabeth A. Klonoff, and Alice Brown-Collins. 1992. "Cultural Diversity and Methodology in Feminist Psychology: Critique, Proposal, Empirical Example." *Psychology of Women Quarterly* 16, no. 2: 145–63.

Luthra, Amit. 2015. "Shaping Lips with Fillers." *Journal of Cutaneous and Aesthetic Surgery* 8, no. 3: 139–42.

Marquardt, Stephen. 2016. "Beauty Analysis." *Marquardt Beauty Analysis.* Accessed March 25, 2016. http://www.beautyanalysis.com.

Patton, Tracey Owens. 2006. "Hey Girl, Am I More Than My Hair? African American Women and Their Struggles with Beauty, Body Image, and Hair." *NWSA Journal* 18, no 2: 24–51.

Peiss, Kathy. 1998. *Hope in a Jar: The Making of America's Beauty Culture.* New York: Henry Holt

Thorpe, JR. "The Ideal Lips Throughout History, From the Ming Dynasty to Kim Kardashian." *Bustle.* Accessed March 25, 2016. http://www.bustle.com/articles/95689-the-ideal-lips -throughout-history-from-the-ming-dynasty-to-kim-kardashian.

LIPSTICK AND LIP TATTOOS

Lipstick has been made and used since prehistoric times from fruit and plant juices. Mesopotamian women crushed semiprecious stones and added them to an animal fat base to develop the first lipsticks. Women in the Indus Valley of India between BCE 3000 and 1500 used a purplish-red dye extracted from seaweed to create lipsticks. Ancient Chinese beauty seekers combined vermilion (which is actually a mercuric sulfide) and plant juices or animal blood to mineral wax and animal fat to create rouge for both the lips and cheeks. In ancient **Egypt**, lipstick was manufactured for use by the elites by crushing the bodies of cochineal insects to derive a carmine color (Lipstick History 2016). Sometimes they also added pearlescent fish scales to the mixture to promote shine. From the eighth until the twelfth century, Arab traders carried solid lipsticks based on the same technology, which allowed for **perfume** sticks to be rolled into special molds without melting (Ibid.). In the Western world, lipstick fell out of favor for everyone but prostitutes during the ultra-conservative medieval period; however, lipstick made a comeback under the reign of Elizabeth I of the **United Kingdom**, who encouraged her courtesans to dust their faces white and paint their lips a bright color. In 1884, the first modern lipstick was introduced by Parisian perfumers. It was made of deer tallow, castor oil, and beeswax and came wrapped in silk paper. By 1915, Maurice Levy, the French cosmetics entrepreneur, had figured out a way to sell lipstick in cylindrical metal tubes that had a tiny lever on the side to move the lipstick up the top of the case. The first swivel-up tube was patented by James Bruce Mason, Jr. of Nashville, Tennessee.

Initially, the use of lipstick in the United States was the most troubling for emerging cosmetic companies to promote. Considered the most artificial cosmetic in everyday use, it was negatively associated with sexual assertiveness (Peiss 1998, 154). A market for women's commodities rose up to underscore the national narrative of love and romance. In the wake of World War II, Max Factor, Jr. cited the efforts of women in other parts of the world to "keep up appearances," suggesting that American women continue to "beautify themselves according to the 'American plan' (Peiss 1998, 239). Women were doing men's work during the war, but **advertisements** from popular **magazines** like *Ladies' Home Journal* encouraged women to continue to wear cosmetics to symbolize "the precious right of women to be feminine and lovely—under any circumstances" (Ibid., 240). Even the All-American Girls Professional Baseball League, organized during the war in the absence of male players, ordered the women ballplayers to take makeup lessons from Helena Rubenstein.

In the meantime, chemists were experimenting with new technologies to make lipstick more durable and longer lasting. Hazel Bishop invented an indelible lipstick that was marketed widely under the tag line, "Stays on you, not on him." The product also promised that the lipstick need not be regularly reapplied, so a woman could "wake up beautiful" (Peiss 1998, 247). Women's sexual allure became more openly and heavily celebrated, to the degree that women were expected to act upon their desire for a man by making themselves beautiful and thus drawing his attention. In 1952, Revlon introduced the Fire and Ice Line of lipstick colors promising results for consumers "who love to flirt with fire, who dare to skate upon thin ice." The advertising campaign is widely credited for changing the sexual resonance of cosmetic advertising to a more frank appraisal of women's sexual agency (Peiss 1998, 249). The Fire and Ice campaign featured a fantasy of a "high class tramp" paired with "a really nice girl." The advertising copy included unexpectedly provocative questionnaires about women's desire for sensual pleasure, their adventurousness, and their iconoclasm: "Do you dance with your shoes off? Do you secretly hope that the next man you meet will be a psychiatrist? If tourist flights were running would you take a trip to Mars?" The Fire and Ice color palette, paired with nail polishes, were dark red and dramatic, changing only slightly from season to season in order to produce an array of beauty product "must-haves." The therapeutic appeal of the cosmetics industry allowed the average American woman to own ten or more tubes of lipstick, each one compelling her to continually interrogate, experiment with, and renew her looks (Peiss 1998, 252).

A chairman of the board for the Estee Lauder cosmetic company coined the term "the lipstick index" to describe the increased sale of cosmetics during the global recession of the early 2000s. He claimed that lipstick sales worked as an economic indicator, inversely correlated to the economic health of the nation. The assumption of such a claim is that during times of economic crisis, consumers will splurge on small luxuries designed to make themselves feel better, at least temporarily (The Economist 2009). Commentators and trend watchers also note a similar rise in the sales of nail polish. A similar phenomenon was noted in the United Kingdom again in 2016, when voters cast ballots to leave the European Union, launching an anxious period of economic instability (Hall 2016).

Lip gloss was first introduced by Max Factor in 1930 as a way to introduce shimmer to the lips of black and white film actresses. Lip gloss allows for more subdued colors and a more natural look, as well as for protection from the sun, wind, and water. In the 1970s, lip gloss got a boost when the Bonnie Bell company added flavor to their lip glosses and marketed them to teenage girls.

In some cultures, in order to accentuate the mouth, it is not the lips that are colored, but the gums. Gingival **tattoos**, or dying the gums, have been common in some cultures since ancient times in order to make the teeth appear whiter and give the smile more of a dazzling effect. In Senegal and other parts of West Africa, the coloring agents for the striking gingival tattoo treatment comes from a powder obtained by burned oil and shea butter (Stewart 2013). The tattoos typically have to be applied over a long period and can be extremely painful. It is also believed that the procedure protects the health of the mouth. Sometimes, a silver tooth is also added to accent the darkened colors of the gums.

See also: Advertising; Egypt; Lips; Magazines; Makeup and Cosmetics; Perfume and Scented Oils; Tattoos; United Kingdom.

Further Reading

The Economist. 2009. "Lip Service: What Lipstick Sales Tell You about the Economy." Accessed October 1, 2016. http://www.economist.com/node/12998233.

Hall, Victoria. 2016. "Why the Beauty Industry Is Booming Post-Brexit." *Telegraph*. Accessed October 1, 2016. http://www.telegraph.co.uk/beauty/make-up/why-the-beauty-industry -is-booming-post-brexit.

Lipstick History. 2016. "Lipstick History and Facts." Accessed October 1, 2016. http://www .lipstickhistory.com.

Peiss, Kathy. 1998. *Hope in a Jar: The Making of America's Beauty Culture*. New York: Owl Books.

Stewart, Dodai. 2013. "Meet the Women Who Tattoo Their Gums Black for a More Beautiful Smile." *Jezebel*. Accessed October 1, 2016. http://jezebel.com/5972634/meet-the -women-who-tattoo-their-gums-black-for-a-more-beautiful-smile.

LONG EARLOBES

Earlobes are commonly pierced in many cultures. Archaeological evidence shows that people have worn wood, stone, horn, bone, fossilized materials such as amber, and bamboo as **jewelry** in ear piercings for thousands of years. Other items used as jewelry, including shells, teeth, or claws, were also used by some cultures to beautify the self by accentuating the earlobe and, sometimes, to symbolize certain exceptional qualities or accomplishments of the individual. Red hornbill earrings, which are long and graceful and extend from the upper lobe to the lower lobe, were traditionally only worn to draw attention to and beautify the accomplishments of Ilongot warriors of the Philippines who had taken a head of another person (Rosaldo 1986).

Many images of the Siddhartha (also known as Gautama Buddha) feature his long, stretched ears. As an aristocratic prince of the Shakya clan of India, the Buddha wore heavy gold earrings during his youth to emphasize his worldly riches and high social status. After his enlightenment under the Bodhi tree at the age of 35, the Buddha practiced asceticism and removed the expensive earrings, allowing his ears to be free of the symbols of earthly wealth, though his earlobes remained stretched.

Over time, heavy earrings may stretch the earlobe, a look that might be preferred or discouraged in the society. In some cultures, intentional earlobe stretching is practiced in combination with piercing using a variety of techniques. "Tapering" is a practice of progressively increasing the size of a hole in the ear which in turn, extends the length of the lobe. Tapering involves the use of a conical rod that is inserted into the existing hole and creates a gradual stretching of the area without the risk of tearing, bleeding, or scar tissue formation. "Scalpelling" is a technique that

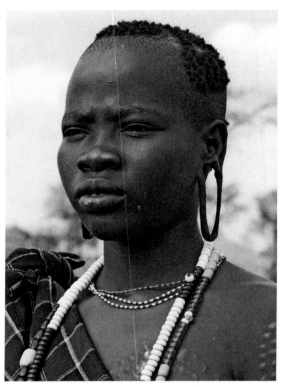

A Mursi tribal woman with elongated earlobes, Mago National Park, southern Ethiopia. (Antonella865/Dreamstime.com)

dramatically increases the size of a piercing without necessarily adding to the length of the lobe. It relies on a scalpel or other sharp implement to cut at the edges of the existing hole in order to increase the diameter of the hole without stretching the ear. "Dead stretching" is another technique designed to lengthen the earlobe through massaging, tugging, or pulling at jewelry present in the piercing. The weight of the jewelry is often progressively increased in order to work with gravity to drag the length of the lobe down to the desired dimensions. In most cultures where stretching is a preferred practice, the process extends over the life course, as the skin naturally sags with age and becomes more amenable to stretching. Care is taken not to rip the flesh but to allow the lobes to descend gradually. With patience and a lifetime of effort, the highest-ranking and eldest members of the group are those with the most exaggerated stretched lobes.

The Maya intentionally stretched their piercings to accommodate ear plugs, which in turn lengthened the lobe. In Western cultures, neotribal aesthetics frequently focus on ear plugs, cylindrical jewelry that penetrates the earlobe and sometimes flares on one or both ends. Intentional earlobe stretching can also be seen among the Mursi of Ethiopia, the Maasai of Kenya and Tanzania, and the West African Fulani. Usually, the ears are fitted with long lengths of beads, which may be removed when not required for ceremonial or ritual occasions. The practice was also historically observed by Karenic women of Myanmar.

See also: Jewelry; Maya.

Further Reading

Rosaldo, Renato. 1986. "Red Hornbill Earrings: Ilongot Ideas of Self, Beauty and Health." *Cultural Anthropology* 1, no. 3: 310–16.

Urban Body Jewelry.com. 2016. "Ear Stretching Guide." Urban Body Jewelry [Web site]. Accessed June 15, 2016. https://www.urbanbodyjewelry.com/ear-stretching-guide.

MAASAI

The Maasai are a pastoralist people of East Africa, living primarily in Kenya and Tanzania. The Maasai concept of wealth, "enkishon," means to be blessed with sons and daughters, especially to care for old age. The central idioms for a successful Maasai life focus on living harmoniously within a large network of kin and raising abundant, healthy cattle.

Male beauty is highly prized by the Maasai. An old Maa expression states, "A man's head is worth an ox." Between the ages of 18 and 35, young warriors (called *moran*) undergo extensive rites of passage that involve painful circumcision and seclusion. This period prior to marriage also involves a prolonged training to be a warrior. Young men live outside the village with other young men, roaming the savannah, rustling any available cattle, and seducing young girls and sometimes the young wives of the village elders.

Highly aware of the value of looking good in order to attract women, young warriors grow their **hair** long as a symbol of youth and vitality, and treat it liberally with a red **pomade** made from a mixture of red ochre and animal fat. They also decorate their bodies with ritual chalk patterns, which may symbolize animals of the savannah, including zebras and lions. Warriors wear a dazzling assortment of beaded belts and necklaces, which they receive as gifts from women. To ward off the cold nights spent outdoors, they wear

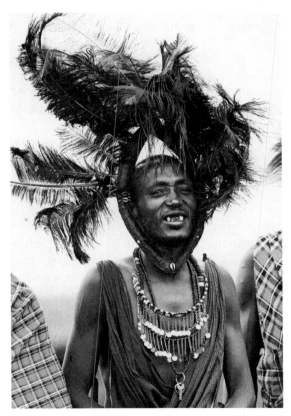

A Maasai warrior in ostrich-feather headdress and decoration, Kenya. Male beauty is highly prized by the Maasai. Young men prepare their hair and wear beaded belts and necklaces to enhance their masculine good looks. (Digistockpix/Dreamstime.com)

thick blankets made of red cotton called *olkarasha*, or *shuka*. For important ceremonies and rituals, warriors who have earned the right also top off their colorful garb with *enjuraru*, a crown made of ostrich feathers, or *olawaru*, a "crown" made from a lion's mane that is worn around the face to resemble the facial hair of the predator.

Many men look back at the years they spent as warriors with nostalgia. As a man matures, he gradually finds himself in the financial position to take a wife and settle down to live within the village. At these *eunoto* ceremonies, held every seven years to mark the maturity of a group of warriors, the heads of the men are shaved and rubbed liberally with ochre and animal fat. Men leave behind the flamboyant trappings of youth and receive much simpler ornaments to wear, including ceremonial "flyswatters" that are symbolic of rank and authority, made of gnu hair (Winkel 2006). Older men, especially those with many wives and offspring, are highly revered, known as *laibon*.

The lives of young girls are quite leisurely. They are not required to do a great deal of work, but they spend time with the attractive young warriors who camp outside the village. Prior to marriage, young girls may engage in intimacies with the warriors, but they must take care not to become pregnant, which could lower their brideprice (Llewelyn-Davies 1974).

Marriages among the Maasai are arranged and ultimately organize important property rights over animals. In Maasai, to be married means "to be led." On her first day in the village, a new bride is blessed by her father-in-law and white clay is applied to her face. She also receives nine perfect cows from her husband's herd to form the core of the herd that her sons will someday inherit.

In preparation for marriage, a girl is excised (undergoes ceremonial clitoridectomy) and her head is shaved. Special branches from sacred trees are brought to her house to mark the place where the girl is recovering from circumcision. She gives away her distinctive *emangeki* **jewelry** (large, flat, circular necklaces made of small glass (or plastic) beads arranged in brightly colored, graphic designs) to her sister in order to mark the transformation of her status from a daughter to a wife. The necklaces may also include buttons or small, hammered pieces of aluminum in distinctive triangular or circular shapes. The colors of the *emangeki* necklaces may contain symbolic messages of beauty or seduction, and wealthy women may come to own many of these necklaces, often given as gifts. For the wedding ceremony, the bride's mother and father are smeared with red ochre. Later, at the climax of the ceremony, the mother will anoint the feet of the guests with butter while the father will put on women's necklaces and ask for the blessings of the male guests.

Girls are often married to men much older than themselves, and so they often pursue romantic liaisons with young warriors. Young women compose songs about their lovers: "My lover has soft lines around his neck. His mouth is strong, his hair is beautiful . . . He doesn't churn about in his sleep, he just lays straight not turning to the wall" (Llewelyn-Davies 1974).

Both men and women of the Maasai observe extensive earlobe stretching, which they accentuate with strands of small, colorful beads in red, black, green, and white. Women with adult sons also wear highly prestigious brass spirals (surutia) to mark their importance within the community. Grandmothers wear red beaded earrings through their upper ears (Winkel 2006).

Similar stylings can also be found among the Maasai's pastoralist neighbors, the Samburu and the Rendile. Like many other indigenous peoples around the world, the legendary photogeneity of the Maasai attracts tourists and presents both economic opportunity as well as unique challenges to the integrity of their cultural identity (Bruner 2001). A wide range of options for interacting with the Maasai exist, from exploitive top-down corporate tours to grassroots eco-lodges that are managed by the people at the village level. It is essential to investigate these options responsibly (Bruner 2001).

See also: Hair; Jewelry; Pomade.

Further Reading

Bruner, Edward M. 2001. "The Maasai and the Lion King: Authenticity, Nationalism and Globalization in African Tourism." *American Ethnologist* 28, no. 4, 881–908.

Llewelyn-Davies, Melissa. 1974. *Disappearing Worlds: Maasai Women*. Film. Royal Anthropological Institute.

Winkel, Bertie and Dos Winkel. 2006. *Vanishing Beauty*. Amsterdam: Prestel.

MAGAZINES

Magazines are periodical publications that typically appeal to a certain group or interest, featuring articles and illustrations. Beauty and fashion magazines represent one of the most dominant markets for magazines in the United States today, with subcategories to appeal to women of different ages, races, and social classes.

Though men typically dominate the media in the United States, women have been active participants in publishing since the beginning of the nation. During the 19th century, the public press increased and women continue to exert clear, if restricted, influence (Sapiro 1999, 244). This period saw the rise of what we know today as the "mass media," and women were successful at attracting a mass readership that was influenced by its publications by exploiting feminine identity and influencing the 19th-century culture of moralism (Douglas 1977). Women contributors both created and reinforced a "cult of true womanhood," which emphasized supposedly "traditional" female qualities, including piety, purity, domesticity, and submissiveness, in the interest of creating ideal wives and mothers.

The early women's magazines in the United States were not feminist or politicized, though they did generally support women's suffrage. Rather, these early women's magazines set standards as the arbiters of good taste in terms of fashion and a well-groomed appearance. One of the first truly mass-circulation magazines was *Godey's Lady's Book* (1837–1897), which was edited by Sara Josepha Hale (1788–1879) who sought to emulate Queen Victoria of England. The magazine is widely credited with being the most influential popularizer of symbolism surrounding the pious "white wedding," following Queen Victoria's choice to wear a white gown for her marriage to Prince Albert in 1840. The magazine was so influential that it petitioned heavily to establish Thanksgiving as a U.S. national holiday, offering recipes and

> "Although beauty may be in the eye of the beholder, the feeling of being beautiful exists solely in the mind of the beheld."
>
> —MARTHA BECK

decorating tips for quintessential Thanksgiving-day foods such as roasted turkey with stuffing and pumpkin pie. Considered the "Queen of the Monthlies" and published in Philadelphia, its circulation reached 150,000 issues by 1860. Though the magazine included poems and essays, it was probably best known for its featured hand-tinted color fashion plates, which included patterns for a stylish garment that could be sewn at home. The magazine was avidly consumed by women across the country. Today, plates from the magazine sell as expensive collector's items.

The first magazine designed explicitly for African American women was Juli Ringwood Coston's *Ringwood's Afro-American Journal of Fashion*, begun in Cleveland, Ohio, in 1891 (Sapiro 1999). The twelve-page journal treated topics of homemaking, etiquette, grooming, and fashion and had a yearly subscription fee of $1.25 (Allen 2005). Many of the magazines aimed at African American women were important for introducing consumers to the products of **Madam C. J. Walker**, the entrepreneur whose innovations revolutionized hair care products for black women.

Today, many—if not most—magazines are aimed at gender-segregated markets (Shapiro 1999), making it possible to speak of "women's" magazines. The so-called "Seven Sisters" are long-running women's service magazines that occasionally offer nutritional or fashion advice, but mostly focus on the role of women as homemakers, including *Better Homes and Gardens*, *Family Circle*, *Good Housekeeping*, *Ladies' Home Journal*, *McCall's* (no longer in publication), *Redbook*, and *Woman's Day*. Fashion and style magazines also target women, with special emphasis on achieving and maintaining a particular appearance. The best sellers in this category are *Cosmopolitan*, *Glamour*, *Harper's Bazaar*, *Vogue*, and relative newcomer *Marie Claire*. Women's magazines, largely successful because of large **advertising** revenues, continue to be shaped by and to sell views of women based on gender, race, and class stereotypes (McCracken 1993). Advertisers require the content of women's style magazines to serve their needs, and many emphasize striving for a standard of beauty that is impossible for most women to achieve or maintain. Women's magazines make a large proportion of women readers feel unhappy with themselves, ugly, or fat (Sapiro 1999, 257). A great deal of psychological and sociological literature suggests that continual exposure to advertisements and magazine spreads that depict difficult-to-achieve idealized forms of beauty can contribute to feelings of dissatisfaction on the part of women consumers and viewers.

There is also a large and lucrative subcategory of the "women's magazine" that features beauty and style advice for teen women. The oldest of these publications is *Seventeen*, which began circulation in 1944. A study of *Seventeen* magazine in 1951, 1971, and 1991 showed that roughly one-third of the content consistently focuses on beauty advice (Budgeon and Currie 1995).

"Men's magazines" also represent a vibrant publishing category. Since the World War II era, "men's magazines" were often synonymous with "adult" pornographic magazines, like *Playboy*. Since then, a new generation of men's magazines (*Maxim, Esquire, GQ, Men's Fitness, Men's Journal*) has emerged combining advice on lifestyle with ideas for fashion and grooming. In some cases, this emerging set of ideals about **masculinity** overlaps with the figure of the **metrosexual** male consumer. Launched in 1987, *Men's Health* is one of several men's "beauty" magazines that focuses on fashion, health, and lifestyle and gives readers a view of masculinity in keeping with an idealized image. As "windows to the future self" (Alexander 2003, 541), the models in these men's lifestyle magazines strike active poses, appearing alongside advice devoted to developing arm, pectoral, and "six-pack" abdominal muscles. Content analysis of the magazine reveals that 23 percent of essays and features deal with creating a hard body and 21 percent give advice on nutrition, diet, and fat reduction (Alexander 2003, 544).

Evidence also suggests that many of the conventions of Western beauty standards presented in U.S.-based magazines are influential in the ways that consumers in other parts of the world perceive beauty (Yan and Bissell 2014). The presence of an "ideal" body type as presented in magazines can predict lower self-esteem in women around the world (Balcetis et al. 2013).

Since its introduction in 1888, the well-known magazine *National Geographic* has set a tone for extensive pictorial representations of other cultures, often paying especially close attention to "exotic" practices of beauty, grooming, or styling that differed from mainstream American ideals. At its peak, *National Geographic* had a global circulation of 12 million copies circulated in nearly 40 local-language editions. Some critics argue that the photographers, editors, and designers of *National Geographic* magazine intentionally select images and text to produce a misrepresentative interpretation of race, gender, privilege, and modernity, particularly in the ways that non-Western women's beauty comes to reinforce notions of difference (Lutz and Collins 1993). Immediately following World War II, many visual representations of non-Western women in the magazine were depicted as dark skinned, bare breasted, sexually licentious, and **exotic** in ways that (re)inscribed troubling distinctions of imperialism, empire, and racism. "Sensual" women, often topless, were photographed dancing or posed with elaborate flower headdresses, to emphasize narratives about a "savage beauty" or "innocent sexuality" in ways designed to eroticize non-Western women and appeal to Western curiosity about **the Other.**

See also: Advertising; Exoticism; Masculinity; Metrosexual; The "Other"; Walker, Madame C. J.

Further Reading

Alexander, Susan M. 2003. "Stylish Hard Bodies: Branded Masculinity in *Men's Health Magazine*." *Sociological Perspectives* 46, no. 4: 535–54.

Allen, Patricia. 2005. "Newly Discovered Magazines Reveal Vital Information on Early Black Women's Issues." *News at Princeton*. March 24. Accessed August 31, 2016. https://www.princeton.edu/main/news/archive/S11/16/94I92.

Balcetis, Emily, Shana Cole, Marie B. Chelberg, and Mark Alicke. 2013. "Searching Out the Ideal: Awareness of Ideal Body Standards Predicts Lower Global Self-Esteem in Women." *Self and Identity* 12, no. 1: 99–113.

Budgeon, Shelley, and Dawn H. Currie. 1995. "From Feminism to Postfeminism: Women's Liberation in Fashion Magazines." *Women's Studies International Forum* 18: 173–86.

Douglas, Ann. 1977. *The Feminization of American Culture*. New York: Knopf.

Lutz, Catherine A., and Jane L. Collins. 1993. *Reading National Geographic*. Chicago: University of Chicago Press.

McCracken, Ellen. 1993. *Decoding Women's Magazines: From Mademoiselle to Ms*. New York: St. Martin's Press.

Sapiro, Virginia. 1999. *Women in American Society*, 4th edition. Mountain View, CA: Mayfield Publishing Company.

Yan, Yan, and Kim Bissell. 2014. "The Globalization of Beauty: How Is Ideal Beauty Influenced by Globally Published Fashion and Beauty Magazines? *Journal of Intercultural Communication Research* 43, no. 3: 194–214.

MAKEUP AND COSMETICS

The human use of pigment to alter the appearance of skin for the purposes of enhancing beauty and creating an impression is thousands of years old. Contemporary "makeup" to hide skin's flaws, redden lips, and darken eyelashes is just the latest version of a practice that may date back as far as 40,000 years (Etcoff 2000. Whether as a health aid, to highlight elements of beauty to appeal more to potential mates, or to project power, cosmetics have both a long history and a significant place in ancient and modern world cultures.

> "I'm no natural beauty. If I'm gonna have any looks at all, I'm gonna have to create them."
>
> —DOLLY PARTON

Some of the earliest uses of makeup were on warriors and soldiers, who sought to project fierceness and power by creating scary designs on their bodies and faces. In Africa and South America, many groups used pigments to cover themselves in bright and distinctive designs when going to war or going hunting (Kent 2004).

Cosmetics have also been used to protect and heal the skin and body. The ancient Egyptian use of a heavy pigment around the eyes, as well as bright colors for eyelids, is believed to have been a way of protecting the eyes from the harsh North African sun (Kent 2004). In this same period, more than 3,000 years ago, the Egyptians used animal fat, olive oil, and nut oils as moisturizers for the skin (Etcoff 2000). This trend only continued, as in later centuries in Europe the use of homemade creams to protect and relieve dry skin became common (Kent 2004).

Women in Asia were among the first to widely use cosmetics for the sole purpose of enhancing beauty and appeal by highlighting and enhancing coloration that was considered "beautiful" in the 12th and 13th centuries. In China, as the beauty norms of the time preferred red lips, cheeks, and nostrils, women used red dye to accentuate those features. As the society also preferred smooth white skin, the ladies made copious use of rice flour to lighten their complexions and hide wrinkles (Kent 2004). This color palette of red and white has also been favored in Japan for centuries, where women as early as the ninth century used rouge made from the extract of safflower to color lips, cheeks, and fingernails (Etcoff 2000).

In the Americas, the first Spanish explorers in the Caribbean encountered both men and women who decorated their bodies with paint, and in what is now

Mexico, Hernán Cortez discovered Aztec women using axin to soothe and color their skin and jojoba oil on their hair. Further contact with the people of South America also revealed that the Quechua (commonly called Inca) people regularly and widely used face powder and lip color (Kent 2004). French explorers in the South Pacific reported that women used blue paint to accentuate their buttocks (Broby-Johansen 1968, 15).

In India and Pakistan, one of the most common cosmetics since the 12th century is a red powder known as *mahindi*, or henna. Henna is mixed with water, oil, or juice and applied to the skin in elaborate designs. The result is a stain that will mark the top layer of skin, and so the designs then last up to four weeks. Whereas henna is most commonly used to beautify the hands and arms of women on their wedding day, in modern times, henna is used for a wide variety of special occasions and as a fashion statement in Southeast Asia (Arthur 2000).

For centuries, cosmetics and makeup tended to be homemade preparations, family recipes handed down from generation to generation, until the late 19th and early 20th centuries, when a makeup industry appeared. "Pearl powder" was used to give the complexion a brilliant glow that also reflected light. However, the product was misnamed, as it was not made from pearls, but rather a subchloride of bismuth that injured the skin by producing paralysis of the blood vessels beneath the surface. Additionally, bismuth reacts violently with sulfur, which was frequently present in the air near a coal fire or gas lighting, causing disastrous effects for ladies of the Victorian era (Downing 2012, 37). In one of the first examples of celebrity endorsements, the curvy 19th-century actress Lillie Langtry put her name to the best-selling "Lillie Powder," a tinted concoction of talc carmine and sienna worked into melted lanolin with a hint of violet perfume and worn to disguise blemishes on the face.

Lipstick was invented and first sold in France in 1910 (Etcoff 2000). Emphasizing plump, youthful **lips** is a common beauty technique in many cultures across time and space. At this time, however, makeup was often considered a threat to morality, and its use was limited to actresses, prostitutes, and other women with lower social standing (Jones 2010).

The use of makeup in the 19th century in Europe and the Americas was often considered vain, provocative, and a sign of loose morals (Kent 2004). This association of cosmetics with vanity and deceit likely springs from the notion that inner beauty is reflected in outer appearance, and that clear white skin, with rosy lips and cheeks is a marker of both health and wealthy family lineage (Nichols 2016). To use cosmetics to mimic those features would be "cheating," a sign

---

Axin

Whereas the natural skin tone of the Aztecs in pre-Colombian Mexico was a brown or bronze color, the most fashionable and desirable shade for a woman's was yellow. Therefore, women in Aztec society often rubbed their cheeks with bitumen, yellowish clay, to achieve that color. From at least the 15th century, Aztec women also produced and used a cosmetic called axin. Axin is a waxy, yellowish ointment that was created by cooking and crushing the bodies of fat-producing insects such as the timber tree fly. The ointment was used on the face to create the yellow shade, but also on the lips and skin to avoid and heal chapping.

of both vanity and dishonesty. Attitudes slowly began to change for older women, but the cultural consensus remained firm that young women and girls should be protected from the vanity and loose morals of cosmetics (Downing 2012, 44).

Mascara was invented in 1913 as an improvement upon lampblack, which had formerly been used to darken eyelashes. T. L. Williams, a young chemist in Philadelphia, is responsible for developing the first cake mascara that would emphasize lashes without smudging or clogging. He named the product "Maybelline," after his sister. By 1917, he had patented and packaged the formula and was successfully selling mascara in great quantities by mail order. The cake mascara, which had to be moistened (sometimes with saliva) could be difficult to apply with the small straight brush, but many admired the exotic results, especially when combined with a flat line of kohl around the edges of the eye and a well-defined brow. The exaggerated smoky eye look of actress Theda Bara as *Cleopatra* in the early 20th century coincided with the discovery of Tutankhamen's tomb in **Egypt** in 1923 and popularized a fashionable silhouette look for women that emphasized a heavily made-up eye. It wasn't until the late 1940s that Helena Rubinstein introduced the first liquid "automatic" mascara that came in a tube with a spiral brush (Downing 2012).

As mentioned, during the late 19th and early 20th centuries, commercially produced cosmetics often contained dangerous substances such as lead or mercury. As the 20th century progressed, the production and sale of makeup by companies developed into a whole global beauty industry that maintained stricter quality control. Over the 20th century, Paris and New York emerged as the two centers of the global makeup and cosmetics trade, and in 2010, a French (L'Oreal) and U.S. (Proctor & Gamble) multinational company were still the biggest on the planet, accounting for more than 20 percent of all global cosmetics sales (Jones 2010).

Today, cosmetics are sold widely in a variety of stores around the world, from department stores and pharmacies to

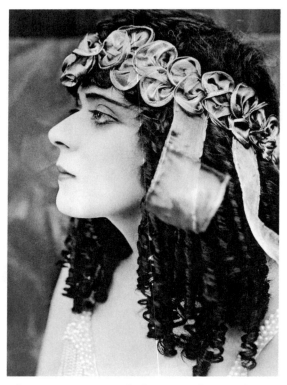

Silent movie actress Theda Bara, whose nickname was "The Vamp," is captured here in the title role of *Cleopatra* (1917). Her dramatic makeup would help inspire a fashion trend in the 1920s that featured heavily made-up eyes. (Bettmann/Getty Images)

shops that specialize in makeup and cosmetics. Additionally, in-person direct sales are still a huge market for cosmetics across the globe. Avon, a direct-sales operation in which women sell to other women (and men) was a $11.3 billion business in 2010, and the South American makeup and perfume company Yanbal reported more than $125 million in revenue in 2006 (de Casanova 2011).

Although the use of cosmetics is often associated in the current century with women, it is worth remembering that paint and color have been used just as widely by men throughout history. In the 1920s, both skin care and hair care products were introduced for men and were widely used in Europe and the United States. The Depression and postwar period dampened the men's market; however, in the late 20th and early 21st centuries there has been a resurgence in the production and sales of men's cosmetics. Multinational companies that target men, such as Unilever, Gillette, or Hugo Boss, market their hair care, skin care, and shaving products as well as their cologne in hypermasculine environments worldwide, such as auto races or bull fights (Jones 2010).

Some of the strongest markets for men's cosmetics are in Asia. Skin care products such as moisturizers and skin whiteners sell very well in Asian nations, and the 21st century found a new trend in Japanese and South Korean men of purchasing colored cosmetics designed to make men look more delicate. Foundation, eyelash tints such as mascara, and lip color for men began to sell well in those nations in the 2000s (Jones 2010). In South Korea, perfectly smooth and light skin was seen to be a prerequisite for landing a job and having professional success for men, an attitude that helped drive cosmetics sales (T. F. 2016).

In the 21st century, the makeup and cosmetics industries are high-tech and fast-moving entities that are continually working to create new and more effective products to help both men and women. Asian companies now lead the way in much cosmetics research, including what are known as BB (blemish balm) and CC (color correcting) creams, which look and feel like tinted moisturizer, while using natural ingredients to even skin tone (Payne 2014). Lip plumpers, or products designed to increase the appearance and size of the lips by using cinnamon or ginger, were also a significant trend in 2016 (Drug Store News 2016). In the meantime, even more fantastical treatments, like an invisible, wearable polymer "skin" worn on the face to cover wrinkles, were in development (Adee 2016).

See also: China; Egypt; India; Perfumes and Scented Oils; South Korea; Wrinkles.

Further Reading

Adee, Sally. 2016. "Paste On Beauty that's Skin Deep." *New Scientist* 230, no. 3073: 8–9.

Arthur, Lisa. 2000. "Henna Salon." *Arts & Activities* 127, no. 5: 27, 66.

Broby-Johansen, Rudolf. 1968 *Body and Clothes: An Illustrated History of Costume*. Translated from the Danish by Erik I. Friis and Karen Rush. New York: Reinhold Book Corporation.

de Casanova, Masi. 2011. *Making Up the Difference: Women, Beauty and Direct Selling in Ecuador*. Austin, TX: University of Texas Press.

Downing, Sarah Jane. 2012. *Beauty and Cosmetics, 1550–1950*. Oxford, England: Shire Library.

Drug Store News. 2016. "Lip Treatments, Plumpers Inflate Sales." *Drug Store News* 38, no. 1: 16.

Etcoff, Nancy. 2000. *Survival of the Prettiest: The Science of Beauty.* New York: Anchor.

Jones, Geoffrey. 2010. *Beauty Imagined: A History of the Global Beauty Industry.* Oxford, England: OUP.

Kent, Jacqueline C. 2004. *Business Builders in Cosmetics.* Minneapolis: Oliver Press.

Nichols, Elizabeth. 2016. *Beauty, Virtue, Power and Success in Venezuela 1850–2015.* New York: Lexington.

Payne, Leah. 2014. "New Beauty Trends." *Alive: Canada's Natural Health & Wellness Magazine* no. 375: 79–83.

T. F. 2016. "Glam Guys." *Teen Vogue* 16, no. 5 (June): 56.

MALE GAZE

In the 1940s, French existentialist philosopher Simone de Beauvoir argued that beauty rituals and elegance were a waste of time for women and required a great deal of money, time, and care, thus deflecting their energies away from other pursuits that might have implications for their quality of life. She observed that whereas male identity was achieved through projects of self-transcendence, for women, the main avenue for self-realization was through the cultivation of their appearance and the appreciation of men. Because women often find themselves in cultural settings where there is no opportunity for creative expression, women instead become self-absorbed in their own looks, cultivating themselves in order to be rewarded by men in their lives for achieving the right kind of attractiveness (Negrin 2008). Because women are admired for their looks rather than their achievements, women become passive objects of what art historians first termed the male gaze.

In his essay "The Eye of the Beholder," social theorist and philosopher Michel Foucault argued, "[T]here is no need for arms, physical violence, material constraints. Just a gaze. An inspecting gaze, a gaze which each individual under its weight will end by interiorizing to the point that he is his own overseer, each individual thus exercising this surveillance over, and against, himself" (1980,155).

Following Foucault, art historian Laura Mulvey coined the term in 1975 to refer to the perspective of the (usually) heterosexual man behind the camera, responsible for the ways that a camera might focus on the sensuous details of a woman's body, including her **cleavage**, her curves, her **buttocks**, or her legs. Looking at others is pleasurable. Looking can create feelings of sexual desire, which Mulvey identifies as "scopophilia" (borrowing this term from Freud).

Mulvey argued that the single male responsible for engineering the direction and the context of the gaze is actually part of a larger cultural perspective on how to view women's bodies. Images of women are often complicit in flattening out the complexity of women's lives to create a **narcissistic** fantasy, wherein the viewer (the subject) is an active participant and the "viewee," typically a woman (the object), is passive. The power relationship of this encounter is entirely one-sided, as the viewer can choose how to gaze at the object, how to use those images for his own purposes or pleasure, and how to render her body into a series of disembodied "parts," which can then be assessed, judged, and evaluated by the viewer. Mulvey says that the filmmaker invites the viewer of the film to see the object (the woman) the same way that he does, through the male gaze, and that through this complicity in looking, the woman may be rendered into an erotic object without desires or feelings or agency of her own. Rather, she is there to be looked at by the male gaze.

Even though it's called "the male gaze," it's important to keep in mind that this term labels a technique of power. It is not necessary to be male, straight, or gay to participate in the power of the gaze or to suffer from the dehumanization that such a technique perpetuates. The male gaze can be easily internalized by other woman, too, as they participate in the framing of the female object as part of a fantasy, even as they identify with that object. Similarly, men can also be objects of the male gaze when deconstructed as sexual objects by other men. Women may also be a dehumanized part of the homosexual male gaze, as demonstrated by crude or misogynistic representations of female artists in the popular media (Cruz 2015).

See also: Butts and Booty; Décolletage; Narcissism.

Further Reading

Cruz, Eliel. 2015. "Male Gays and the Male Gaze." *The Advocate*. Accessed October 1, 2016. http://www.advocate.com/commentary/2015/01/26/op-ed-male-gays-and-male-gaze.

De Beauvoir, Simone. 1949. *The Second Sex*. New York: Random House.

Foucault, Michel. 1975. *Discipline and Punish: The Birth of the Prison*. Translated by Alan Sheridan. New York: Pantheon.

Foucault, Michel. 1980. "The Eye of the Beholder." In: *Power/Knowledge: Selected Interviews and Other Writings 1972–1977*, edited by Colin Gordo. New York: Vintage.

Mulvey, Laura. 1975. Visual Pleasure and Narrative Cinema. *Screen* 16, no. 3: 6–18.

Negrin, Llewellyn. 2008. *Appearance and Identity: Fashioning the Body in Postmodernity*. New York: Palgrave Macmillan.

MANICURE

A manicure is a cosmetic treatment of the hands, especially the fingernails. Manicures involve moisturizing of the skin and nails; maintenance of the cuticle and nail bed; and trimming, shaping, polishing, or other adornment of the nails. In the United States, manicures are often performed at nail **salons**, which report more than $6 billion in sales annually (Kang 2010, 38). The growth in the number of nail salons in the United States by 60 percent between 1993 and 2003 indicates that American women are increasingly heading to nail salons to enjoy the self-pampering luxury of a "mani-pedi," the combination manicure and pedicure in a spa-like environment. Increasingly, as part of the efforts of **manscaping**, Western men are also enjoying professional manicures to present a clean, crisp, tidy look.

For centuries, henna was used to accentuate and tint the fingers, toes, and palms across the ancient world of Turkey, India, and Egypt. Women in North Africa, **India**, and the Middle East used henna (**mehendi**) to color their nails a deep orange/red color. Since ancient times, Egyptian women rubbed their hands in rich oil and then stained their nails using henna. Henna comes from the mignonette tree and is prepared by drying and powdering the flower of the plant. The resulting powder is a greyish-green, but the dye yields a shade of orange on fabric, skin, and hair which deepens to a darker, richer shade of red. They dye of henna is temporary: it wears off after several weeks. Henna treatments continue to be used today, especially in bridal celebrations.

In ancient Babylon, men manicured and colored their nails using kohl. Darker hues were reserved for the most elite, and those with fewer resources settled for a greenish color. Archaeologists have uncovered manicure sets made of pure gold. During the Ming Dynasty (1368–1644) in China, elite men and women preferred very long, talon-like nails, tinted with a mix of egg whites, wax, and vegetable dye to create black nails.

Archaeologists reveal that in pre-Columbian Peru, many Inca used sharpened sticks and natural dyes to create small images on their fingernails for ceremonial occasions. The most popular of these images was that of the eagle, a bird revered among the Inca (PopSugar 2010).

Care of the nails also signifies health and life. Because nails are assumed to continue to grow after death, long nails have also been associated with the avoidance of mortal decay characteristic of the "undead," including zombies, vampires, and revenants. (In fact, nails do not continue to grow, but dehydration of the corpse causes the skin around the nails to retract and shrink back, creating an unsettling effect of extended length on the fingernails of the deceased.) In **Greek** mythology, Eros cuts the fingernails of the sleeping Aphrodite and scatters them on the beaches around the world. The Fates then collected these by-products of the world's most divine "manicure." The Greek word for "fingernail" is shared with the word of the semiprecious "onyx."

In China, the Zhou dynasty (BCE 1046–256) pioneered the use of artificial nails. Gold and silver dust was used to create colors worn by nobility. Artificial nail tips that could be worn over the top of the finger were produced from metals and then painted with enamels with inlays of gemstones. Many of these nail tips contained extremely detailed cloisonné work (PopSugar 2010).

Nail polish applied directly to the surface of the nail with a small brush was invented in **China** as early as BCE 3000. During the Ming Dynasty (1368—1644), nail polishes contained egg whites, gelatin, beeswax, vegetable dyes, and Arabic gum to create a long-lasting polish. In the West, nail polish (also called "nail varnish") was not commonly used until the mid-20th century. Clean, unstained hands were linked with good hygiene and moral purity. Women in the 1800s used lemon juice or vinegar to whiten their nail tips. Commercial products like buffers, emery boards, and bleaching powders were also available so that women could maintain a scrubbed look that belied the necessity of doing any manual labor.

The durability and luster of commercially available nail polishes were given a bump in the 1920s when the technology used to create car paint was adopted for the manufacture of nail polishes. The early colors were available in shades of pink, red, coral, and peach to complement shades of **lipstick**.

The half-moon manicure was a popular style in the 1920s and 1930s, when women painted only the center of the nail with deep crimson colors, leaving the half-moon cuticle and also the tips of the nails bare, or tinted from the underside with a white-nail pencil (Sauners 2011).

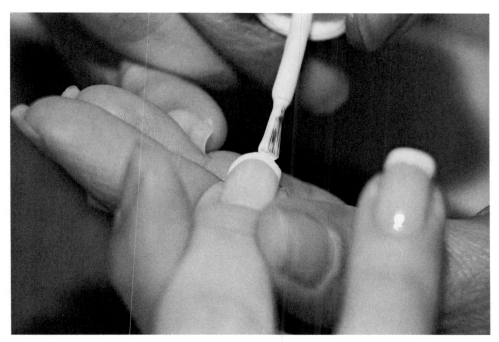

The French tip manicure is often chosen for its versatile simplicity and clean, professional look. (Sophieso/Dreamstime.com)

Another manicure type that was popular during the era, the French tip manicure (sometimes called a "pink-and-white" manicure) is an enhancement of the natural, unpolished nail. To achieve the look, the nail bed is painted a neutral skin tone or light pink color, while the tips of the nails are painted a stark white. The overall effect is a clean look, favored by many models for the versatility of the manicure in print. This manicure style experienced a revival in the 1970s thanks to the cosmetic company ORLY, who reinvented the classic-looking nail treatment for the Parisian runway (Valenti 2014).

Deep red nail polish became a style must-have for American women in the 1950s when Revlon launched its "Fire and Ice" **advertising** campaign, which paired nail colors with **lipsticks**. The groundbreaking advertising campaign raised eyebrows because it overtly linked **cosmetics** with sexuality with clever copy enticing consumers with lines like, "For you who love to flirt with fire/Who dare to skate on thin ice" (Peiss 1998). The polishes were easily accessible and affordable to almost everyone, sold in drug stores across America.

Since the 1980s, the range of nail colors available has proliferated to include virtually all colors, including the "Brush-On Peel-Off" innovation Tinkerbell Cosmetics marketed to young girls. Called "Bo-Po," this ingenious advancement did not require toxic nail polish remover to take it off the nails. The iconic Chanel cosmetic line went retro in 1995 when it introduced its "Vamp" line of deep red to black nail polishes, priced at a steep $15 per bottle to create a market for high-end polishes and the success of cosmetic companies that featured nontraditional colors like Urban Decay and Hard Candy (Forde 1998). In the 1990s, this wider range of colors allowed for a growing acceptance for straight men to paint their nails black, sometimes as part of a counterculture lifestyle scene characterized by grunge or punk.

Acrylic nails were invented when U.S. dentist Frederick Slack fixed a broken nail using aluminum foil and a dental acrylic used for bonding teeth in 1954. He later collaborated with his brother to take out a patent for acrylic nail forms or tips, which can be temporarily bonded to the nail bed through the use of polymer acrylics, allowing the wearer to adopt much longer, more durable nails that can be shaped and styled in a wide variety of ways. The acrylic nail tips can be removed using a solvent like acetone, or the wearer may choose to allow the tip remain affixed as the nail itself naturally grows from the cuticle, opting to get resulting space at the base of the nail bed "filled" to maintain the manicure for as long as possible. Another technique for extending the length and shape of the nail is through the use of a fiberglass or silk wrap. In this technique, the fiberglass or silk bonds directly to the nail through the use of acrylic polymers and can protect it from peeling or splitting. The wrapped nail "grows" with the length of the natural nail and cannot be safely removed without damaging the nail underneath.

If enameled nails were originally designed to beautify the hands and to attract the attention of men, the tide soon turned as women began to consider manicures as a self-pampering ritual.

See also: Advertising; China; Greece; India; Lipstick and Lip Tattoos; Makeup and Cosmetics; Manscaping; Mehendi; Salon.

Further Reading

Forde, Katherine. 1998. "History of Nail Art. Love To Know." Accessed July 28, 2016. http://fashion-history.lovetoknow.com/alphabetical-index-fashion-clothing-history/history-nail-art.

Kang, Mailiann. 2010. *The Managed Hand: Race, Gender, and the Body in Beauty Service Work.* Berkeley, CA: University of California Press.

Mulvey, Kate, and Melissa Richards. 1998. *Decades of Beauty: The Changing Image of Women, 1890–1990s.* New York: Hamlyn.

Peiss, Kathy. 1998. *Hope in a Jar: The Making of America's Beauty Culture.* New York: Henry Holt.

PopSugar. 2010. "The Colorful History of Nail Polish." *PopSugar* [Web site]. July 8. Accessed July 28, 2016. http://www.popsugar.com/beauty/History-Nail-Polish-2010-07-08-080032-9041578#photo-9041578.

Sauners, Jenna. 2011. "How to Do a 30s-Style Moon Manicure." Jezebel [Web site]. August 12. Accessed July 28, 2016. http://jezebel.com/5830193/how-to-do-a-30s-style-moon-manicure.

Sciacca, Noelle. 2016. "The Nail Files: A Visual History of Fingernail Fashion." *Mashable* [Web site]. January 14. Accessed July 28, 2016.http://mashable.com/2016/01/14/fingernail-history/#16HFsi0DEkq7.

Shapiro, Suzanne. 2014. *Nails: The Story of the Modern Manicure.* New York: Prestel.

Valenti, Lauren. 2014. "Telling Talons: The History of the Manicure." *Marie Claire* [Web site]. May 14. Accessed July 28, 2016. http://www.marieclaire.com/beauty/makeup/a9570/history-of-manicures.

MANNEQUIN

Wooden, wax, or plastic figures have been used to display and sell clothing and shoes for hundreds of years. The word "mannequin" comes from the Dutch word *maneken*, or "little man," an indication of how we expect the forms to represent us as humans (Iarocci 2013).

When researchers opened the tomb of the ancient Egyptian pharaoh Tutankhamen, they found a wooden torso with a head bearing the king's likeness placed next to the chest in which the king's wardrobe was carefully packed away (Oatman-Stanford 2013). This is one of the earliest examples of human forms being used to showcase the clothing of a person, in this case probably to help the king select his outfit for the day. The early mannequin would also likely have been used by his tailor to measure and fit clothes to his body more precisely, a practice still common with the forms used to make custom clothing (Oatman-Stanford 2013).

The use of these tailor's or dressmaker's models eventually turned, in the middle of the 19th century, into a way to display clothes for sale by showing how they would look on human bodies. With the advent of garment factories and large quantities of premade clothes replacing custom-made fashions, retailers increasingly used mannequins to display their products in new large plate-glass windows that were lit for evening shoppers by modern electric lights (Oatman-Stanford 2013).

The size and shape of mannequins, however, has changed greatly worldwide and across time. In the early 20th century, mannequins more accurately reflected the actual body size of European and U.S. citizens. One figure produced in the Depression era of the 1930s, for example, was the size 18 Bertille, one of the most popular models (Haywood 2013).

The size 18 Bertille can be seen as more than just an accurate reflection of women's bodies, however. The size 18, during a time of scarcity and hunger, was also a figure that suggested wealth and plenty (Haywood 2013). In this way, the heavier, more voluptuous figure is an example of how mannequins in the 20th and 21st centuries often represent aspirational body ideals, showing what consumers want to look like, even if they don't, in fact, match that body type.

As international beauty ideals changed, so have mannequins. Researchers studying the evolution of the female mannequin form in Japan, Italy, and Malaysia found that from the 1920s to the 1960s, the size of arm, hip, and thigh circumferences reduced dramatically, reflecting new trends preferring slimmer models and actresses such as the British model Twiggy (d'Aulaire and d'Aulaire 1991). Some retailers, such as Old Navy, have made the effort to include the representation of other skin colors and ethnicities (other than Caucasian) in their mannequins or forms that represent older people, but this is the exception, rather than the rule (d'Aulaire and d'Aulaire 1991).

The body sizes and shapes being produced to display clothing in the late 20th and 21st centuries continue to present a vision of the human form that is fit, slim, and "sophisticated." In 1991, researchers found that although the average size of women in the United States was a size 14, mannequins were still being produced at an "optimal" size 8 or size 6. For men, mannequins have become progressively more muscular, based on Greek and Roman heroic sculpture

Twiggy

London in the 1960s was international center of youth culture. The music of the era, from the Beatles to The Who, defines the soundtrack of the 1960s, and the fashion of the era, spread and popularized by models like Twiggy, is still the visual representation of the 1960s. Twiggy (born Lesly Hornby) was one of a select group of models that included Jean Sharpton and Penelope Tree that made 1960s mod and hippie fashion famous around the world. Twiggy is known and remembered for an extremely thin frame (which gave her the nickname, looking like a twig), a shaggy, boyish mop of blonde hair, and extraordinarily large round eyes normally adorned with elaborate false eyelashes. Her popularity spawned numerous fan-based products, from her own Barbie doll, to lunchboxes, to specific mannequins made to look like her.

and looking "more like Arnold Schwarzenegger than in the past" (d'Aulaire and d'Aulaire 1991.)

This change toward exaggerated and idealized beauty norms is perhaps nowhere more notable in the 21st century than in Venezuela, where the most popular and best-selling mannequins are those with the extreme proportions of bust and waist that reflect the nation's widespread acceptance and expectation of plastic surgery. The forms in many Venezuelan store windows, with "bulging bosoms," a "cantilevered buttocks," a "wasp waist," and "long legs," are evidence of the Venezuelan's fantasy of what a woman can and should look like, and plastic surgeons report that women come in seeking to look like the mannequins they pass every day (Neuman 2013).

See also: Egypt; Plastic Surgery; Venezuela; Weight.

Further Reading

d'Aulaire, Emily Ola, and Per Ola d'Aulaire. 1991. "Mannequins: Our Fantasy Figures of High Fashion." *Smithsonian* 22, no. 1: 66.
Haywood, Sharon. 2013. "Model Behaviour." *Herizons* 27, no. 2: 24.
Iarocci, Louisa, editor. 2013. *Visual Merchandising: The Image of Selling.* New York: Ashgate.
Neuman, William. 2013. "Mannequins Give Shape to a Venezuelan Fantasy," *New York Times.* November 7. Accessed January 8, 2016. http://www.nytimes.com/2013/11/07 /world/americas/mannequins-give-shape-to-venezuelan-fantasy.html?_r=0.
Oatman-Stanford, Hunter. 2013. "Retail Therapy: What Mannequins Say About Us." Accessed October 3, 2016. http://www.collectorsweekly.com/articles/what-mannequins -say-about-us.

MANSCAPING

Whereas the presence of copious amounts of male body hair is a symbol of virility and masculinity in some cultures, recent trends in Europe and the United States demonstrate a preference for the removal of male body hair on certain parts of the body. This practice is sometimes called "manscaping."

In the mid- and late 20th century, male sex symbols and those men who represented aspirational images of male beauty and appearance often displayed noticeable and thick head and body hair. During this time period, luxurious facial hair was also common on male celebrities. Highlighting the visual connection between hair, power, and masculinity, hirsute men often portrayed hypermasculine, strong, sexually promiscuous, and violent characters (Immergut 2008). The association with facial hair, power, and violence is strongly connected with the tradition of the "villain mustache," where the "bad guy" is often identified easily in 20th-century film by his mustache (McKay 2010).

In the 21st century, the majority of celebrity men who represent the male ideal of appearance worldwide are clean shaven, not just on their faces, but also on their chests and back. From the Bollywood star Shah Rukh Khan, to the Chinese actor Jackie Chan, to "The Rock," Dwayne Johnson, the heartthrobs and heroes of 2015 had hairless chests.

There are many theories about why this trend has taken hold in the 21st century. Some scholars suggest that the removal of hair is part of trying to look younger, and therefore more virile and powerful (Immergut 2008). Others suggest that the strict grooming of facial and body hair and the removal of that hair are indicators of social class. Like manicured nails, tightly controlled hair on the face, head, and body is a marker of a white-collar office job, one where the man does not work with his hands (Cassutt 2007). Manscaping is one grooming technique often sought out by the **metrosexual**, young, urban men with disposable incomes who care deeply about their appearances.

Another explanation for the recent preference for hairless chests is the way in which smooth skin showcases muscular development that might be hidden by hair. As the beauty standard for men has become increasingly lean and muscular in the shoulders and chest, a phenomenon often called "progressive muscularity," more attention has been paid to the extent to which a man's chest, back, and shoulder muscles are defined.

The ideal is for a man to be "shredded" or "ripped." These terms refer to the visual ideal of the combination of large muscles and low body fat where each individual muscle is visible (Smith 2016). In order to showcase this work and muscle definition, then, body builders both remove their body hair and oil their bodies, while increasingly, other men around the world emulate that ideal by manscaping.

See also: Bodybuilding; Hair Removal; Metrosexual; Progressive Muscularity.

Further Reading

Cassutt, Melissa. 2007. "Concern with Looks, Fading Taboos Fuel Rise of 'Manscaping.'" *The Gazette (Colorado Springs, CO)*. September 17. Accessed July 14, 2016. *Newspaper Source*.

Immergut, Matthew. 2008. "Manscaping: The Tangle of Male Body Hair, Nature and Culture." *Conference Papers—American Sociological Association* (2008 Annual Meeting 2008). Accessed July 14, 2016.

McKay, Brett. 2010. "The 12 Most Infamous Mustaches of All Time." Art of Manliness. November 10. Accessed July 14, 2016. http://www.artofmanliness.com/2010/11/10/the -12-most-infamous-mustaches-of-all-time/.

Smith, Stephanie. 2016. "Trainer Q&A: How to Increase Muscle Definition." *Men's Fitness*. Accessed July 18, 2016. http://www.mensfitness.com/training/build-muscle/trainer-qa -how-to-increase-muscle-definition.

MASCULINITY

Anthropological and other cross-cultural research indicates that preferred body images vary among cultures as well as within cultures across groups and time (Bailey 2008, 14). Outward signs of health, wealth, power, and strength often help define the parameters of what is considered "beautiful."

Male facial beauty in New Ireland of Melanesia includes an emphasis on a large flat nose, pierced earlobes, side whiskers, and a large mouth with strong teeth. In the Iatmul region of New Guinea, people prefer long noses to flat noses in their assessment of a beautiful face (van Damme 1996, 33).

> "The three wishes of every man: to be healthy, to be rich by honest means, and to be beautiful."
>
> —PLATO

In the Western world, the idealized slender, muscular male bodies of ancient Greece and Rome are iconic from their frozen forms on marble statues, murals, and other art forms. Men of the ancient world were often represented nude, and the male body was generally revered and considered more attractive than the female body. The "Daedalic style," named for Daedalus of Crete, emerged in BCE seventh century, characterized by a broad-shouldered, narrow-hipped body and remained the standard of male beauty until the 18th century (Grogan 1999).

By the end of the 19th century, the ideal male body changed due to the rise in sports culture. In 1921, Charles Atlas (born Angelo Siciliano in Italy in 1892) won the "World's Most Beautiful Man Contest," solidifying the American connection between musculature and male beauty, which continued with such (imported) muscular actors of the 1980s as Arnold Schwarzenegger, Jean-Claude Van Damme, and Dolph Lundgren. Atlas was described as muscular, smooth, well proportioned, and extremely masculine. He rose to fame with an apocryphal story about a bully who kicked sand into his face at the beach and a well-**advertised** line of training products designed to help fellow "97-pound weaklings" develop muscles and make the ladies swoon.

As a response to the perception that masculinity is framed in a muscular version of the male body, some researchers argue that a particular form of **body dysmorphia** for Western men manifests itself as "muscle dysmorphia," a condition where individuals report an obsessional preoccupation with their muscularity to the point where their social or occupational functioning may be severely impaired (Pope et al. 1999, 66). Men suffering from this disorder may refuse to be seen in public without their shirts on for fear of being judged too "small," or they use anabolic steroids or other performance-enhancing drugs to address the persistent anxiety they feel about their muscularity.

In much of contemporary global society, being seen as sufficiently "masculine" is tied strongly to not being seen as "too feminine." Contemporary Western male clothing is often marked by its neutral nature and not intended to attract attention (Negrin 2008). Western men also typically do not ornament themselves with as much jewelry or use as many cosmetic products as women do. Deviations in dress or appearance that reflect the feminine are immediately suspicious, and so many Western men over the past few decades have avoided colorful embellishments to their clothing (Pitcher 1963).

This division between looking "masculine" and "feminine" as a marker of attractiveness for men, however, is not universal. In cultures such as South Korea, "flower boys," or young, very feminine men who wear makeup and bright colors, are considered extremely attractive, and in Europe and the United States, sales of cosmetics and beauty products for men rise every year (AP 2012).

Adding to the slippage between hypermasculine and more feminine preferences, since the 1990s, the preferred male body type in the United States is more slender and streamlined than the "muscle man" of the previous era. Based on analysis of men's **magazines**, Euro-American men are under increased social pressure to conform to the muscular, well-toned shape expected of idealized men, including Brad Pitt and Channing Tatum. The United States is arguably a culture where beauty matters more than ever before for men. Instead of women being judged less for their looks, now it is the case that men are increasingly subjected to the same measure (Negrin 2008, 48). As men continue to become more image conscious, some clinicians have noticed a rise in male eating disorders and other pathologies that used to be exclusively associated with women.

An increasingly complex set of societal expectations for men in terms of beauty and physical attractiveness is on the rise. Men in the 21st century must navigate conflicting messages and norms for what makes a man "beautiful." As Morgan Spurlock investigates in his 2012 documentary *Mansome*, in the age of beard competitions, manscaping, bodybuilding, and male grooming products, it can be hard for men to build individual masculine identities and achieve the social norm of beauty (Spurlock 2012).

See also: Advertising; Bodybuilding; Body Dysmorphic Disorder; Magazines; Metrosexual; Progressive Muscularity; South Korea.

Further Reading

Alexander, Susan M. 2003. "Stylish Hard Bodies: Branded Masculinity in *Men's Health* Magazine." *Sociological Perspectives* 46, no. 4: 535–54.

AP. 2012. "The 'Flower Boys' of SOUTH KOREA WHO SPEND MORE on Beauty Products than Any Other Men in the World." Accessed October 11, 2016. http://www.dailymail.co.uk/news/article-2204587/The-flower-boys-South-Korea-spend-beauty-products-men-world.html#ixzz4MnXtB8HA.

Bailey, Eric. 2008. *Black America, Body Beautiful: How the African American Image Is Changing Fashion, Fitness and Other Industries*. Westport, CT: Praeger.

Barber, Kristin. 2016. *Styling Masculinity: Gender, Class and Inequality in the Men's Grooming Industry*. New Brunswick, NJ: Rutgers University Press.

Benitez-Eves, Tina. 2012. "The Male Factor." *Gifts & Decorative Accessories* 113, no. 9: 70.

Black, Jonathan. 2009. "Charles Atlas: Muscle Man." Smithsonian [Web site]. August. Accessed January 29, 2017. http://www.smithsonianmag.com/history/charles-atlas-muscle-man-34626921/?c=y%3Fno-ist

Bordo, Susan. 2000. *The Male Body: A New Look at Men in Public and Private*. New York: Farrar, Strauss, and Giroux.

Grogan, Sarah. 1999. *Body Image: Understanding Body Dissatisfaction in Men, Women, and Children*. New York: Routledge.

Negrin, Llewellyn. 2008. *Appearance and Identity: Fashioning the Body in Postmodernity*. New York: Palgrave Macmillan.

Pitcher, Evelyn Goodenough. 1963. "Male and Female." *The Atlantic*, 211: 87–91.

Pope, Harrison G., Roberto Olivardia, Amanda Gruber, and John Borowiecki. 1999. "Evolving Ideals of Male Body Image as Seen Through Action Toys." *International Journal of Eating Disorders* 26, no. 1: 65–72.

Spurlock, Morgan. 2012. *Mansome*. Film. Directed by Morgan Spurlock. Electus Films.

Van Damme, Wilfried. 1996. *Beauty in Context: Towards an Anthropological Approach to Aesthetics*. Leiden, Netherlands: EJ Brill.

MAYA

A civilization and culture that dates back to at least BCE 1800, the Maya are an indigenous group that still lives in the southern part of Mexico as well as in Guatemala, Belize, Honduras, and El Salvador. As a networked, complex, scholarly civilization of astronomers, farmers, architects, and priests, the Mayan civilization peaked in about the year 600 CE, seeing a decline in population and the abandonment of their great cities by 900 CE, before the arrival of the Spanish (History 2009). Though the structure of the civilization declined for unknown reasons in the first century, nearly a million people of Mayan ancestry and ethnicity still live in Mexico and Central America (Walker 2012).

During the height of the civilization, the major cities of the Maya held hundreds of thousands of people in well-organized and planned urban areas that included temples, schools, a sophisticated agricultural system, and modern-style plumbing and sewage systems that were hundreds of years more advanced than those in use in Europe during the same time period (Walker 2012).

In addition to this advanced urban planning, the Maya were highly skilled and advanced architects and artists. The Maya had the only pre-Colombian written language known in the Americas that corresponded directly to the spoken language and represented the language through a beautifully intricate set of hieroglyphs on scrolls, on walls, and in temples (Walker 2012). Much of what we know about the beauty standards of the ancient Maya comes not only through the archeological study of remains and the contents of tombs, but also through looking at the complex, intricate representations of life that the Maya left painted and carved in their public spaces.

The ancient Maya also participated in an elaborate set of beauty practices and body modification. Archeologists studying the remains of high-ranking members of Mayan society have found a number of clues as to what constituted "beauty" for the ancient civilization. These findings are then reinforced by the images of the Maya found in paintings and reliefs.

One common practice for members of the upper class was headbinding, in which the parents of infants placed a flat block or stone on the baby's soft cranium so that it would grow flat, with a defined ridge directly above the eyebrows slanting back, creating a long line from the tip of the nose to the back of the head. Very high-ranking

Maya would wear nose pieces made of precious stones that sat on the nose and followed this line up past the hairline (Miller 2009).

The ancient Maya also believed that crossed eyes were beautiful, and parents often hung a bead between the eyes of babies to draw their attention and to make them permanently cross-eyed. This practice was in honor of the god of the sun—since humans must squint to see the sun, the Maya believed that the sun god also squinted to see them. The crossed eyes represented this double gaze between the Maya and their god (Miller 2009).

The Maya also practiced tooth filing, using tools to change the shape of each tooth in a variety of ways. Teeth were modified into points, like fangs, into "T" shapes, or drilled with small holes so that pieces of jade or other precious stones could be hung from them (Linn 2006). Women would also modify their teeth so that jewels could be inlaid into the outer surface (Miller 2009). Jewels and jewelry in the forms of necklaces, earrings, and bracelets were used by men and women in the ancient period.

Both the male and female ancient Maya of the upper classes also used cosmetics, painting their bodies in vibrant, abstract designs, designs that were reflected in their clothing as well, which featured intricately woven and embroidered designs. The color blue-green, with its association with jade, the sea, and the plant life, was considered the most desirable and beautiful color, and is sometimes called "Mayan sacred blue" (Miller 2009).

Although the beauty practices of the ancient Maya of a centuries-old civilization are compelling and fascinating, it is important to remember that nearly a million Maya people live and continue to engage in beauty work today. In the 21st century, modern Maya culture continues to be particularly well known for its production and use of both jewelry and elaborately woven textiles.

Modern-day Maya people living in Mexico and Central America still produce and wear the types of vibrantly colored, embroidered, and patterned cloth visible in ancient carvings and paintings. Each village often has its own design, and the pattern and color of a woman's dress or a man's pants can identify the wearer in terms of origin, marital status, and social class. More than 150 different, distinct patters of textile are used by contemporary Mayans in Guatemala today (Dwyer 2005).

This use of traditional clothing is a powerful symbol of heritage and tradition, but can be a symbolic marker of the rural upbringing of the wearer, often associated with a lack of education or sophistication. In the 21st century, many modern Maya people seeking professional employment in larger cities have stopped wearing traditional textiles for everyday use and have adopted the imported European style of business wear in order to find more professional success. In many of these cases, however, these people still wear their traditional clothing for ceremonial occasions (Dwyer 2005).

The tension between European standards of beauty and traditional indigenous work and beauty norms is similar in this case to many areas of Latin America where native peoples struggle to manage the expectations of participation in a global economy and society with the desire to maintain the specificity of their local traditions. Weaving, especially, for Mayan women, continues to be a source of income, as the

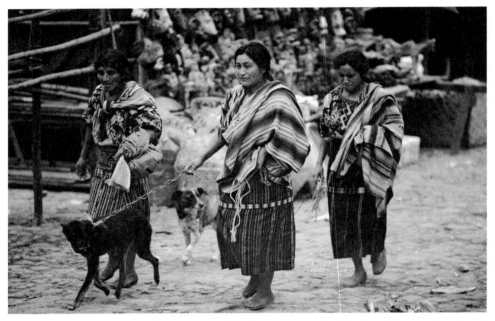

Maya women wearing everyday traditional clothing, western highlands of Guatemala. (David Mcnew/iStockphoto.com)

textiles are highly prized for their beauty, both by Guatemalans and international art collectors and fashion designers, but also as a way to maintain their indigenous heritage (De La Cruz 2010).

See also: Body Modification; Headbinding; Mexico; Pageants—Indigenous Pageants; Tooth Chipping.

Further Reading

De La Cruz, Sonia. 2010. "Weaving the Life of Guatemala: A Participatory Approach to Cross-Cultural Filmmaking." *Conference Papers—International Communication Association* 1. Accessed July 21, 2016. *Communication & Mass Media Complete*, EBSCOhost.

Dwyer, Deborah. 2005 "The Rainbow Textiles of the Guatemalan Highlands." *Piecework* 13, no. 2: 52–55.

History.com. 2009. "Maya." Accessed July 21, 2016. http://www.history.com/topics/maya.

Linn, Virginia. 2006. *Pittsburgh Post*. "Revisiting Mayans." *Pittsburgh Post—Gazette*. November 5: F-1.

Miller, Mary. 2009. "Extreme Makeover." *Archaeology* 62, no. 1 (January): 36–42.

Walker, Tim. 2012. "What Have the Mayans Ever Done for Us." *The Independent* December 19: 35.

MEHENDI (HINA, HENNA)

Mehendi is the art of temporarily marking the hands or feet of women in elaborate lace-like designs, usually as part of a preparation for a rite of passage or other festive occasion. The practice is most commonly found in North Africa, India, and the

Middle East. The word "mehendi" (sometimes spelled "mehndi") comes from Sanskrit and appears in the earliest Hindu Vedic ritual texts. The design stains the skin and nails, and can last for several weeks.

In order to create the design on the skin, the leaves of the henna plant (*Lawsonia inermis*, also known as the mignonette tree) are cultivated from a bush. Henna paste is prepared by grinding up the leaves and adding oil to create the "ink." Historically, the paste is carefully applied from a cone-shaped bag with a small hole or funnel-shaped tip or tiny rod at the end; today, henna paste is often applied with a syringe. The paste is left to dry and then it is removed, leaving a deep red stain on the surface of the skin. Sometimes a top layer "fixative" made of water, rose sugar, ground cloves, and lemon juice is also dabbed onto the henna design after its application to make the image last longer.

As a botanical product, henna paste also has prophylactic and healing properties. It may also be used for its natural cooling properties as a skin conditioner or to reduce the itching of a rash. Henna may be used to counter fever, hair loss, and ringworm. The combination of the beautifying capacity, as well as the possibility of healing, lends the henna plant a rich folkloric history, including the idea that it is a carrier of *baraka*, which means divine blessing (Kapchan 1993). These blessings are desired by brides, which is why mehendi applications are central to marriage preparations in some parts of the world.

In Morocco, a bride is literally inscribed as a carrier of social symbols that can be read by members of the society. The bride is the visible embodiment of the meanings of feminine beauty that exist within the society. Geometric and floral patterns are ritually applied to the backs of her hands and tops of her feet following the natural lines of her features on the day before her wedding, called on *nhar al-henna* ("day of henna," also sometimes called *nhar an-nquash*, "the day of engraving"). First, the bride is purified by soaking for several hours in a public **bath**. The process of marking the bride with these gender-specific body ornaments and symbols can take up to eight hours, and the designs are usually made by a professional henna artist, called an *nqasha*. The patterns usually lead the eye in a path through intricate lines that culminate in a triangular-shaped filigree above the wrist or the ankle. Male palms are also dabbed with henna at the marriage ceremony, though they do not receive the elaborate designs on the backs of their hands. In general, male henna designs are much less intricate and much smaller than the designs of women. Women may also gather together to apply mehendi designs in a more secular event called a *hefla*, or party held by women for women. The process of applying the henna and waiting for the design to emerge is one of the few self-initiated events that allow for feminine celebration in the general public (Kapchan 1993). It allows women to express their own version of feminine aesthetics, signifying important values about what it means to be a woman in the society. Whenever possible, a Moroccan woman also paints herself with henna just prior to the birth of a child, believing that if she dies in childbirth she will enter heaven as a bride (Kapchan 1993).

In India, mehendi designs were originally associated with the Vedic tradition of "awakening the inner light." Designs were created to represent the sun on the palm,

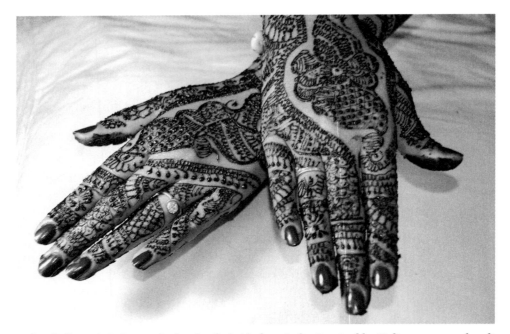

Mehendi (henna) design on the hands of a bride from India. Inspired by Vedic custom, mehendi designs on the palm represent the sun, signifying inner light, and radiating out into the world. For brides, symmetrical floral designs capture the sense of sunlight or radiating energy. (Stock Shooter/Dreamstime.com)

signifying inner light, and radiating out into the world. Symmetrical floral designs also capture the sense of sunlight or radiating energy. This Vedic custom remains important in the context of the Indian Hindu marriage ceremony.

Henna has also flourished in Islamic countries. The recognizable, hennaed "Hand of Fatima" wards off the evil eye and is found over door lintels, on taxis, in market stalls, and in most other public places. Each finger represents a pillar of Islam (faith, charity, prayer, fasting, and the profession of Allah), and so may be decorated with specific henna designs. Henna designs in the Arabic tradition are usually identifiably different from those in India. Whereas Indian mehendi designs involve paisley and lacy patterns composed of fine, thin lines, Arabic henna designs are usually large, floral patterns that are focused on the hands and the feet. The designs are more abstract and less dense than Indian design, featuring trailing floral and vine motifs.

Henna is also worn throughout a number of regions of northern and west Africa. Designs on the African continent are generally large, bold, and geometric. Henna-stained nails are considered especially attractive.

Western celebrities like Madonna and Gwen Stefani began to wear henna decorations, sometimes called "henna tattoos," in the 1990s, prompting critics to chastise these celebrities for cultural appropriation and cultural insensitivity. No stranger to religious controversy surrounding her provocative music videos, Madonna brought strong criticism from a Hindu group called the World Vaishnava Association, who objected to her sacrilegious use of henna marriage patterns, a black sari, and a Tilak facial adornment which signified purity in her sexually charged performance at an awards ceremony (Kaufman 1998). In Western cities, modern henna decorations are sometimes sought out by young people in ways comparable to tattoo designs, but, of course, mehendi is far less permanent.

See also: Bathing and Showering; Tattoos.

Further Reading

Kapchan, Deborah. 1993. "Moroccan Women's Body Signs." In: *Bodylore*, edited by Katharine Young, 3–34. Knoxville, TN: University of Tennessee Press.
Kaufman, Gil. 1998. "Madonna Blasts Back at Critical Hindu Group." MTV News. September 16. Accessed July 27, 2016. http://www.mtv.com/news/501729/madonna-blasts-back-at-critical-hindu-group.
Kumar, Dolly. 2012. "Fashion and Beautification in India: Expression of Individuality." Paper presented at the 2nd Global Conference on Beauty: Exploring Critical Issues, Mansfield College, Oxford University. Accessed July 27, 2016. http://www.academia.edu/25826501/Fashion_and_Beautification_in_India_Expression_of_Individuality.

METROSEXUAL

Coined in the **United Kingdom** in 1994, the term "metrosexual" refers to a straight man, usually living in an urban, postindustrial, capitalist culture with a high degree of disposable income, who is especially meticulous about his grooming and appearance and spends a significant amount of time and money on shopping to reinforce his personal style. The term did not really rise to international prominence until 2002, when Salon identified football superstar David Beckham as the quintessential "metrosexual" (Simpson 2002). Shortly after, influential essays about the rise of the metrosexual as a new marketing segment changing contemporary notions about **gender** ran in Australia and the United States.

Traditionally, the stereotype argues, heterosexual men were boring and uninspired consumers. **Masculinity** was defined through a narrow range of options about the gender **performances** available to straight men in public: masculine men were expected to be strong, unemotional, and fearless. They were expected to demonstrate competence through certainty, confidence, and assertiveness. The range of fashion choices for professional men since the last century has been limited to suits and neckties in a dull palette of blue, grey, and black. When persuaded to shop, men bought beer, cigarettes, and possibly condoms. They expected the women in their lives to buy the rest of the products used to keep up a household. The emerging metrosexual contradicted the basic premise of traditional heterosexuality in the West by subverting the norm of the **male gaze**—that only women are looked at and only men do the looking. The metrosexual demographic enjoyed being pampered and splurging for luxurious moisturizers, **manicures**, and **pedicures**. Metrosexual men also pay close attention to their personal grooming giving rise to the phenomenon of **manscaping**. They also buy quality brand-name clothing and accessories, persuading other young men to study them with envy and desire. Gay men were the original test market for **advertising** campaigns, but the straight single man living in the metropolis and taking himself as his own **narcissistic** love-object soon became the target of companies seeking larger range (Simpson 2011). Unlike the vaguely questionable and sexually ambiguous "dandy" of previous eras, the metrosexual is a straight man who cares deeply about his appearance and is in the financial position to consume and model products or services that mark him as a fashionable man.

In the **United States**, an important moment for the dissemination of metrosexual aesthetics came from the popular reality television program *Queer Eye for the Straight Guy,* which aired from 2003–2007 on the Bravo Network. Proceeding with the stereotypical premise that gay men have superior taste in matters of fashion, style, and personal grooming, each week, a team of five gay male "lifestyle experts" performed a "make better" (rather than a conventional "makeover") on a straight man by improving his wardrobe, offering advice on grooming, and redecorating his home. Although some criticized the overly simplistic generalizations the program made about sexual identity, it was surprisingly well received and won an Emmy award for Outstanding Reality Program in 2004.

See also: Advertising; Gender; Male Gaze; Manicure; Manscaping; Masculinity; Narcissism; Pedicure; Performance/Performativity; United Kingdom; United States.

Further Reading

Khoo, Michele, and Kavita Karan. 2007. "Macho or Metrosexual: The Branding of Masculinity in FHM Magazine in Singapore." *Intercultural Communications Studies* 16, no. 1: 34–46.

Miller, Toby. 2005. "A Metrosexual Eye on Queer Guy" *GLQ: A Journal of Lesbian and Gay Studies* 11, no. 1: 97–101.

Pompper, Donnalyn. 2010. "Masculinities, the Metrosexual, and Media Images: Across Dimensions of Age and Ethnicity." *Sex Roles* 63: 682–95.

Shugart, Helene. 2008. "Managing Masculinities: The Metrosexual Moment." *Communication and Critical/Cultural Studies* 3: 280–300.

Simpson, Mark. 2002. "Meet the Metrosexual." *Salon.* July 22. Accessed October 1, 2016. http://www.salon.com/2002/07/22/metrosexual.

Simpson, Mark. 2011. *Metrosexy: A 21st Century Self-Love Story.* Seattle: Amazon Digital Services.

MEXICO

When Hernán Cortez arrived in what is now Mexico in 1521, he found a thriving civilization that had dominated the area for 300 years (Lopez Hernández 2012). The Aztec, also known as Mexica people, had built and managed an empire that stretched across the region, managed from a capital of nearly 300,000 citizens in Tenochtitlan, the city that is now known as Mexico City (Quick 2014). The size of the Aztec empire along with the flourishing population, traditions, and knowledge of its people still influence social norms of beauty in modern-day Mexico. Together with the traditions of the Spanish, brought by Cortez and those who followed him, Mexican beauty and beauty practices are a mix of European and indigenous values and ideas.

The Mexican flag today has in its center the image of an eagle eating a snake, an Aztec symbol that forms part of the legend of the founding of Tenochtitlan. This image, however, is only one way that indigenous heritage is present in Mexican culture. At least 90 percent of the population in Mexico today is of indigenous or *mestizo* (mixed European and indigenous) descent, and the traditions of the Aztecs, Maya, and other tribes can be seen in everything from the visual arts to fashion and jewelry design (Camp 2011).

This history of indigenous peoples conquered by European soldiers and of the struggle to maintain and accept indigenous identity in the 20th and 21st centuries is of particular relevance in the construction of social norms

---

María Félix

María de los Angeles Félix Guereña, known professionally as María Félix, is the most famous actress in the history of Spanish-language cinema. Known by the nicknames "La Doña" [The Lady] and "María Bonita" [beautiful María], Félix made 47 films in Mexico, Argentina, Italy, Spain, and France. Félix was discovered while at the University of Guadalajara, where she was crowned the Queen of Beauty. Her famous beauty led her to model for many of the world's greatest painters, including José Clemente Orozco and Diego Rivera, and the French fashion house Hérmes designed a collection just for her. The modern "beauty czar" and director of the Miss Venezuela pageant has been noted as saying that all women need work. For him there has only ever been one perfect beauty: María Félix.

---

of beauty and appearance. Arguably, nearly all modern-day Mexicans are descendants of both indigenous and European ancestors. However, traditionally, the power of the European conquest has privileged European norms of beauty in appearance, ranging from skin color, to hair color and texture, to fashion. The modern state of beauty norms in Mexico represents a struggle for identity and a social norm of beauty (Chavez 2012).

The colonial period in Mexico, through the mid-19th century is marked by the dominance of European ideals of fashion, beauty, and appearance. As the Spanish had dominated in wealth and power, as in other Latin American nations, white skin, European features, and long, wavy hair continued to be understood as indicators of beauty and success. The assumption of European superiority in all areas was the norm through the early 20th century.

Attitudes toward the specific primacy of European and North American ideals, however, began to turn in the 1920s, many influenced by philosopher José Vasconcelos's influential essay "La raza cósmica" [The Cosmic Race]. This essay, published in 1925, proposed a vision of an aspirational race of people that are a mix of the best of the indigenous and European bloodlines. Vasconcelos called this group "the cosmic race" (Celarent 2014). This idea was revolutionary in the way it recognized the value of Mexican indigenous traditions and culture, and proved important in the way it influenced art and style, particularly in the work of such famous muralists as Diego Rivera and José Clemente Orozco. Vasconcelos's ideas started a dialog on the place of indigenous values and image in the nation, a conversation that continues today.

The Mexican Civil War of 1936–1939 (known as the Mexican Revolution) revealed tensions between the traditionally Euro-dominant ideology and the reality of indigenous Mexicans of the period, and the time since has continued to show the push and pull between acceptance of traditional European and indigenous visions of beauty, mixed with the influence of other global ideals from the United States and abroad. Indigenous pageants in the early and mid-20th century often competed with imported styles of beauty such as burlesque to form modern notions of appearance and image (Sluis 2010).

In the 20th century, across Mexico, indigenous pageants became a popular way to celebrate and promote traditional beauty ideals of the native peoples of the nation. In festivals and pageants across Mexico, beginning in the 1920s, "*indias bonitas*," or "pretty Indians," began to be selected as representatives of native "Mexicaness" and traditional indigenous beauty values (Sluis 2010). These pageants and contests judged young indigenous women on their physical features, but also on the traditional dress, jewelry, and hairstyles that identified them as native.

Other important cultural figures, like the artist Frida Kahlo, worked to specifically challenge social norms of beauty by embracing their indigenous heritage. Kahlo not only explored themes of racial and ethnic mixing and traditional visions of beauty in her painting, she also embraced indigenous dress and fashion in her daily life (Garrido 2012). Kahlo, the daughter of a German father and *mestizo* mother, often painted herself in both European and indigenous dress. One of her most famous portraits is of "Two Fridas," one dressed in Tehuana clothing, the other in a Spanish-style dress. Kahlo's image in photographs and self-portraits, wearing native clothing and jewelry, is embraced by Mexicans in many areas of culture. Indeed, the image of Frida in the 20th century is still a hugely influential cultural and style icon.

In the 21st century, the tensions between indigenous and European values of beauty continue to be felt by men and women in Mexico. Norms of beauty are often associated with wealth and success, with members of any culture seeking to conform to the standards and appearance of the richest, most powerful members of any group (Etcoff 2000). In Mexico, this continues to mean pressure to look "more white." Research demonstrates that those Mexicans with the darkest skin tone have the lowest socioeconomic status, and that mobility between social classes is often associated with the ability to appear or to be recognized as "more white" (Flores and Telles 2010).

In the second decade of the 21st century, the official discourse of the Mexican state still follows the ideology of Vasconcelos in promoting *mestizaje*, or an ideal of a beautiful mixed race. The reality of many Mexicans, however, is that this narrative still privileges being "whiter" rather than "darker" (Moreno Figueroa 2013). To consider oneself beautiful in the Mexican context, according to scholars working in the nation, is a relative matter, where each individual evaluates their own appearance on that whiter to darker scale. For modern Mexicans, and especially women, the rules of what constitutes beauty continue to work around images of skin, hair, and trappings of wealth that have been in play for a hundred years.

See also: Brazil; Burlesque; Maya; Pageants—Indigenous Pageants; Venezuela.

Further Reading

Camp, Roderic A. 2011. *Mexico: What Everyone Needs to Know*. Oxford, England: Oxford University Press, 2011.

Celarent, Barbara. 2014. "La raza cósmica / The Cosmic Race/A Mexican Ulysses: An Autobiography." *American Journal of Sociology* 120, no. 3: 998–1004.

Chávez, Daniel. 2012. "From Miss Cristera to the Desert Within: Towards a Contemporary War of Images in Mexico." *Studies in Hispanic Cinemas* 9, no. 1: 63–79.

Etcoff, Nancy. 2000. *Survival of the Prettiest: The Science of Beauty*. New York: Anchor.

Flores, René, and Edward Telles. 2010. "Social Stratification in Mexico: Disentangling Color, Ethnicity and Class." *American Sociological Review* 77, no. 3: 486–94.

Garrido, Edgard. 2012. "Frida Kahlo's Wardrobe Goes on Exhibit in Mexico City; Iconic Artist was Famed for Traditional, Flowing Dresses that Disguised Her Injured Legs." November 26. Accessed July 21, 2016. http://www.nydailynews.com/life-style/fashion/frida-kahlo-wardrobe-exhibit-mexico-city-article-1.1208081.

López Hernández, Miriam. 2012. *Aztec Women and Goddesses*. Mexico City: Cacciani S.A. de C.V.

Moreno Figueroa, Monica G. 2013. "Displaced Looks: The Lived Experience of Beauty and Racism." *Feminist Theory* 14, no. 2: 137–51.

Quick, P. S. 2014. *Awesome Aztecs*. Luton, England: Andrews UK.

Sluis, Ageeth. 2010 "Bataclanismo! Or, How Female Deco Bodies Transformed Postrevolutionary Mexico City." *The Americas* 66, no. 4: 469–99.

MOKO TATTOOS

When notorious British explorer Captain Cook and his naval crew arrived in New Zealand in 1769, they were struck by the arresting facial tattoos of the indigenous Maori people they met there. Called *ta moko*, these facial tattoos are distinctive for their highly symbolic, curvilinear design, which can spread extensively across the cheeks, forehead, nose, and chin of adult men. Women's designs are typically confined to the chin and **lips**.

Moko tattoos are unique and highly personal, conveying both status and affiliation. To prepare for the moko design, the face was divided by the moko artist into four quadrants: the right side of the face indicates information about the father's rank and lineage, and the left side of the face conveys the same information about the person's mother and her lineage. Artists further divide the face into sections in order to give balance and symmetry to the design. The design around the eyelids was known as *rewha*, and the spirals around each nostril were known as *pongiangia*. Each design is as unique as each individual, and obviously moko is the process of a lifetime, usually applied as a rite of passage to mark some significant change in one's personal status. Information can be added as an individual advances in rank, prestige, or position.

The Maori were also known for their exquisite wood carving, which possibly initially inspired moko tattoos to be carved into the skin with a sharpened stone tool made from albatross bones called *uhi whaka tataramoa*. Different sizes of chisels were made to complete the delicate work around the eyelids, the wider spirals around each nostril, and the multiple serrations of a "shading tool," used to color larger surfaces like thighs and shoulders. The chisels were rumored to have first come to humans from the magical realms of Rarohenga (the underworld). After the design was cut into the flesh, it was rubbed with specially prepared pigments made of local materials to accentuate and maintain the design. The "ink" was traditionally made from a mixture of *ngarehu* (burnt timbers), *awheto* (a fungus valued as an herbal remedy), and the soot of burnt kauri gum (a resin from local trees). The pigment was stored in an elaborately carved wooden vessel known as an *oko*, which was passed down from one generation to the next and frequently buried when not in use. A great deal of ceremony surrounded the creation of moko tattoos. The highly trained tattooists who created and implemented the designs and the craftsmen who made the *uhi* chisels were considered sacred persons. The process of completing a moko design took a long time and was excruciatingly painful, inviting potentially deadly medical complications from infection and sepsis. Tattooing in the South Pacific was widely practiced at the time of Cook's expedition. In fact, the English word "tattoo" is drawn from this region. Neighboring Polynesian ethnic groups in Samoa, Hawaii, and Tahiti also practiced extensive tattooing through the use of a puncture method. After Europeans introduced metal to the region, all these regional techniques combined to allow for innovation in technique and design.

Across the South Pacific, many indigenous cultural groups historically felt that human heads were sacred and the seat of *mana*, the magical energy that animates all living things. The moko design of a deceased relative lived on as Maori family

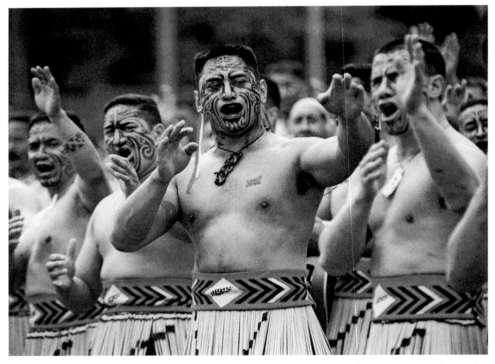

Maori warriors and dancers wearing moko tattoos rehearse the traditional kapa haka. Moko tattoos are highly personal, conveying both status and affiliation. (AP Photo/David Cheskin)

members dried and preserved the tattooed heads (called *Mokomokai*) of high-ranking people to maintain their memory after death. The practice began to fade in the late 19th century, though women continued receiving moko through the 20th century (King and Friedlander 1992).

Today, a cultural revival promotes more active moko designs, especially among New Zealand youth, who see the practice both as a beauty practice and as an important link to their cultural identity. Those with contemporary tattoos often state that they seek a connecting of *whakapapa* (spiritual) philosophies and a deeper spiritual connection with the heritage (Monahan 2009). Designs are typically done with contemporary tattooing equipment. True moko designs continue to be considered sacred by the Maori because of their deep significance to identity and lineage. As with many markers of the beauty of non-Western **Others**, the recent appropriation by non-Maori, Western celebrities, including Robbie Williams, Mike Tyson, Ben Harper, and the male models at a 2007 Jean Paul Gaultier fashion show, has been considered controversial. As a gesture of generosity and consolation to non-Maori individuals who would like to wear "traditional" designs, the Maori offer a generic design known as *kirituhi* ("drawn skin"), which maintains a distinctive Maori flavor but can be applied without offense to anyone, at any time, for any reason.

See also: Lips; Masculinity; The "Other."

Further Reading

King, Michael, and Marti Friedlander. 1992. *Moko: Maori Tattooing in the 20th Century*, 2nd edition. Auckland, New Zealand: David Bateman Publishing.

Monahan, Kate. 2009. "Myth and the Moko." Stuff. Accessed November 22, 2015. http://www.stuff.co.nz/167499.

New Zealand Herald. 2007. "Revival of Moko." Accessed November 22, 2015. http://www.nzherald.co.nz/nz/news/article.cfm?c_id=1&objectid=10484537.

Nikora, Linda Waimarie, Mohi Rua, and Ngahuia Te Awekotuku. 2005. "Wearing Moko: Maori Facial Marking in Today's World." In: *Tattoo, Bodies, Art and Exchange in the Pacific and the West*, edited by Nicholas Thomas, Anna Cole, and Bronwyn Douglas, 191–204. Chicago: University of Chicago Press.

MONROE, MARILYN

Perhaps best known from an iconic set of images where the busty **blonde** wears a white halter dress and bright red lipstick, Marilyn Monroe represents one of the United States' most compelling and tragic figures. She remains immediately recognizable even decades after her death (Steinem 1986).

Imitated in every generation since the height of her fame in the 1950s, the internationally celebrated superstar was born Norma Jeane Mortensen in 1926. The world's most famous platinum blonde was originally a brunette. While working as a factory worker in 1950, she bought a bottle of peroxide to lighten her hair for a screen test (Gattis 2016).

Monroe began modeling during the "bombshell" era where the standard of beauty dictated a buxom, **hourglass shape**. The average Miss America winner during the 1950s had bust–hip–waist measurements of 36-23-36 (Grogan 2008, 19). Women's clothing of the 1950s also deliberately highlighted large **breasts** with tiny waists and slim legs. The 5'5" Marilyn Monroe became the first *Playboy* centerfold in December 1953, showcasing her own 36-22-34 figure from photographs taken five years earlier, when she was a relatively unknown model. Some credit the overwhelming success of the gentleman's **magazine** to this lucky photo spread, which featured a nude Marilyn lying upon a background of red velvet, thus legitimizing nudity by featuring the most famous woman in America.

The roles Monroe played embodied an impossible, contradictory masculine hope for a woman who is both innocent and sensuously experienced at the same time. Monroe was beautiful, but somehow managed to use her vulnerability to appear as a compliant child-woman. Watching Marilyn Monroe, the viewer worries about what might hap-

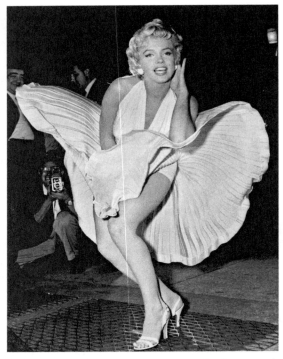

Marilyn Monroe poses over the updraft of New York subway grating while in character for the filming of *The Seven Year Itch* in Manhattan on September 15, 1954. The former Norma Jean Baker modeled, and starred in 28 movies grossing $200 million. Sensual and seductive, but with an air of innocence, Monroe became one of the world's most adored sex symbols. (AP Photo/Matty Zimmerman)

pen to her. Though she was photographed thousands of times, it is still possible to see the self-consciousness in her poses. The viewer feels a need to protect and preserve her beauty. Some have credited Monroe's enduring legacy to the ways she captured the secret desires of men for an undemanding, beautiful woman and the secret fears of women that they will be continually asked to achieve the impossible standard of giving without receiving anything in return and that they might appear dependent, a joke, in danger of becoming a victim (Steinem 1986).

Many commentators have written about the ways that Monroe's beauty prompted others to want to save her. At the height of her fame, she received 5,000 fan letters a week from both men and women who wrote to her because of the "sadness they saw in her eyes" (Kashner 2008). Monroe's death in 1962 at the age of 36 remains an enduring controversy. She died of an overdose that may have been suicide or may have been an accidental side effect of being prescribed sleeping pills and tranquilizers. Her death made front-page news throughout the world and launched a string of conspiracy theories about her alleged relationships with Robert Kennedy and his brother, President John F. Kennedy.

Following her death, many **feminists** began to write about Monroe's life and the ways her career held "a mirror to the exaggerated ways in which female human beings are trained to act" (Steinem 1986). Those portrayals could be seen as embarrassing, sad, and revealing about the ways that society demands women to be "female impersonators." Many feminists also wrote empathically about the lesser known corners of Monroe's life that are shared by many women in the postindustrial age: allegations that Monroe may have been sexually abused as a child; her difficult childhood under the care of a schizophrenic mother; the lack of seriousness and respect that was largely denied her throughout her career; the ways that modeling forced her to suppress her inner self to become an interchangeable "pretty girl"; the ectopic pregnancy that underscored her infertility and inability to become a mother; and the two disastrous marriages to famous men that she tried to have while living a life in the public eye (Steinem 1986).

See also: Blondes and Blonde Hair; Breasts; Feminism; Hourglass Shape; Magazines.

Further Reading

Gattis, Lacey. 2016. "The Best Hair Color Transformations of All Time, From Marilyn Monroe to Jennifer Lawrence." *Vogue*. September 21. Accessed October 11, 2016. http://www.vogue.com/11119225/best-hair-color-transformations-makeovers-of-all-time-marilyn-monroe.

Grogan, Sarah. 2008. *Body Image*, 2nd edition. New York: Routledge.

Kashner, Sam. 2008. "The Things She Left Behind." *Vanity Fair*. Accessed October 11, 2016. http://www.vanityfair.com/news/2008/10/marilyn200810.

Steinem, Gloria. 1986. "The Woman Who Will Not Die." *American Masters*. Accessed October 11, 2016. http://www.pbs.org/wnet/americanmasters/marilyn-monroe-marilyn-monroe-still-life/61.

Summers, Anthony. 1985. *Goddess: The Secret Lives of Marilyn Monroe*. New York: Macmillan.

MOUSTACHE. *See* Facial Hair.

NARCISSISM

Narcissism is characterized by manipulativeness, selfishness, and vanity. Narcissists feel entitled to special treatment in all areas. Their belief in their greatness, beauty, power, and intelligence cannot be swayed, and the narcissist will become defensive and aggressive if these self-perceptions are challenged.

The term "narcissism" comes from a tale by Ovid, the ancient Roman poet and author. Narcissus was a beautiful young boy who spurned a series of lovers and admirers, one of whom curses him to "love what he cannot enjoy." Narcissus saw his reflection in a pool of water as he leaned down to drink and fell in love with the beautiful face that he saw (his own). He was cursed to only love his own image and could never love anyone else (Janan 2007). The tale of Narcissus ends with him dying of thirst because he cannot drink without disturbing the image from which he cannot look away (Burton 2012).

In modern society, narcissists need not be exceptionally attractive. Narcissists are usually preoccupied with attaining the "perfect" image, while not having any capacity to listen to, care about, or understand others (Behary 2013). Some common characteristics include self-absorption (everything is about them), entitlement (makes the rules and breaks the rules), demeaning, put-down behavior, demanding behavior, distrustful behavior, perfectionist behavior (for others, everything must be perfect), superiority and snobbishness, lack of remorse, and lack of empathy.

Because members of society respond to both attractiveness and confidence, narcissists often find a way to be in charge of organizations and decisions, convincing others to give them special privileges that they may not deserve. Studies have found that narcissists are more successful in job interviews, more likely to become leaders, and preferred by the opposite sex.

Narcissists can be fashionable, charming, and confident, but long-term attempts to work with them often fail. Because a narcissist has an insatiable need for attention and praise, they may be difficult to get along with. Narcissists often end up being fired, sued, divorced, or thrown out because those surrounding them have "had enough" (Behary 2013).

Descriptions of the characteristics and traits of narcissists, as well as the social problems they cause, are certainly not limited to North American or Western cultural values. Studies in nations such as China reveal that those with narcissistic traits believe themselves to be much more attractive and agreeable than the way others see them (Zhou, Zhang, Yang, et al. 2015).

Although narcissism is present in both men and women, it is more common in men, and some believe that 20th-century changes in the way that men's appearance is evaluated have exacerbated the prevalence of narcissism in men. Both modern conceptions of metrosexuality and progressive muscularity are related to narcissistic attitudes in men, who seek, in self-absorbed fashion, to create a perfect image of themselves to show others (Collis, Lewis, and Crisp 2016).

See also: Bodybuilding; Metrosexual; Progressive Muscularity; Vanity.

Further Reading

Behary, Wendy. 2013. *Disarming the Narcissist: Surviving & Thriving with the Self-absorbed.* Oakland, CA: New Harbinger Publications.

Burton, Neel. 2012. "Thinking About Love: The Myth of Narcissus." *Psychology Today.* Accessed September 29, 2016. https://www.psychologytoday.com/blog/hide-and-seek/201203/thinking-about-love-the-myth-narcissus.

Collis, Nathan, Vivienne Lewis, and Dimity Crisp. 2016. "When Is Buff Enough? The Effect of Body Attitudes and Narcissistic Traits on Muscle Dysmorphia." *Journal of Men's Studies* 24, no. 2: 213–25.

Janan, Micaela. 2007. "Narcissus on the Text: Psychoanalysis, Exegesis, Ethics." *Phoenix* 61, no. 3/4: 286–95.

Psychology Today. 2016. "Narcissistic Personality Disorder." Accessed September 29, 2016. https://www.psychologytoday.com/conditions/narcissistic-personality-disorder.

Young, Emma. 2016. "All About Me." *New Scientist* 231, no. 3081: 26.

Zhou, Hui, Bao Zhang, Xiaoyang Yang, and Xiao Chen. 2015. "Are Chinese Narcissists Disagreeable? Evidence from Self- and Peer-Ratings of Agreeableness." *Asian Journal of Social Psychology* 18, no. 2: 163–69.

NOSE JOBS

The International Society for Aesthetic Plastic Surgery (ISAPS) defines rhinoplasty (more commonly known as a "nose job" or "nose surgery") as a procedure that "reshapes the nose by reducing or increasing the size, removing a hump, changing the shape of the tip or bridge, narrowing the span of the nostrils, or changing the angle between the nose and upper lip" (ISAPS 2015b). This procedure is often undertaken to improve breathing in patients, but is also one of the world's most common aesthetic surgeries.

In 2014, rhinoplasty was overall the fourth most common cosmetic surgical procedure performed worldwide, after eyelid surgery, breast augmentation, and liposuction. Among men, however, nose surgery was the second most common aesthetic procedure. Although Iran has gained some notoriety for the number of rhinoplasties performed in that nation, the percentage of citizens having rhinoplasty in Iran was still significantly lower than in other nations (Davis 2008). In 2014, more than 800,000 nose surgeries were reported in nations around the globe, with South Korea leading the list of nations performing the most rhinoplasties, with 102,597 surgeries performed. The other nations where rhinoplasty was most commonly performed in 2014 were Brazil, the United States, Mexico, and Japan. (ISAPS 2015a).

Rhinoplasty has been practiced since at least the 1920s, when cosmetic surgery began to gain widespread traction as a way to improve not only a person's appearance, but also their mental health and level of self-esteem. Early advertisements and reporting on the procedure in the United States, for example, extolled the virtue of "modern surgery" on the nose to "remedy the looks and appearances of individuals who enjoy good physical health but are weighed down psychologically by some deformity of appearance" (Haiken 1999, 126).

Since that time, nose surgeries have been undertaken worldwide not only to correct what are considered "deformities" of the nose, but also to allow people to conform to a globally standardized norm of beauty that privileges a thin, pointed, well-defined nose that communicates a white, Euro-descended appearance. This process is often termed "caucasianization," the adopting of the beauty norms and aesthetics of Caucasian people (Lin 2001). Three groups that are cited as regularly receiving nose jobs and other procedures for the purpose of adopting Caucasian beauty norms are African Americans, Asians, and people of Jewish Heritage (Haiken 1999).

The American actress Fanny Brice was among the first celebrities to publically undergo cosmetic rhinoplasty in 1923. Although the actress herself denied it, most of her contemporaries and many scholars believe that the decision to undergo the procedure was an attempt to look "less Jewish" (Haiken 1999, 182). After the very public example of Ms. Brice in the United States, the first group to show a widespread movement to undertake cosmetic surgery in order to reduce elements of their physical appearance deemed "ethnic" was Jewish persons, often in pursuit of a more "Roman nose" (Haiken 1999, 182). Though this trend continued for generations of American Jews, in the second decade of the 20th century, studies show that young Jewish American women have been undergoing rhinoplasty in fewer numbers, a trend credited to increased ethnic pride among American Jews (Rubin 2012).

As the effort to "caucasianize" a nose has declined among the Jewish population of the United States, other U.S. groups and populations worldwide are undergoing surgeries in greater numbers. In Asian populations both in the United States and abroad, for example, patients influenced by globalized images of Western beauty seek nose implants to create a more pointed, and less wide nose (Haiken 1999). In Latin American nations, pursuit of what is known as the perfect "*nariz perfilada*" [defined nose] often leads to aesthetic rhinoplasty to communicate a more desirable race and class status (Gulbas 2008, 231). Indeed, in some Latin American nations, surgeons openly discuss cosmetic surgery as a specific "correction of negroid nose" (Edmonds 2010, 144).

Rhinoplasty is performed as an outpatient procedure under general anesthesia. The surgery generally takes an hour or more. After the surgery, there is usually bruising and stuffiness in the nasal passages. Permanent risks associated with rhinoplasty can include infection, but the main risk is an unsatisfactory appearance of the new nose (for example, unevenness) that may require further surgery (ISAPS 2015b).

See also: Class; Eyelid Surgery; Plastic Surgery.

Further Reading

Davis, Rowenna. 2008. "Nose No Problem." *New Statesman* 137, no. 4887: 21.

Edmonds, Alexander. 2010. *Pretty Modern: Beauty, Sex and Plastic Surgery in Brazil*. Durham, NC: Duke University Press.

Gulbas, Lauren. 2008. "Cosmetic Surgery and the Politics of Race, Class and Gender in Caracas, Venezuela." PhD diss. Southern Methodist University.

Haiken Elizabeth 1999. *Venus Envy: A History of Cosmetic Surgery*. Baltimore: Johns Hopkins University Press.

ISAPS. 2015a. "Global Statistics." Accessed August 20, 2015. http://www.isaps.org/Media/Default/globalstatistics/2015%20ISAPS%20Results.

ISAPS. 2015b "Rhinoplasty." Accessed August 25, 2015. http://www.isaps.org/procedures/rhinoplasty.

Lin, Shirley. 2001. "In the Eye of the Beholder?: Eyelid Surgery and Young Asian-American Women." Accessed August 27, 2015. http://www.alternet.org/story/10557/in_the_eye_of_the_beholder%3A_eyelid_surgery_and_young_asian-american_women.

Rubin, Rita. 2012. "A Nose Dive for Nose Jobs." Accessed August 27, 2015. http://www.tabletmag.com/jewish-life-and-religion/101732/a-nose-dive-for-nose-jobs.

OBESITY

Evolutionary biologists suggest that obesity was an important adaptive feature to maintain optimal health for those living in times of poverty and food scarcity. The seasonal aspects of feast and famine may have conditioned early humans to value the fertility promised by a rounder, more filled-out shape (Shipton 1990). A psychological study at the University of Liverpool found that the hungrier a person was, the more desirable they found heavier women, prompting researchers to speculate that resource availability may intersect with aesthetic preference (Swami, Poulogianni, and Furnham 2006).

However, rarely is a culture's notion of the perfect body in agreement with the population's actual shape or size (Savacool 2009, 17). Most of the time, the cultural standards for beauty comprise a narrow range of acceptable body shapes and sizes (Grogan 2008, 5). Countries ravaged by famine or disease may prefer heavier bodies; in the United States, where 3,900 calories are consumed every day for every man, woman, and child, the cultural preference is for slim bodies.

A recent study measured cultural attitudes toward obese people in six countries and compared this to the population's actual body size. They found that although the United States ranked second highest in body mass index (BMI), it also ranked second highest in the belief that fatness is not a culturally acceptable aesthetic. The study also found that respondents in the study ranked fear of becoming fat as one of their most significant fears and that they equated fatness with laziness or lack of intelligence. The perception of the respondents was that overweight people "didn't care" about living a healthy lifestyle (Savacool 2009, 43).

NAAFA, the National Association to Advance Fat Acceptance, was created in 1969 explicitly to contest popular notions of beauty in the United States (Gimlin 2002, 111). Members of the organization argue that they are discriminated against both socially and professionally by the broader society. They point to the considerable barriers they face buying clothes, gaining access to common spaces such as the theater or on public transportation, and inferior treatment by health professionals and insurance companies. NAAFA's policy documents charge society with regarding its fat members as not only physically ugly, but also suspect them of possessing immoral character flaws and a lack of personal discipline. Members of NAAFA suffer from cruel jokes and verbal assaults, causing them to endure feelings of guilt and worthlessness (Ibid.). The goals of NAAFA, which sponsors a number of social events designed to introduce members to individuals who are attracted to heavy people, include pursuing anti–size discrimination legislation and investigating the negative treatment of fat people within a wide range of institutional policies and practices.

Among the cattle-herding Bodi of Ethiopia, men gorge on large quantities of a mixture of cow's blood and milk to compete to see who can become the "fattest" (Afritorial 2013). Families enter unmarried men for the challenge who live in isolation for six months and avoid movement and sexual relations for the duration of the competition. The blood is derived from the cattle of the family, who are not killed but bled each day to provide the nutritional supplement. Men must be able to drink the blood and milk mixture quickly, before it coagulates. Obviously, the ability of the young man to bulk up on this diet depends on the number of cattle owned by the family lineage and also the ability of the family to care for the livestock in such a way that they are robust and able to shed blood regularly in pursuit of the young man's enlargement. The result of six months of gorging displays itself in a large, round belly, which the man will eventually shed as he resumes his normal way of life.

The mark of beauty for Ndebele women in South Africa focuses on well-rounded lower bodies, especially through the buttocks, hips, and thighs. Traditional fashion encouraged women to wear large beaded hoops around their waists and legs called *golwani*. These *golwani* were designed to look like "rolls of fat" and were often stuffed with rubber or other materials to enhance the size and appearance of the buttocks. Large buttocks were an essential sign of womanliness and the central focus of dances, where women contracted their buttock muscles in rhythm with the music (Savacool 2009, 79).

The curvy hourglass shape of a woman is preferred in Jamaican culture, where the Coca-Cola bottle shape is a reference for a woman's ideal body (Savacool 2009, 90). Large body size is an important indicator of status and wealth, thinness is pitied, and heavier women are considered more attractive. Enthusiasm for fuller figures can be traced to Jamaican folk notions about the body, especially the belief in "vital fluids" necessary to make life. Being flush and swelling with ripeness, like a fruit, was thought to be a good indicator of healthy men and women, with the body literally bursting with life. The vital fluids concept remains important to Jamaican folk medicine and lifestyle regimens, as people seek to balance the sense of fullness with management of adult sexuality and attractiveness. Until fairly recently, Jamaican women proudly discussed weight gain, an implication of being well loved and successful in life. Women welcomed the opportunity to show curvy bodies in the dance halls, and they also welcomed a mature lifestyle that accommodated a well-rounded adult woman.

Gender also mediates the degrees to which obesity is accepted as positive or attractive. For civil servants in contemporary Cameroon, a mark of success is the inability to fasten one's shirt collar because of a fat neck, proudly called *le cou plié* (de Garine 1995, 46). Sumo wrestlers, of course, are valued for the girth and size, though the look of the Sumo is not necessarily widely sought as a standard of beauty among the Japanese.

If standards of obesity and attractiveness exist outside of the Western set of expectations for a slender, fit body, it is also important to note that the hegemony of American media actively spreads Western standards of beauty to other parts of the world. Medical anthropologist Anne Becker conducted a series of studies with Fijians about body image beginning in 1989. She found that in Fiji, a preference for larger bodies was driven by an equation that body size was correlated to personal wealth. Her initial team of researchers visited fishing villages and encountered a culture where the average body mass for women was 29.8. (In the United States, a BMI score of 30 or higher is considered obese.) Becker and her team reported that there were virtually no concerns on the part of the people about body size or body shape: people acknowledged that a larger body was considered healthy and a sign that one was able to eat well. No one in the initial study expressed insecurity about their bodies or felt any motivation to change the way they looked (Becker 1995).

With fully two-thirds of male and female adults in Becker's sample considered "overweight," the team collected remarks and appearances on the general shape of others. They discovered that when favorably impressed, Fijians described a person as *juba vina* (well formed) to refer to a full body. Additionally, Fijians were active and enjoyed life. The traditional Fijian styles of dance emphasized movements of the belly and hips, similar to native Hawaiian dancing, and so the ideal Fijian body accentuated an awareness of these regions on a woman's body.

Becker returned to Fiji in 1998 to restudy the fishing community where she had lived (and gained twenty pounds) a decade earlier. She found that up to 15 percent of the young girls in her original study were now plagued by eating disorders and feelings of self-loathing about their bodies. Becker blames the rapid social change on the introduction of television to the island, enabled by the country's new infrastructure of electrical and television cable. For the first time, the average Fijian had access to television and began to measure themselves against the standards of the bodies that they saw displayed there.

See also: BBW; Weight; Wife Fattening.

Further Reading

Afritorial. 2013. "The Bodi: Where Big Is Beautiful." Accessed July 21, 2016. http://afritorial.com/tribe-the-bodi.

Becker, Anne. 1995. *Body, Self, and Society*. Philadelphia: University of Pennsylvania Press.

Chernin, Kim. 1985. *The Hungry Self: Women, Eating, and Identity*. New York: Harper Perennial.

De Garine, Igor. 1995. "Sociocultural Aspects of the Male Fattening Sessions among the Massa of Northern Cameroon." In: *Social Aspects of Obesity*, edited by Igor de Garine and Nancy J. Pollock, 45–70. Amsterdam: Gordon and Breach Publishers.

Gimlin, Debra. 2002. *Body Work: Beauty and Self-Image in American Culture*. Berkeley, CA: University of California Press.

Grogan, Sarah. 2008. *Body Image: Understanding Body Dissatisfaction in Men, Women, and Children*. New York: Routledge.

Savacool, Julia. 2009. *The World Has Curves: The Global Quest for the Perfect Body*. New York: Rodale.

Shipton, Parker. 1990. "African Famines and Food Security: Anthropological Perspectives." *Annual Review of Anthropology* 19: 353–94.

Sobo, Elisa J. 1994. "The Sweetness of Fat: Health, Procreation, and Sociability in Rural Jamaica." In: *Many Mirrors*, edited by Nicole Sault, 132–54. New Brunswick, NJ: Rutgers University Press.

Stearns, Peter N. 1997. *Fat History: Bodies and Beauty in the Modern West.* New York: New York University Press.

Swami, Viren, Katia Poulogianni, and Adrian Furnham. 2006. "The Influence of Resource Availability on Preferences for Human Body Weight and Non-human Objects." *Journal of Articles in Support of the Null Hypothesis* 4: 17–28.

ORIENTALISM

Relying on a critical reading of historical works of art and literary analysis, Edward Said's 1978 pivotal book *Orientalism* offers a powerful critique of the way the Western world perceives and defines the East.

Said's analysis explores the imaginary landscape of the 13th and 14th centuries, in the wake of Marco Polo's highly sensationalized tour of China and when some intrepid European traders ventured as far east as the Silk Road to explore "strange new worlds." As these stories took on more resonance, attracting more and more curiosity, it was essential that Europeans establish themselves as the standard by which the story be told. The West is the "Occident": it is the norm, the standard, the fixed point at the center of the universe. The Orient, by design, is the **Other**: the exact opposite of everything in the West. The East was imagined to be exotic, foreign, deviant, and abnormal. Whereas Western men believe themselves to be godly, good, moral, virile, and powerful rulers of empire, they emphasize the markers of difference as signs of decadence or immorality, especially in the ways that "Orientals" look, dress, or behave. Travel writers collected texts about strange religions, martial arts, mysticism, magic, bright colors, unusual foods, barbaric practices, and incomprehensible languages (Fang 2014). Everything that was familiar, comfortable, or safe could be jeopardized in Asia, which came to be seen as alien, Other. Importantly, Said points out that this **social construction** of the nature of the East was created primarily to serve and reinforce the West's own moral conception of itself as superior and dominant.

However, difference carries fascination. Explorers to the East were fixated on how Eastern people, especially women, looked. Completely out-of-context stories about the insatiable sexual appetites of harem girls, dragon ladies, and **geisha** circulated. As time passed and travelers found it easier to reach foreign cities like Constantinople, a wide range of lush, ultra-realistic paintings of "harem" women, alternately described as courtesans, odalisques, and prostitutes, began to appear in salons across Europe, stoking the curiosity about "the Orient" and providing dubious hypersexualized narratives about women living there. Paired with these notions of the lotus-eating, sexually aggressive woman were stereotypes of barbaric, cowardly, and effeminate men.

Although many may admire the silk gowns or "exotic" stylings of the far East, depicting diminutive, "dainty," or fierce "Asian" models in advertising or alluring promotional materials, some Orientalist framings are also (a subtle or not-so-subtle) form of racism (Fang 2014). The strategic positioning of the "Oriental" object continues to construct Eastern cultures as "civilizations" with strikingly different ideologies and rhetoric that make their people incompatible in Western contexts (Smith 2013). Cherokee activist Andrea Smith writes about this differentiation between culture and civilizations that is used over and over in Western political rhetoric that is designed to exclude and keep Easterner immigrants out of "democratic" countries because of assumptions about their innate differences, inferiority, and fundamentalist incompatibility with Western logic.

See also: Exoticize; Geisha; The "Other"; Social Construction of Beauty.

Further Reading

Fang, Jenn. 2014. "What Is Orientalism, and How Is It Also Racism?" *Reapprorpriate.* Accessed October 1, 2016. http://reappropriate.co/2014/04/what-is-orientalism-and-how -is-it-also-racism.
Said, Edward. 1978. *Orientalism.* New York: Vintage.
Smith, Andrea. 2013. "Heteropatriarchy and the Three Pillars of White Supremacy. Women's Empowerment and Leadership Development for Democratization." Accessed October 1, 2016. http://www.weldd.org/resources/heteropatriarchy-and-three-pillars-white -supremacy.

THE "OTHER"

Philosophers since Hegel have made use of the notion of the "Other" to describe the peculiar and hard-to-describe-in-words phenomenon of self-consciousness. The abstract notion unfolds from the combined perspective of the "Self," that objective part of the person which is able to observe and act, and the "Other," that part which is subjective, passive, and unknowable. The Other is an alien social entity to the Self, which exists externally to the Self, and must be present in order to validate the Self. In 1949, French philosopher Simone de Beauvoir applied the concept more directly to patriarchal systems where the Woman is treated as the Other in relation to the primary subject, Man. De Beauvoir wrote, "[A] man represents both the positive and the neutral, as indicated by the common use of Man to designate human beings in general; whereas Woman represents only the negative" (de Beauvoir 1949).

Another use of the term "Othering" comes as a reaction to the proliferation of categories dealing with "racial types" and the highly dubious "scientific" representation of non-Western women during the colonial era. An early version of the term appears in Orientalism, a study of the ways in which political powers, philosophers, medical professionals, and artists had "othered" people from Eastern regions (more generally called "The Orient") in order to draw an arbitrary divide between the West and the East, the "self" and the "Other." With this theoretical structure of difference in place, it became easier for Western writers to begin drawing binary comparisons between themselves as the enlightened world and the "Other" as underdeveloped, chaotic, and archaic. With this structure in place, unequal imperialistic relationships could justify the continual subordination of the "Other" in order to exploit labor, land, and natural resources.

Feminist scholars since de Beauvoir have found the concept of "Othering" useful in describing and analyzing the mechanisms of power that supported male-dominated systems of cultural imperialism. Highly sought French picture postcards of Algerian women during the colonial era displayed women and girls in fetching poses devised by the photographer, although sometimes they were also posed in ways that showed them being dominated or dehumanized (Corbey 1988). In these artifacts of the colonial era, the viewer is granted permission to consume the naked body of the "native" through symbolic acts of cultural violence based in a legacy of colonization, which assumes the right to depict others in a way that does not honor their humanity, but relegates them to objects associated with erotic fantasy.

Basically, these colonial representations **fetishized** the experience of viewing an exposed body within a context of power, domination, and sexualization. Feminist performance artist Coco Fusco labeled this supposedly scientific fascination a conflation of "pornographically inflected voyeurism with ethnography—the voyeurism involved in turning us into ethnographic objects on display. Looking at naked women of color in *National Geographic* constitutes the first pornographic experiences for a lot of American boys" (Lavin 1994, 82).

Representations such as those that appeared in "scientific" journals like *National Geographic* depicted many more naked women than men. The images, especially of bare-**breasted** African women, drew the curious and potentially lascivious attention of the Western world. An early and influential text was Carl Heinrich Stratz's *Die Rassenschönheit des Weibes* ("Racial Beauty of the Woman"). Stratz was a German gynecologist and photographer. His best-selling text featured a wide collection of photographs of naked and seminaked non-Western women and was published in 22 worldwide editions between 1901 and 1941.

See also: Breasts; Exoticize; Orientalism.

Further Reading

Boskovic, Aleksander. 2001. "Out of Africa: Images of Women in Anthropology and Popular Culture." *Etnolog* 11: 177–83.

Corbey, Raymond. 1988. "Alterity: The Colonial Nude." *Critique of Anthropology* 8, no. 3: 75–92.

De Beauvoir, Simone. 1949. *Second Sex*. New York: Vintage.

Lavin, Maud. 1994. "What's So Bad about 'Bad Girl' Art?" *Ms Magazine* March/April: 80–83.

OTOPLASTY

Otoplasty, or "ear surgery," is a procedure to either reduce the size of the ears or to "pin the ears back" on patients whose ears stick out perpendicularly from their heads. The International Society of Aesthetic and Plastic Surgery describes otoplasty as a surgery that "sets prominent ears back closer to the head and/or reduces the size of large ears" (ISAPS 2015b). One of the significant differences between this particular form of plastic surgery and others is that it is commonly performed on children between the ages of four and fourteen.

Otoplasty is one of the oldest known forms of plastic surgery, with recorded instances of the procedure dating as far back as BCE 7th century in the famous treatise of the Indian surgeon Sushruta in his treatise *Sushruta Samhita* (Saraf and Parihar 2006). Whereas the surgeries described by Sushruta covered deformed or injured earlobes, the first recorded purely cosmetic surgery on the earlobes occurred in 1881 in Europe (Adamson and Litner 2011).

One of the reasons that otoplasty is both performed on children and may covered by insurance is the effect of a "Dumbo ears" appearance on the self-esteem of young people. The bullying and teasing that accompany protruding ears are widely recognized, and the surgery to correct this particular difference in appearance is more commonly acceptable than some other cosmetic procedures. Another factor is the relatively noninvasive nature of the procedure, which is often performed on an outpatient basis (Pham 2010).

Although otoplasty is a procedure generally used to create a more pleasing appearance of the ears and reduce the instance of bullying or low self-esteem, some recent developments have necessitated the procedure for adults for whom ears that stuck out too far were a danger and a threat to their physical health. In 2002, two physicians working with U.S. Army soldiers deployed in the field found that soldiers with protruding ears were suffering serious abrasions on their ears from the weight of the Kevlar helmets that they wore in the field for protection. Doctors Salgado and Mardini performed otoplasty on a number of these soldiers and were able to report not only a relief of the symptoms caused by the helmets, but also cosmetic improvement in the appearance of the soldiers (Salgado and Mardini 2006).

Otoplasty is an outpatient surgery with few associated risks. These risks may include infection or excessive scarring, but the biggest risk associated with otoplasty is an unwelcome cosmetic result, fake-looking ears, mismatched ears, or a recurrence of the protrusion of the ears that can require additional surgery (ISAPS 2015b).

See also: Plastic Surgery.

Further Reading

Adamson, Peter, and Jason A. Litner. 2011. *Aesthetic Otoplasty: Thomas Procedures in Facial Plastic Surgery*. Shelton, CT: People's Medical Publishing House.

ISAPS. 2015a. "Global Statistics." Accessed November 19, 2015. http://www.isaps.org/Media/Default/global-statistics/2015%20ISAPS%20Results.pdf.

ISAPS. 2015b. "Otoplasty." Accessed November 19, 2015. http://www.isaps.org/procedures/ear-surgery.

Pham, Thailan. 2010. "Teenage Plastic Surgery." *People* 73, no. 13: 107.

Salgado, Christopher J., and Samir Mardini. 2006. "Corrective Otoplasty for Symptomatic Prominent Ears in U.S. Soldiers." *Military Medicine* 171, no. 2: 128–30.

Saraf S., and R. Parihar. 2006. "Sushruta: The First Plastic Surgeon in 600 B.C." *The Internet Journal of Plastic Surgery* 4, no. 2. Accessed November 19, 2015. http://ispub.com/IJPS/4/2/8232.

P

PAGEANTS, INDIGENOUS

Although the concept of the beauty pageant is a well-recognized global phenomenon that brings together women from different nations to be judged under a single vision of world beauty and poise, an alternative type of pageant, the indigenous, or Indian pageant, celebrates and rewards more specifically local standards of traditional and cultural heritage. From Hawaii to Guatemala, there are many competitions designed to teach, maintain, and celebrate indigenous culture.

Beauty contests and pageants are well-recognized vehicles for the affirmation and dissemination of a society's values (Ballerino Cohen, Wilk, and Stoltje 1996). Beauty pageants and contests are often used to create and display symbolic beauty; an image that reflects the group's collectively held identity and rewards adherence to social norms of beauty, virtue, and the moral ideals. In the case of Indian pageants, this process is used to celebrate, promote, and preserve cultural traditions that the groups see as threatened and in danger.

Many indigenous pageants evaluate not only the physical appearance of the contestants, but also their ability to engage in traditionally "authentic" practices and skills prized by the culture. The ability to weave or throw pottery can be as important to victory as traditional dress and hairstyle. The pageants can be a defiant gesture of the continuing power and vigor of indigenous culture (Konefal 2009).

In Guatemala, a nation with many Maya Indians, the election of the *Rab'in Ajaw* [Indian Princess] takes place at a national festival every July. The event, the National Folklore Festival, was originally organized in 1969 as a way to preserve and celebrate Mayan heritage and tradition (Schackt 2005). Seeking to preserve traditional dress and weaving techniques, the organizers developed the idea of electing an "Indian Princess" who would demonstrate not only the appearance of "authentic" Mayan culture, but also the ability to make and design her own costume (Schackt 2005).

Participants in the *Rab'in Ajaw* must make their own traditional clothing, showing their knowledge of traditional craft skills. The women who participate must also, however, show adherence to indigenous norms of modesty. Mayan Indian codes of decency for women insist that a woman's lower half always be covered, from waist to ground. A swimsuit competition, therefore, would be unthinkable. It is, however, characteristic of some Maya towns on the coast, where it is very hot, for women to wear only the skirt and to go bare breasted. This standard, then, is acceptable, if not preferred, for the contestants from those areas (Schackt 2009).

The idea of an "Indian Pageant" designed to preserve indigenous traditions is not confined to Latin America. The Indian nations of the United States and Canada also participate in a similar event. The United States has hosted the "Miss Indian World" competition annually at the Gathering of Nations powwow in Albuquerque, New Mexico, since 1984 (Gatewood 2014). In 2016, 24 contestants from 24 different indigenous tribes in North America competed (Madalena 2016). In the words of one contestant, it was a way to "introduce my tribe to the world" (Gatewood 2014).

The "Miss Indian World" pageant does not advertise itself exclusively as a "beauty pageant." Rather, it calls itself a "culture pageant," designed to showcase the lives, work, knowledge, and traditional appearance of young Indian women from the United States and Canada. The idea of selecting one young woman to represent the cultural values of the group is common in beauty pageants and has particular relevance for some American native nations. In Quechua, the language of the people commonly called Inca, for example, women are known as "*tage*," an honorific describing a woman's role as not only the reproducer of people

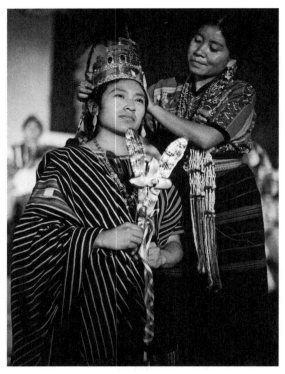

Rosa Lidia Aguare Castro receives the *Rab'in Ajaw*, or Indian Princess, crown from last year's winner Sara Dalila Mux Mux, at the Rab'in Ajaw National Folkloric Festival and Indian beauty contest in Coban, Guatemala, July 30, 2011. Unlike traditional beauty contests, the panel of judges not only value the participants' leadership skills, but their commitment to the rescue and maintenance of Maya values. The contestants, whose ages range from 14 to 26 years, go through numerous rounds of competition, including a speech that must be given in their native dialect and Spanish. (AP Photo/Rodrigo Abd)

through childbirth, but also the reproducer of customs, values, and traditions. A woman is "*tage*" in the way she accumulates and dispenses her knowledge of her people's culture and values (Barrig 2001).

Participants in the Miss Indian World contest compete in five categories: traditional dance, traditional talent, essay, personal interview, and public speaking. Each category is judged based on the cultural knowledge of the contestant's home tribe and her ability to present that information to others (Miss Indian World 2016). In keeping with her symbolic nature as a representative of her tribe and indigenous culture, each competitor must also agree to a code of conduct that is strict in communicating the morals and values of the position. The young woman must not be a mother and may not, under any circumstances, engage in "Unacceptable socializing with a companion in public." No public displays of affection are allowed. She must refrain from the use of alcohol or cigarettes and not use strong or "profane language."

These rules, similar to those of any beauty pageant anywhere, help underline and emphasize the symbolic nature of the "Queen": to serve as a visual symbol of morality, virtue, beauty, and worth for the culture she represents.

See also: Maya; Pageants—International, National, and Local; Pageants—Transpageants.

Further Reading

Ballerino Cohen, Colleen, Richard Wilk, and Beverly Stoltje. 1996. *Beauty Queens on the Global Stage: Gender, Contests and Power.* New York, Routledge.

Barrig, Maruja. 2001. *El mundo al revés: Imágenes de la mujer indígena.* Buenos Aires, Argentina: CLASCO.

Gatewood, Tara. 2014 "Miss Indian World at 30." *Native Peoples Magazine* 27, no. 2: 38.

Konefal, Betsy. 2009. "Subverting Authenticity: Reinas Indígenas and the Guatemalan State, 1978." *Hispanic American Historical Review* 89, no. 1: 41–72.

Madalena, Leandra. 2016. "2016 Miss Indian World Contestants." April 16. Accessed July 22, 2016. http://www.gatheringofnations.com/2016-miss-indian-world-contestants.

Miss Indian World 2016. "2017 Official Miss Indian World Application." Accessed July 22, 2016. http://www.gatheringofnations.com/miss-indian-world-information.

Schackt, Jon. 2005. "Mayahood Through Beauty: Indian Beauty Pageants in Guatemala." *Bulletin of Latin American Research* 24, no. 3: 269–87.

PAGEANTS—INTERNATIONAL, NATIONAL, AND LOCAL CONTESTS

The 21st-century system of international beauty contests and pageants, from Miss Universe to Miss World, began as an unrelated system of local competitions in several different countries. Whereas what we would now recognize as a beauty contest first became common worldwide in the mid-20th century, the process of selecting one woman to serve as the symbolic representative of a culture's values—the "Queen" of morality, hard work, and beauty—goes back much further.

Most scholars who study the phenomenon of the beauty pageant divide the practice into two categories: the beauty contest, which is a simple effort, whether in person or via mail or the Internet, to allow voters to choose the winner of a competition based on the criteria that the contest sets. An example of this type of beauty competition would be the first "Señorita Venezuela" [Miss Venezuela] ever elected in 1905. This competition served as a marketing plan for a national cigar company. In that year, the manufacturer handed out postcards with the images of beautiful women in tobacco shops. Customers collected the cards, then sent the one that they chose as the most beautiful back to the company. The girl represented on the most cards as received by the manufacturer was selected as "Miss Venezuela" (Nichols 2016).

> "Taught from infancy that beauty is woman's scepter, the mind shapes itself to the body, and roaming round its gilt cage, only seeks to adorn its prison."
>
> —MARY WOLLSTONECRAFT

This type of contest, with public voting, is slightly different from the modern idea of the beauty "pageant," in which the competition itself appears surrounded by an elaborate production, or show. In a "pageant" the performance of the contestants is much more central to their success (as opposed to a simple photograph), and the judging of the contest is not usually undertaken by the general public, but rather a select group. This type of spectacle has a long tradition, especially with regard to the evaluation of female beauty. We can trace the roots of the public celebration and critical appraisal of the female form back to the rituals associated with goddess worship and the selection of priestesses in ancient Mesopotamia (Wember 2009).

In each of these cases, whether contests or pageants, the effort of displaying and selecting, choosing, and evaluating male and female beauty is commonly understood as a way that societies teach, reinforce, and maintain common cultural values. Some researchers go so far as to propose the beauty pageant as a way that a culture helps construct its own identity, while instructing members on the importance of adherence to the norms being represented. In this way, a beauty pageant or beauty contest is a public act of civic participation (Du Toit 2009).

For many women, especially in developing nations, the process of working through the local, national, and international beauty pageant process is a way for advancement and success in their personal and professional lives. Women without physically safe home regions (such as nations at war), those whose families are impoverished, and those women without access to higher education or resources for their families make up a number of the contestants in international contests, which often supply training, education, scholarships, and cash prizes. As one contestant from a war-torn nation confided to a trainer at the Miss Universe competition, "You can have my foot, I'll give it to you. Just get me out of my country" (Dominus 2016).

Many local and national beauty pageants began worldwide as searches for a local "bathing beauty," often with an associated desire to promote tourism to the location where the pageant was held. The Miss America pageant was born in 1921 in the oceanside town of Atlantic City as a contest of local women in bathing suits, and the Miss England pageant started with a search for the local "Bathing Beauty Queen" in the seaside resort city of Morcambe (Cooke 2004). In other areas of the world, the election of the Queen of Carnival, the pre-Lenten celebration also known as Mardi Gras, was one of the first types of public beauty pageants. In Latin America and the Caribbean, the first contests, like the one mentioned earlier in Venezuela, were publicity stunts for local or national businesses, beginning the strong link between pageantry and economic consumption (Barnes 2006). In time, these local contests became national and then international, with the first Miss Universe pageant taking place in 1952 and the first Miss World event happening in 1951.

Although the foundational events that prompted the creation of the international competition may have started as searches for local bathing beauties, the national and international competitions of the 21st century often place emphasis on different sets of values and morals, while still reinforcing globalized social norms of beauty, which often privileged a Euro-descended appearance over local traditions or phys-ical features.

Many nations over time have used the spectacle of the beauty pageant to iden-tify and reinforce the cultural values deemed most important for women in the nation. In 1930s Argentina, for example, the prototypical local and national beauty pageants were organized to select "The Prettiest Little Worker." These pageants allowed each working community, from vineyard workers to dairy farmers, to pick the woman who represented for them the ideal combination of beauty, a strong work ethic, and firm family values (Lobato 2005). This type of pageant was important for the Argentine project of national identity building as the former colony sought to project a "modern" image and participate in the global stage. The values of hard work, family loyalty, and adherence to global, Euro-descended beauty norms helped Argentina place itself in the wider economic, cultural, and political arena (Nichols 2014).

Indeed, the desire to appear "modern" and conform to global beauty standards, which inevitably are based in European visions of body type, facial features, and hair, is seen across the globe. In the Caribbean, through the 20th century, local and national pageants continued to devalue Afro-descended features and traditional cul-ture while seeking to aspire to globalized European and North American appear-ances (Barnes 2006).

In Africa, in order to be successful in the Miss Universe or Miss World competi-tion, local and national groups had to stop selecting candidates that conformed to local beauty norms and find young women who the local culture did not necessarily feel were beautiful, but who would validate local beauty by conforming to globalized norms. The first African Miss World, Agbani Durego in 2001, from Nigeria, was the product of a specific campaign by the orga-nizers of the Miss Nigeria pag-eant (called "The Most Beautiful Girl in the World). In the cam-paign, the pageant made a con-scious effort to reject local beauty norms that called for a "Coke bottle–shaped" body and look for a tall, slim beauty that would fit in with the rest of the world's representatives. The result was a winner, but one who was not particularly attractive to Nigeri-ans (Onishi 2002).

It is undeniable that in the 21st century, the contestants for the premier international beauty

---

Miss Landmine

One controversial 21st-century pageant was "Miss Landmine." The first "Miss Landmine" was a project organized by a Norwegian filmmaker in cooperation with the government of Angola, a heavily mined nation. The pageant's ideal was to help create awareness while challenging social norms of beauty and raising the self-esteem of those injured and disfigured by mines. The pageant in Angola was controversial, as observers debated whether the format of the pageant was appro-priate, especially in the context of a European outsider coming in to police "beauty" in the nation. The second "Miss Landmine," which was planned to be held in 2009 in another heavily mined nation, Cambodia, was cancelled by the government at the last minute and ended in a secret international Internet vote to select the winner.

contests, Miss Universe and Miss World, all look remarkably similar. A quick look at the slate of contestants for any year will reveal women from 90 or more nations around the globe who are the same height, with the same body type, same hair texture and style, and remarkably similar facial features. This is, perhaps, why different, competing contests and pageants have appeared, including indigenous pageants, pageants for the disabled, and pageants for women who carry more weight than global beauty norms would expect.

See also: Argentina; Pageants—Indigenous; Pageants—Transpageants; Venezuela.

Further Reading

Barnes, Natasha. 2006. *Cultural Conundrums: Gender, Race, Nation, and the Making of Caribbean Cultural Politics*. Ann Arbor, MI: University of Michigan Press.

Cooke, Rachel. 2004. "Girls, Girls, Girls." *New Statesman* 133, no. 4692: 38.

Dominus, Susan. 2016. "Game of Crowns." *Marie Claire (US Edition)* 23, no. 4: 196.

Du Toit, Herman C. 2009. *Pageants and Processions: Images and Idiom as Spectacle*. Newcastle upon Tyne, England: Cambridge Scholars Publishing.

Lobato, Mirta Zaida, editor. 2005 *Cuando las mujeres reinaban: Belleza, virtud y poder en la Argentina del siglo xx*. Buenos Aires, Argentina: Biblos.

Nichols, Elizabeth Gackstetter. 2014. "Ultra-Feminine Women of Power: Beauty and the State in Argentina." In: *Women in Politics and Media: Perspectives from Nations in Transition*, edited by Maria Raicheva-Stover and Elza Ibroscheva. London: Bloomsbury.

Nichols, Elizabeth Gackstetter. 2016. *Beauty, Virtue, Power and Success in Venezuela 1850–2015*. New York: Lexington.

Onishi, Norimitsu. 2002. "Globalization Makes Slimness Trendy." *The New York Times*. October 3. Accessed July 22, 2016. https://www.globalpolicy.org/component/content/article/162/27589.html.

Vunileba, Amelia. 2006. "Miss Pearl Vies for Crown." *Fiji Times*. August 1. Accessed July 22, 2016. http://www.fijitimes.com/story.aspx?id=378275. Newspaper Source, EBSCOhost.

Wember, Michelle. 2009. "Makers of Meaning: Plays and Processions in the Goddess Cults of the Near East." In: *Pageants and Processions: Images and Idiom as Spectacle,* edited by Herman Du Toit. Newcastle upon Tyne, England: Cambridge Scholars Publishing.

PAGEANTS—TRANSPAGEANTS

Although some regions and nations have beauty pageants for men, "Mr. Venezuela," for example, the phenomenon of the beauty contest worldwide is overwhelmingly an event for female people. Therefore, it is not surprising that members of transgender communities, those people born with masculine sex organs who experience themselves as female, also increasingly participate in pageants designed to showcase their feminine forms.

For many transgendered persons, the act of showing the world the gender of the body that they feel inside is known as "bringing out the body," or in Spanish "*sacar el cuerpo*," a process of revealing what has been hidden. For persons born with male bodies, this is the process of "bringing out" their female bodies (Ochoa 2014).

The process of bringing out the female body is common globally among transgendered people, and what most transgendered women are seeking to show is the global norm of feminine beauty: the long hair, large breasts, slim waist, and clear skin

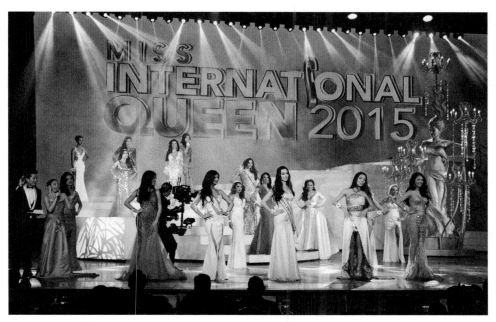

Contestants perform during the Miss International Queen 2015 beauty contest in Pattaya, Thailand, on November 6, 2015. Miss International Queen is the world's largest beauty pageant for transgender women from all around the world. (Piti A. Sahakorn/LightRocket via Getty Images)

that characterize the ideal of feminine appearance in such pageants as the Miss Universe contest or on a fashion catwalk. To achieve this transformation, people in some nations, such as the United States, must navigate the medical system to gain access to hormones, plastic surgery, and pharmaceuticals. In other nations with less regulatory apparatuses, individuals have more and less controlled access to the kinds of products and practices that will allow them to display a more traditional version of the female body (Ochoa 2014).

This body, sought and displayed by both the "Misses" of traditional beauty pageants and the transgendered bodies on view in a transpageant, can be described as a type of "spectacular," hyperfeminine version of femininity whose purpose is to be viewed, judged, and evaluated by other members of society (Ochoa 2014). In each case, the woman is seeking to show and be rated on how well she conforms to the highest local, national, or global standard of feminine beauty. Indeed, for members of transgendered communities, the opportunity to participate in the global social norm of beauty for women can be a way for those participants to find belonging in an international community that accepts them in a way that their local culture may not.

In the island nation of Tonga, the national transpageant is known as "Miss Galaxy" and takes place during the annual Heilala festival, which is also the venue for the more traditional national beauty and culture pageant for persons born female, the Miss Heilala Pageant (Vi 2016).

The "Miss Galaxy" pageant, a two-day event incorporating music, costumes, and dance performances, is an opportunity for the transgendered members of Tongan society to publically express and perform their female identities (Besnier 2002). Whereas the nontransgender national pageant, Miss Heilala, is as much an indigenous pageant as a beauty contest in its celebration of Tongan language and culture, the Miss Galaxy pageant is markedly global in approach. Transgendered Tongan people, known as *fakaleitl*, find in the English-language pageant and the idea of a global standard of transgender and feminine beauty a way to fit in to an international culture (Besnier 2002). This allows transgender people to find both acceptance and celebration of their work and identity in a way that is dismissed or taboo in Tongan society.

This access to an international community accepting the identity and appearance of transgendered individuals is a common reason for women to enter transpageants. Participants in the first annual Miss Trans Israel pageant, for example, related both shocking stories of abuse at the hands of their families and local cultures when they revealed their desire to transition to a female body, but then also the strong sense of belonging and community in the transpageant culture. This community broke down significant barriers in the deeply divided nation. "Here," one participant said, "I don't feel Muslim, Jewish, Christian. All of the people are together and the transsexual [people], they love together" (Jabari and Bruton 2016).

Once competitors win local or national transpageants, there are a number of international competitions that they may then proceed to, all very similar in format and staging to Miss Universe or Miss World. The Miss International Queen competition is perhaps the largest and longest-running international transpageant, founded in 2004. Miss International Queen brings more than 20 contestants from around the world to compete in Thailand each year, crowning a winner and awarding more than 10,000 dollars and the option of free cosmetic surgery as a grand prize (Nichols 2014).

See also: Injections; Pageants—Indigenous; Pageants—Local, National and International; Plastic Surgery.

Further Reading

Besnier, Niko. 2002. "Transgenderism, Locality, and the Miss Galaxy Beauty Pageant in Tonga." *American Ethnologist* 29, no. 3: 534–66.
Jabari, Lawahez, and F. Brinley Bruton. 2016. "Christians, Muslims and Jews Compete at Israel's First Transgender Pageant." May 27. Accessed July 25, 2016. http://www.nbcnews.com/feature/nbc-out/christians-muslims-jews-compete-israel-s-1st-transgender-pageant-n580751.
Nichols, James. 2014. "Isabella Santiago, Transgender Beauty Contestant, Crowned Miss International Queen 2014." Accessed July 25, 2016. http://www.huffingtonpost.com/2014/11/11/isabella-santiago-transgender_n_6140880.html.
Ochoa, Marcia. 2014. *Queen for a Day:* "Transformistas, Beauty Queens and the Performance of Femininity in Venezuela." Durham, NC: Duke University Press.
Vi, Siosaia. 2016. "Miss Heilala." Accessed July 25, 2016. http://miss-heilala.tripod.com.

PEDICURE

Manicures are beauty treatments for the hands, which often include hydration with lotions, massage, and nail polish. Similarly, a pedicure is a practice designed to beautify or care for the feet and toenails. Pedicures often also include hydration and nail polish, but often focus more on the exfoliation of dead and rough skin. Pedicures in the 21st century are often touted for their health benefits of relaxation and stress relief. Most professional pedicures take place in a spa-like setting where the customer feels pampered.

Both manicures and pedicures are depicted in the carvings and visual representations of the ancient **Egyptians**, indicating the long history of the practice (Maines 2016). For many centuries, the practice of having professional nail care was limited to elites in the United States and Europe and was a sign of wealth. It was only in the late 20th century in the United States that a group of Asian immigrants revolutionized the salon nail business by offering professional services for lower prices (Morris 2015).

By the early 21st century, pedicures formed a key part of a multibillion-dollar industry. In 2015, there were more than 125,000 nail salons in the United States alone. The biggest growth in nail salon patronage was in women older than 35 years old and in men who are in the United States increasingly seeking out manicures and pedicures (Nails Magazine 2015). In general, pedicures made up 29 percent of the $7.7 billion of revenue of all nail salons, the highest revenue-generating service (Nails Magazine 2013).

The American Podiatric Medical Association (APMA), an organization of physicians who specialize in feet and foot care, recognize the value of a pedicure for helping feet both look and feel better. The doctors have specific recommendations, however, many of which are concerned with the possible infections a person can contract from the nail salon. To avoid these, physicians recommend scheduling pedicures earlier in the day when the salon foot baths are cleaner, bringing your own pedicure utensils, and refraining from shaving your legs before the treatment, as small cuts can allow bacteria to enter the skin (APMA 2016).

The APMA does recommend soaking feet in warm water before exfoliating the rough skin of calluses with a pumice stone, foot file, or scrub. The organization also cautions that toenails should never be rounded, as this can lead to ingrown nails, but should be cut straight across. The APMA also recommends hydration with a softening lotion (APMA 2016).

Nail Salons

The nail salon industry in the United States is dominated by Vietnamese Americans, a fact linked to the United States' involvement in the 1960s war in Vietnam. After the war, many refugees who had supported the American forces were resettled in camps in northern California. At one of these camps in the early 1970s, the American actress Tippi Hedren visited and made an impression on many of the women with her long, manicured nails. Hoping to provide a way to succeed in the United States and get an economic leg up, Ms. Hedren flew in her personal manicurist and recruited a local beauty school to teach twenty women—both the wives of military officers and some military officers themselves—how to do manicures and pedicures. Those twenty women revolutionized the salon manicure industry in the United States, and by 2015, 51 percent of all nail technicians in the United States and 80 percent in California were of Vietnamese descent.

Beyond the basic foot care recommendations of the APMA and the application of nail polish to toenails, another, less common, but still popular service worldwide is the *Garra rufa*, or doctor fish, pedicure. The *Garra rufa* are a species of small, toothless fish native to **South Korea** that survive by eating the dead skin cells of other animals. In a doctor fish pedicure, clients soak their feet in a bath of warm water full of the fish, which gently eat away the dead skin cells, leaving the new, healthy skin untouched. Clients report that the treatment tickles, rather than hurting, but can make some uncomfortable (Baute 2010) Although this type of pedicure is particularly popular in Canada and the **United Kingdom**, some physicians warn that because the fish can't be disinfected between clients, there is a greater risk of the transmission of infections.

See also: Egypt; Manicure; South Korea; United Kingdom.

Further Reading

APMA. 2016. "Pedicure Pointers: The Do's and Don't's of Fabulous Feet." Accessed October 7, 2016. http://www.apma.org/Learn/HealthyFeetTips.cfm?ItemNumber=9859.

Baute, Nicole. 2010. "The Right to Bite? Popular Pedicure Raises Red Flags." *Toronto Star (Canada)*. Accessed October 7, 2016. *Newspaper Source*, EBSCOhost.

Maines, Heidi. 2016. "The History of Manicure & Pedicure." Accessed October 6, 2016. https://www.leaf.tv/articles/the-history-of-the-manicure-pedicure/.

Morris, Regan. 2015. "How Tippi Hedren Made Vietnamese Refugees into Nail Salon Magnates." Accessed October 7, 2016. http://www.bbc.com/news/magazine-32544343.

Nails Magazine. 2013. "2012–2013 Industry Statistics." Accessed October 7, 2016. http://files.nailsmag.com/Market-Research/NAILSbb12-13stats.pdf.

Nails Magazine. 2015. "2015–2016 Nails Big Book: Everything You Need to Know About the Nail Industry." Accessed October 7, 2016. http://files.nailsmag.com/Feature-Articles-in-PDF/NABB2015-16stats.pdf.

PERFORMANCE/PERFORMATIVITY

In 1959, sociologist Erving Goffman published *The Presentation of Self in Everyday Life*, which argued that all participants in social interactions are actively engaging in practices to minimize embarrassment of themselves and others for the sake of forging, maintaining, or improving social relationships. Later, some scholars would begin to call this set of ideas about intentional self-positioning, appearance, and mannerisms "impression management."

Using "dramaturgical analysis" derived from the study of theater, Goffman offered the "front stage-backstage" metaphor to reveal how individuals, thought of as "actors," sometimes hide their true selves in order to "perform" the most positive version of the self and to maximize the desired impression in a given social setting. The performance may be enhanced by beautification rituals, cosmetics, costuming, or any other modification to the appearance. Importantly, Goffman notes that it is essential that the "actors" involved in any given social situation agree upon the context and the social rules that govern their social interactions. In this way, individuals create social occasions that others may participate in without having to relearn the social rules, and in so doing, individuals collaboratively create social norms that they reenact over and over to **construct** ideal models of behavior. These behavioral norms are reinforced by a social system of rewards and consequences.

Decades later, in her influential text *Gender Trouble* (1990), feminist philosopher Judith Butler tweaked the notion of embodied performance to suggest that "performativity" represented a productive way to look at the complex multiple ways that **gender** is enacted throughout the life course. In short, Butler said, behavior creates gender. She argued that rather than a biological category of identity, all experiences and behaviors of "gender" are actually part of an elaborate performance, learned and modified since childhood, and enacted within social settings where individuals are continually aware of the "regulative discourses" that limit uninhibited expression. Butler argued that the conflation of the categories of sex, gender, and sexuality in Western societies often collapses into a sense that only a narrow range of behaviors are "natural" and that other behaviors could be subject to discipline, coercion, or even violence. In this way, Butler explained, cultural understandings about womanhood (or manhood) include a very specific and narrow range of ideas about how women should look, how they should move, how they should act, and how they should desire, to name only a few cultural expectations. Butler prescribed an opening or a freeing of the idea of identity, allowing for more cultural acceptance of more transformative and flexible performances of gender.

Butler's scholarship gave rise, in part, to the field of study called Queer Theory, wherein the rigid coupling of gender, sex, and sexuality is destabilized, critiqued, and challenged. In an era of increasing awareness of gender fluidity and the ways in which our gender identities are continually performed, celebrity RuPaul quipped, "We are born naked. The rest is **drag**."

See also: Drag; Gender; Social Construction of Beauty.

Further Reading

Butler, Judith. 1990. *Gender Trouble: Feminism and the Subversion of Identity.* New York: Routledge.
Goffman, Erving. 1959. *The Presentation of Self in Everyday Life.* New York: Anchor Books.
Jagose, Annamarie. 1996. *Queer Theory: An Introduction.* New York: New York University Press.

PERFUMES AND SCENTED OILS

The sense of smell is one of the most evocative ways to connect a person to an emotional response (Humphries 2011), and smelling good is big business. Approximately $20 billion is generated every year by industrially manufactured smells, including scents that fragrance our everyday products, colognes, and perfumes (Burr 2003). Virtually all of the smells that are made today come from six corporations that carefully protect the production and sale of the specific scent molecules that trigger the human sense of smell and taste and give their brands a distinct odor (Burr 2003, 38).

The expense and energy expended to smell great did not begin in the current era. Egyptian love poetry rapturously describes the enticing scent of the beloved. In the ancient world, it is likely that perfumes and scented oils were also used in part to minimize body odor. **Bathing and showering** were of tremendous importance to many of the world's ancient cultures, but personal hygiene became sketchy in medieval Europe. The reek of the unwashed bodies of explorers during the Age of Discovery is commented upon in the annals of history by both Asians and Native Americans (Sandbeck 2010, 14).

Frankincense, opopanax, and myrrh were fragrant plant resins that were highly desirable, suitable as gifts for royalty, and considered luxury commodities among the elite. Cedar and cypress were two other plant-based fragrances that were used in perfumes, soaps, and oils. Longer-lasting fragrances relied on oil-based fixatives. Many of the legendary perfumes of the ancient world relied on a viscous, black, stinky substance called ambergris (produced in the stomachs and intestines of squid-eating male sperm whales and then expelled in a manner similar to vomit) as a base for enriching and intensifying their exotic scents. Much of the Portuguese expansion to the Indian Ocean in the 15th century was an effort to corner the market on this valuable commodity, which can cost up to $10,000 per pound. Chemists explain that ambergris molecules are lipophilic (fat-loving), which means they adhere to skin more durably and thus make a richer, longer-lasting perfume.

Besides ambergris, other important bases designed to "fix" perfumes, slow their evaporation, and make the scent more long lasting include animal products made from civet musk, deer musk, or castoreum. Civet musk is an oily substance produced in a glandular pouch located between the anus and genitals of civet cats, which are native to Asia and eastern Africa. The civet cat, which looks a bit like a mongoose or a weasel, is a nocturnal mammal native to most of sub-Saharan Africa, which came to be "farmed" for their oily musk. Each civet cat secretes up to four grams of musk each week. Civet farms exist today in Indonesia.

Deer musk is an oily substance that is produced in a small sac located in the preputial gland of the male musk deer of the Himalayas and Central Asia. This dark-purplish secretion is often described as the most complex scent on earth, evoking something like the smell of a baby's skin. Deer musk was used widely in ancient India as a medicine in the Ayurvedic system to treat a variety of cardiac, mental, and neurological disorders. The collected glands, or "musk pods," of approximately forty deer are required to make one kilo of usable-quality deer musk, making the substance highly valuable. Deer musk was introduced to the Western world by a sixth-century explorer. The perfumes made with this powerful fixative soon came to be widely desired for their supposed aphrodisiac properties. Deer musk are now an endangered species.

Castoreum is a yellowish secretion produced in the perianal glands of both European and North American beavers. It is combined with urine by the animal in order to "mark" territory. The strong scent is sometimes allowed to age and mellow for several years before use in fragrances. Castoreum evokes the scent of "leather" and is used in earthy-toned perfumes that also feature tones of honey or tobacco, or in sprays designed to suggest a "new car" smell. Classic perfumes that use castor as a key tincture are Shalimar, Emeraude, and Chanel Antaeus.

The luxury trade in ancient perfumes connected royalty and elites from Egypt, China, Rome, Iran, Greece, India, and all points in between. Archaeologists find evidence of precious perfume bottles in most classical sites. Among the most famous perfumers in the world are the Muslim merchants and artisans located along Mumbai's Mohamedali Road called "attarwallas."

Perfumers rely on five key families of scents arranged in what is known as the "fragrance wheel." These families include Oriental, woody, floral, fresh, and aromatic *fougère* (or fernlike). Advertisers spend enormous amounts of money to persuade consumers that the odors of the human body should be disguised. In the 1960s, breakthroughs in chemical technology allowed for the "molecular blacksmithing" (Burr 2003, 48) of synthetic raw materials, allowing for a profusion of new odors and a cost reduction in the production of fine-quality perfumes that could be added to everyday household products (for example, furniture polish or scratch-and-sniff stickers) and less expensive colognes, deodorants, and other products.

Perfumes are designed to make the person wearing them more attractive to those around them. Some research in evolutionary psychology seems to demonstrate that human pheromones can influence behaviors, especially around the issue of gender. Pheromones contain subtle chemical signals that can be detected through the sense of smell. In 1971, Martha McClintock published an important study noting that women who lived together in close quarters experienced synchronization of their menstrual cycles. In a similar study, researchers showed that strippers earned higher tips when they were ovulating. The relatively small study asked eighteen professional lap dancers to record their menstrual cycles and tips. Their data suggest that ovulating dancers earned an average of $185 more per five-hour shift (Miller, Tybur, and Jordan 2007).

Some pheromones seem to be integrally involved in sexual attractiveness and promote positive reactions from members of the opposite sex. In one experiment, researchers asked male volunteers to wear a plain white T-shirt for several days. The researchers also recruited a similar number of female volunteers with a variety of genetic backgrounds. After two days of continuous wear, the T-shirts were placed in a box equipped with a "smelling hole." The women volunteers were then asked to rank the odor of the boxes according to intensity, pleasantness, and sexiness. Overall, the women preferred the scents of the T-shirts worn by the men who had different genetic profiles than their own (WGBH 2001).

The implication, of course, is that certain human odors may be advantageous to appearing sexy, and so, not surprisingly, some cosmetic companies are trying to cash in on the appeal of pheromones by suggesting that their products contain ingredients that make the wearer irresistible to members of the desired sex. A great example of this appealing approach can be seen in the Axe Body Spray advertisements, although there are plenty of high-end pheromone-based colognes available on the market. Some pheromone-based products are specifically designed for a gay and lesbian market.

See also: Bathing and Showering.

Further Reading

Burr, Chandler. 2003. *The Emperor of Scent: A True Story of Perfume and Obsession.* New York: Random House.

Graber, Cynthia. 2007. "Strange But True: Whale Waste Is Extremely Valuable" *Scientific American,* April 6. Accessed November 9, 2015. http://www.scientificamerican.com /article/strange-but-true-whale-waste-is-valuable.

Humphries, Colleen. 2011. "A Whiff of History." *Boston Globe.* Accessed November 9, 2015. http://archive.boston.com/bostonglobe/ideas/articles/2011/07/17/a_whiff_of_history.

McClintock, Martha K. 1971. "Synchrony and Suppression Among a Group of Women Living Together in a College Dormitory Suggest that Social Interaction Can Have a Strong Effect on the Menstrual Cycle." *Nature* 229: 244–45.

Miller, Geoffrey, Joshua M. Tybur, and Brent D. Jordan. 2007. "Ovulatory Cycle Effects on Tip Earnings by Lap Dancers: Economic Evidence for Human Estrus?" *Evolution and Human Behavior* 28, no. 6: 375–81.

WGBH. 2001. "Sweaty T Shirts and Human Mate Choice." *PBS.org.* Accessed November 9, 2015. http://www.pbs.org/wgbh/evolution/library/01/6/l_016_08.html.

PIERCING

The piercing of body parts for decoration and display is a worldwide practice that goes back thousands of years. Mummies have been found with the elongated earlobes that indicate the use of heavy earrings, and historical and archeological records show that people have used shells, bones, feathers, and metallic objects as piercings for virtually every part of the face: ears, noses, lips, eyebrows, and tongue. Piercings are a way to enhance beauty and visual appeal, but also may serve an important social function as markers of wealth, class, race, and gender (Etcoff 2000).

Social norms regarding body piercings vary from culture to culture and from subculture to subculture. Whereas piercing of female ears may be the norm in both U.S. and Latin American society, the age at which this procedure happens varies widely. In many Latin American nations ear piercing happens to infants in the hospital, but for many U.S. women, ear piercing is a preteen rite of passage (Konttinen 2001). The number of piercings varies as well. In many European and North American cultures, multiple piercings of the earlobe may be accepted as the norm or understood as rebellious and taboo. In some cultures, these same rules of ear piercing apply for men, or there may be a whole different set of norms regarding male members of society.

In Europe and the United States one or perhaps two piercings of the earlobe are considered part of the cultural norm for women, whereas men's ear piercing is considered an act of rebellion and nonconformity, sometimes associated with homosexuality or lack of good judgment. Cultural arbiters in the United States, such as men's magazines, assert that although piercings may happen for men in college, part of "dressing like an adult" is getting rid of all piercings (Lawler 2015). Other piercings, of the nose or lip, for example, are also likely to identify the person as one who refuses to blend in, a choice that can have negative repercussions (Seiter and Sandry 2003).

Piercings for men are considered rebellious and outside the norm in many Western cultures; however, other cultures allow and celebrate piercings for men as part of social norms of adornment. In India, ear piercing for men is widely accepted and

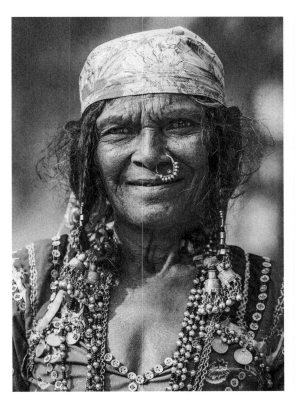

A Banjari woman wears a traditional nose ring, Hampi, Karnataka, India. The style and social significance of nose rings differs from region to region in India. (Aliaksandr Mazurkevich/Dreamstime.com)

practiced as a religious ritual (Swayam 2001). In Kenya, Maasai men wear elaborately beaded ear ornaments that both pierce and cover the ear, stretching the earlobe in a way considered both beautiful and a mark of wealth. Indeed, both men and women of the Maasai practice ear "stretching," in which more weight is added gradually to the piercing to stretch the skin of the ear into a "donut" shape. This allows the wearer to display more wealth, an important piece of display for the nomadic Maasai, for whom body wealth is the ultimate form of portable wealth (Copeland 1998).

Whereas a few piercings are considered part of the norm of appearance in the United States and Europe, in a nation such as India a nose piercing for women is a well-established element of beauty norms (Swayam 2001). In India, where the practice of piercing is centuries old, nose piercings for women have special cultural significance. Indeed, as diverse as Indian culture and subcultures are, so, too, are the traditions of nose piercing. There are several different types of nose rings worn by women in different areas of the nation, from those that only pierce the left nostril, to those that pierce the septum, or middle part, of the nose. The rings that women wear in their noses also vary, from simple studs, to long and elaborately decorated rings that cover part of the mouth (Jagannathan 2016).

Traditionally, nose piercing for women was a part of the marriage preparations and ceremony and marked a woman as married. In these traditions, the nose stud or ring are important symbols of the woman's status and may not be removed until the death of the woman's husband. The size, metal, and jewels involved in the nose piercing additionally communicate the wealth of the family. In the 20th century, however, the piercing is often simply decorative or is often rejected as an outdated symbol of submission and ownership (Thomas 2007).

Beyond merely visual appeal, piercings may also communicate and provide tactile appeal. Piercings of the nerve-rich sexual organs or areas such as the nipple, for example, provide constant stimulation and allow a potential viewer to imagine the sensations being experienced. This type of piercing is often found as part of the fetish fashion movement (Etcoff 2000).

It is perhaps the combination of the sensual with the visual that has made body piercings taboo in many cultures and limited the amount of acceptable piercings in others. Several forms of Orthodox Judaism consider piercing against God's will as a violation of the natural state of the body and because of its association with idolatry (Moment 2009).

Some researchers also theorize that European, North American, and Asian sub-cultures that embrace rebellious forms of piercing or stretching are using practices considered more "uncivilized" in their home society to reject the conventions that they grew up with (Liotard 2001). This, generally, is effective. In more than one cul-ture, researchers have found that wearing jewelry outside the social norm correlates with lower perceived levels of attractiveness, hireability, and credibility (Seiter and Sandry 2003).

See also: Fetish; Goth and Gothic; India; Jewelry.

Further Reading

Copeland, Lib I. 1998. "A Hole New Look: The Punctuated Ear Lobe." *The Washington Post.* July 11. Accessed July 13, 2016. http://ezproxy.drury.edu:2048/login?url=http://ezproxy .drury.edu:2143/docview/4083829 84?accountid=33279.
Etcoff, Nancy. 2000. *Survival of the Prettiest: The Science of Beauty.* New York: Anchor.
Jagannathan, Shakunthala. 2016 "Traditional Jewelry of India." Accessed July 12, 2016. http://www.utc.edu/faculty/sarla-murgai/traditional-jewelry-of-india.php.
Konttinen, Janet. 2001 "Wit & Wisdom." *Baby Talk* 66, no. 2: 27.
Lawler, Moira. 2015. "11 Essential Rules to Dressing like an Adult." Accessed July 13, 2016. http://www.menshealth.com/style/11-essential-rules-start-dressing-like-adult.
Liotard, Phillippe. 2001. "The Body Jigsaw." *The Unesco Courier* 54: 22–24.
Moment Magazine. 2009. "Ask the Rabbis: Are Tattoos and Body Piercings Taboo?" Accessed July 12, 2016. http://www.momentmag.com/are-tattoos-and-body-piercings-taboo.
Thomas, Suravi. 2007. "Nose Ring." *Teen Ink* 19, no. 1: 41.
Seiter, John S., and Andrea Sandry. 2003. "Pierced for Success?: The Effects of Ear and Nose Piercing on Perceptions of Job Candidates' Credibility, Attractiveness, and Hireability." *Communication Research Reports* 20, no. 4: 287–98.
Swayam, S. 2001. "Nangli Ear Studs." *Ornament* 24, no. 4: 54.

PLASTIC SURGERY

The commonly used term "plastic surgery" covers surgical and nonsurgical medical procedures that repair or reconstruct different parts of the body, either as part of a treatment for an injury or medical condition, or for cosmetic and aesthetic reasons. Therefore, plastic surgery procedures are generally grouped into "reconstructive" and "cosmetic" types, though the line between those designations worldwide can become blurred.

The history of plastic surgery can be traced at least as far back as BCE 600 in India, where Hindu texts describe early methods of nose reconstruction. The man consid-ered the world's first surgeon, the Indian doctor Sushruta, described various proce-dures in his treatise *Sushruta Samhita* that today we would recognize as plastic surgery (Saraf and Parihar 2006). The modern versions of plastic surgery, then, are generally considered to have been reborn in response to the devastating and widespread injuries and anxieties of people after World War I (Haiken 1999).

In the 21st century, reconstructive plastic surgery is generally considered to be an operation to repair birth defects, to repair the damage from accidents or diseases, and to reconstruct body parts removed as part of treatments for illnesses such as cancer. This type of plastic surgery is defined by the American Society of Plastic Surgeons (ASPS) as a procedure on "abnormal structures of the body caused by congenital defects, developmental abnormalities, trauma, infection, tumors or disease." A few examples of surgery generally grouped in this area would be breast reconstruction after a mastectomy, cleft palate repair, or skin cancer removal (ASPS 2015b).

The other designation, "cosmetic" or sometimes "aesthetic" plastic surgery, is a term for a group of procedures generally considered to not be of strict medical necessity, but rather designed to improve the appearance of a person's body. The ASPS defines cosmetic procedures as "surgical and nonsurgical procedures that reshape normal structures of the body in order to improve appearance and self-esteem." Some procedures generally grouped in this category are breast augmentation, liposuction, and laser hair removal (ASPS 2015a).

Procedures characterized as "reconstructive" are, worldwide, taught more frequently as part of the standard education for doctors and surgeons, and are more frequently covered by private or state-provided medical insurance (McInnes et al. 2012). In Canada, the United States, and many European nations, procedures considered "cosmetic" are also then considered elective, and

> "She got her looks from her father. He's a plastic surgeon."
> —Groucho Marx

therefore not generally taught in medical schools or covered by health plans. This divide means that international statistics on cosmetic and aesthetic surgery are notoriously incomplete, because nations do not track "elective" cosmetic procedures in the same way that they monitor "medical" surgeries. Therefore, researchers depend on professional organizations such as the International Society of Aesthetic and Plastic Surgery to collect and publish data regarding cosmetic procedures.

Despite the widespread differentiation between "reconstructive" and "cosmetic" procedures, for many, the dividing line is not clear. The ASPS, for example, characterizes "scar revision," in which the appearance of a scar is minimized, as a type of reconstructive surgery, though the goal of the procedure is to "provide a more pleasing cosmetic result" (ASPS 2015c). On the other side, some cosmetic surgeons would argue that improving a patient's appearance directly affects their psychological health, making the procedure "reconstructive" of the patient's mental state (Edmonds 2010). Whatever an individual, insurance company, or nation's opinion of the dividing line between "reconstructive" and "cosmetic" procedures, both share the same set of practitioners (doctors) and the same end goal: to improve the appearance of the patient.

Because of the ambiguous line between what is strictly "medically necessary" and what is just for "vanity," it is not surprising that attitudes about the necessity of cosmetic surgery vary worldwide. Indeed, many nations cover cosmetic or aesthetic procedures as part of their national health plans. In Brazil and Venezuela, for example, cosmetic procedures are free to the public in state hospitals (Edmonds 2010, Gulbas 2008). In other nations the government offers tax breaks to those who seek cosmetic surgery. In South Korea, for example, plastic surgery procedures are tax free for national and tourist patients (Kim and Cho 2015). Even in nations such as the United States, many charitable organizations exist to provide surgeries to those made uncomfortable by the bullying of others due to their appearance, seeking to transform "young, shy children into proud, self-confident youngsters" (Romo 2015).

Critics of the use of surgery to correct "ugliness" as a psychological and physical deformity in need of correction point out that the danger of a diagnosis of "inferiority complex" or "low self-esteem" risks reinforcing social norms of beauty as tied to class and race. Prescribing plastic surgery to alleviate the feeling of inferiority of someone who does not conform to the social norm of Caucasian, Anglo-Saxon beauty can reproduce and replicate a definition of beauty that assumes that only the "white" standard is beautiful. Although many cosmetic surgeons claim that the standards of beauty that they conform to are based only on individual preferences, many studied indicate that the vast majority of procedures, from rhinoplasty to otoplasty, are designed to help individuals conform to white, Western beauty ideals (Haiken 1999).

Generally, Brazil and the United States lead international statistics on the total number of plastic surgeries performed in the world, but this is not a complete picture of how important these procedures are in a nation (ISAPS 2015). Another way of looking at the prevalence of the practice in a nation is to see what percentage of citizens of a country had surgeries. Looking at the issue in this way, other nations also reveal significant interest in cosmetic procedures. In 2012, one report indicated that the nations with the most plastic surgeries by percentage of their population were, in order, South Korea, Greece, Italy, Brazil, Colombia, the United States, and Taiwan (Conley 2012).

See also: Breast Augmentation and Reduction Surgeries; Class; Eyelid Surgery; Nose Jobs.

Further Reading

ASPS. 2015a. "Cosmetic Procedures." Accessed September 8, 2015. http://www.plasticsurgery.org/cosmetic-procedures.html

ASPS. 2015b. "Reconstructive Procedures." Accessed September 8, 2015. http://www.plasticsurgery.org/reconstructive-procedures.html.

ASPS. 2015c. "Scar Revision." Accessed September 8, 2015. http://www.plasticsurgery.org/reconstructive-procedures/scar-revision.html.

Conley, Mikaela. 2012. "Nip/Tuck Nations: 7 Countries With Most Cosmetic Surgery." Accessed September 8, 2015. http://abcnews.go.com/Health/niptuck-nations-countries-cosmetic-surgery/story?id=16205231.

Edmonds, Alexander. 2010. *Pretty Modern: Beauty, Sex and Plastic Surgery in Brazil*. Durham, NC: Duke University Press.

Gulbas, Lauren. 2008. "Cosmetic Surgery and the Politics of Race, Class and Gender in Caracas, Venezuela." PhD diss. Southern Methodist University.

Haiken Elizabeth. 1999. *Venus Envy: A History of Cosmetic Surgery*. Baltimore: Johns Hopkins University Press.

ISAPS. 2015. "ISAPS International Survey on Aesthetic/Cosmetic Procedures Performed in 2014." Accessed August 20, 2015. http://www.isaps.org/Media/Default/globalstatistics /2015%20ISAPS%20Results.pdf.

Kim, Cynthia, and Myungshin Cho. 2015. "Korea's Giving Tax Breaks on Nose Jobs." Accessed September 8, 2015. http://www.bloomberg.com/news/articles/2015-08-18 /korea-s-giving-tourists-tax-breaks-on-nose-jobs.

McInnes, Colin W., Douglas J. Courtemanche, Cynthia C. Verchere, Kevin L. Bush, and Jugpal S. Arneja. 2012. "Reconstructive or Cosmetic Plastic Surgery? Factors Influencing the Type of Practice Established by Canadian Plastic Surgeons." *Canadian Journal of Plastic Surgery* 20, no. 3: 163–68.

Romo III, Thomas. 2015. "Little Baby Face Foundation." Accessed September 8, 2015. http://www.littlebabyface.org.

Saraf S. and R. Parihar. 2006. "Sushruta: The First Plastic Surgeon in 600 B.C." *The Internet Journal of Plastic Surgery* 4, no. 2. Accessed November 19, 2015. http://ispub.com/IJPS /4/2/8232.

POMADE

Originally made of bear fat, hair pomade is a greasy or waxy substance, usually used to style the **hair**. Pomades are usually associated with hairstyles worn by men, often applied and then styled with the use of a comb. Pomade gives a characteristic shiny or slick appearance. Because of the desired thick consistency that allows the hair to stay in place, it may take a few washes to rinse pomade out of the hair completely. Pomade is usually oil based and was historically made from petroleum jelly, lanolin, beeswax, tallow, gum arabic, pine resin, or lard. Some pomades include fragrance or pigments intended to darken the hair. Pomade can be used on hair, beards, or mustaches in order to achieve a desired effect.

In the 19th and early 20th centuries, men often cultivated a great deal of **facial hair** and wore handlebar moustaches, so named for their similarity to the curved handles of a bicycle. (This style is also known as a "spaghetti moustache" for its association with gentlemen of the era from Italy.) In order to groom and cultivate the longer hair required for the look, especially at the extremities, men applied a stiff pomade, sometimes called a "moustache wax," as a grooming aid to shape and control their moustache. These specialty pomades needed to be very durable, but worked best at room temperature in order to be pliable enough to style the look. When worn without pomade or grooming, this type of mustache may droop, causing it to be called a "walrus moustache," where long whiskers fall over the mouth. Handlebar moustaches and moustache wax have made a visible comeback in recent years as an iconic look for the "hipster" subculture.

Hollywood leading men of the classic silver screen era like Rudolph Valentino and Clark Gable embodied the sleek, shiny, sophisticated look possible with pomade. These styles often feature a sharp, crisp part and an elegant taper to the back of the head. The iconic Brylcreem brand, an emulsion of water and mineral oil stabilized with beeswax, was introduced to stylish gents to control unruly hair in England in 1928. Murray's Pomade was introduced by C. D. Murray, an African American barber from Chicago, in 1925. Originally intended for black clients to achieve a "classic wave" look, the product was soon discovered by white customers to provide hold, lift, and shine to longer hair trying to achieve the gravity-defying hairstyles that became popular during the era. Heavy and greasy with a consistency like Vaseline, Murray's pomade was designed to stay in the hair for a long time. Some recommend washing with Coca-Cola to remove the product buildup in the hair (McKay and McKay 2011).

The male version of the "pompadour" hairstyle is a masculinized and much-tamed version of the elaborately tall hairstyles of women stretching back to the courts of 18th-century France. During that era, women piled their hair high upon their heads, supporting the style by propping it up on wire frames with bits of straw or fabric to support the look. Later, women rolled their hair over a mound of padding known as a "rat" (Sherrow 2006). For men, the pompadour was a style that achieved a similar amount of lift to the hairstyle. A classic man's pompadour is combed back off the forehead without a part and then controlled with pomade to create a mound that rises from the top of the face, creating a shiny focal point for the hair and creating the illusion of a lengthened face. The style was popularized in the United States during the 1950s by appealing young superstars like Elvis Presley, James Brown, and James Dean.

Another variation of the "pompadour" style is known as the "quiff," which also used pomade to hold the hair in a tall, central sweep above the forehead, but then tapers off into very short hair at the back, closely trimmed at the sides. Quiff styles are also worn as a version of British punk subculture.

A third version of the man's classic pompadour is the colorfully named "D.A.," or "duck's ass," style. Also popular during the 1950s, this style featured hair swept up above the forehead and held with grease and then flattened evenly using the teeth of a comb to a central point at the nape of the neck to resemble the feathers of a duck's posterior. To keep the style looking crisp, young men sporting pompadour hairstyles frequently carried combs tucked into their back pockets in order to redistribute and shape their pomaded hair throughout the day. This masculine preening behavior was frequently spotlighted by the Fonz, a well-known character from the 1970s sitcom *Happy Days*, about teenagers in the 1950s.

Both pompadour styles, the "DA," and the quiff, were favored by young men known as "greasers," so-called for the obvious

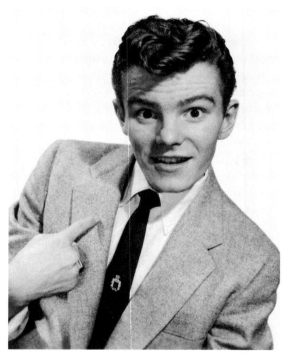

Teenager with a heavily pomaded "D. A." pompadour, 1950s. (ClassicStock/Alamy Stock Photo)

amounts of pomade used to support their hairstyles. "Greasers" representing the disaffected working-class youth of the mid-20th century in the United States, were often depicted wearing leather jackets and jeans, and were sometimes associated with delinquency or high rates of crime. The "greaser" look resurfaces periodically in youth aesthetics, most notably in rockabilly and biker subcultures. These styles are also popular in Korea, India, and China, usually immediately evoking a counterculture vibe due to their association with the classic pompadour look.

Today's pomades are water based and easier to remove from the hair. Punk and contemporary hairstyles that rely on "spikes" may also use pomade as a styling tool.

See also: Facial Hair; Hair.

Further Reading

McKay, Brett, and Kate McKay. 2011. "Your Grandpa's Hair Products: 5 Old-School Hair Grooms to Give You that Cary Grant Shine." *Art of Manliness*. February 16. Accessed October 11, 2016. http://www.artofmanliness.com/2011/02/16/your-grandpas-hair -products-5-old-school-hair-grooms-to-give-you-that-cary-grant-shine.

Sherrow, Victoria. 2006. *Encyclopedia of Hair: A Cultural History*. Westport, CT: Greenwood Press.

Suwarnaadi. 2010. "A Brief History of Hair Pomade." *Cool Men's Hair*. August 10. Accessed March 12, 2016. http://coolmenshair.com/2010/08/brief-history-of-hair-pomade.html.

PROGRESSIVE MUSCULARITY

Men in the 21st century are increasingly presented with idealized images of slim, yet muscular physiques that highlight a triangle-shaped body with wide shoulders and well-developed arms with a slim waist and hips. This model of body image, often seen in representations of superheroes, has become increasingly pronounced over time, giving rise to the concept of "progressive muscularity"—a slow movement toward an ever more muscular, yet lean, physique. This can lead to widespread issues of body dissatisfaction, especially in men, and a psychological condition called "muscle dysmorphia."

Comparisons of the images of superheroes, and the action figure toys that represent them over time, suggest how young men learn to seek increasingly defined physiques. A 1999 study measured the waist, chest, and bicep circumference of G. I. Joe action figures from 1973 to 1998 and extrapolated them to life-size male figures. The study found huge increases in the size of chest and bicep muscles of the figures over time. These changes, the equivalent of a more than 100 percent increase in the size of the arms, led researchers to note that whereas the 1973 G. I. Joe had realistic muscles, a life-size G. I. Joe from 1999 would have larger biceps than any real-life body builder in history. The study also highlighted the increased muscle definition in the abdominal area of these toys (Pope et al. 1999).

These findings mirror what anyone might note about the differences in the representation of a comic book and movie figure, such as Batman from the first issue of the comic in 1939 or the television program in the 1960s to 21st-century film and print representations of the superhero. Visual representations of superheroes over time show how the "super" male body has become increasingly muscular and defined, with lower and lower levels of body fat.

The concept of leanness and weight loss is often linked with the idea of having well-defined muscles, as each muscle is more clearly visible when less body fat is present. Body builders who seek to increase their muscle mass and decrease their body fat in order to showcase their musculature diet regularly to achieve this goal (Thompson 2016). Some researchers use a test called the BIG, or Body builder Image Grid, to show young men different images of men with different levels of muscular development and body fat. When surveyed, a group of U.S. college men overwhelmingly selected the very lowest amounts of body fat and highest amounts of muscularity as ideal (Mayo and George 2014).

Whereas discussions of body dissatisfaction often center around women's concerns about being thin, having perfect breasts, or having smooth skin, for young men, body image can be an equally problematic challenge. As some men have noted, "[I]t's just as hard to be Ken as it is to be Barbie," highlighting how difficult it is for real men to achieve the lean, muscular build of the famous doll and clearly the build of G. I. Joe (David 2012).

In 2014, a study of U.S. college students found that 70 percent of men reported body and weight dissatisfaction (Pritchard and Cramblitt 2014). The study noted that around the world, from Australia to China to Italy, young men viewed media images of muscular, slim men and compared their own physiques to the ones on display. This research suggested that publications such as men's health magazines and films (as well as toys such as action figures) helped young men understand and internalize the image of muscular, slim men as ideal (Pritchard and Cramblitt 2014).

This kind of unhappiness with fitness, slimness, and tone can lead some young men into a disorder called "muscle dysmorphia," a type of body dysmorphia in which young men (or women) become excessively preoccupied with their body image and muscle mass, believing themselves to be too small or weak, leading them to participate in unhealthy behaviors such as compulsive bodybuilding or weightlifting, eating disorders, or use of anabolic steroids (Thompson 2016).

See also: Bodybuilding; Eating Disorders; Weight.

Ectomorph, Mesomorph, and Endomorph Body Types

Those seeking to decrease body fat and build muscle are often counseled to understand their "somatype." There are three basic categories that describe a person's musculature, levels of body fat, and their ability to change these. Ectomorphs have slim, delicate frames with fast metabolisms and find it hard to gain either muscle or fat. Mesomorphs have strong, rectangular-shaped bodies; well-defined muscles; and the ability to gain and lose both fat and muscle more readily than ectomorphs. Endomorphs have rounder, shorter, and stockier bodies with less well-defined muscles. Endomorphs find it easy to gain fat, but harder to gain muscle. Although some argue that these categories are not descriptive enough, many continue to use them in weight loss or bodybuilding programs.

Further Reading

David, Jarrett. 2012. "Men Have (Body) Issues Too!" Accessed June 9, 2016. https://jarrettdavid.wordpress.com/2012/08/31/men-have-body-issues-too.

Mayo, Carrie, and Valerie George. 2014. "Eating Disorder Risk and Body Dissatisfaction Based on Muscularity and Body Fat in Male University Students." *Journal of American College Health* 62, no. 6: 407–15.

Pope, Harrison G., Roberto Olivardia, A. Gruber, and John Borowiecki. 1999. "Evolving Ideals of Male Body Image as Seen Through Action Toys." *International Journal of Eating Disorders* 26: 65–72.

Pritchard, Mary, and Brooke Cramblitt. 2014. "Media Influence on Drive for Thinness and Drive for Muscularity." *Sex Roles* 71, no. 5/8: 208–18.

Thompson, J. Kevin. 2016. "Body Image, Body Building and Cultural Ideals of Muscularity." Accessed June 9, 2016. http://thinkmuscle.com/articles/thompson/body-image-and-bodybuilding.htm.

R

RED HAIR/GINGER

Red hair, sometimes referred to as "ginger," is the rarest naturally occurring hair color and ranges in shade from strawberry blonde to auburn. Conventional wisdom associates red hair with fiery, passionate, and temperamental personalities. Studies also show that people with red hair are more sensitive to pain than other people.

Hair color derives from the percentage of certain types of cells, called melanocytes, within the follicles of the hair. Dark hair has more densely packed melanocytes and high levels of a pigment called eumelanin. Lighter hair, including blonde and red, contains more of the iron-rich pheomelanin pigment (Sherrow 2006). Red hair usually accompanies lighter colored eyes and fair skin, often with freckles.

Red hair is a recessive genetic characteristic, and naturally occurring red hair is displayed by less than 2 percent of the world's population.

Though many assume that the high percentages of redheads in the British Isles and along the Scandinavian coasts are the origin of red hair, genetic tests actually indicate that red hair originated in central Asia and to the haplogroup known as R1b. The origins of this haplogroup are still controversial; however by the Bronze Age, members of the group sporting red hair had reached Europe, though some red-headed members of the group remained in central Asia. Tarim mummies in Xinjiang, located along the ancient Silk Road in northwest China, are shown to have high percentages of individuals with red hair (Killgrove 2015). The Udmurts, a Uralic tribe living in the northern Volga basin of Russia, also demonstrate a high incidence of red hair.

In the remote and closed communities of the British Islands, the rate of incidence for red hair is high. Geneticists at Trinity College in Dublin argue that it is likely that many of those in Ireland with red hair are related to a powerful dynasty of chieftains established by the notorious "Niall of the Nine Hostages," a prehistoric king of Ireland in the late fourth century whose offspring dominated Ireland for six centuries (Moore et al. 2006). In Ireland, nearly 10 percent of the population has red hair; in Scotland, about 13 percent. In Wales, up to 15 percent of the population demonstrates red hair. About 40 percent of the population of the British Islands carries the recessive gene necessary to produce a ginger-haired offspring; for red hair to occur, both parents must carry the gene (Eupedia 2016).

During the Elizabethan period, the Virgin Queen's hair inspired a vogue for red-gold hair. Men and women across the **United Kingdom** dyed their hair and beards to emulate her; others sported wigs in bright shades of red and purple (Downing 2012).

Red hair had another popular revival in Renaissance Italy when artists like Titian used red-gold shades to paint hair. People of the age used bleaches and caustic dyes, including alum, sulfur, and rhubarb, to achieve a variety of shades of red hair. Some hair-lightening recipes were made from costly imported saffron, wine, or horse urine. After creating a paste of the required materials, the person seeking redder hair would sit in the sun to activate the chemical reaction. The fascination with red hair continued into the pre-Raphaelite era when poets and painters depicted heroines with flowing, fiery hair on large canvases (Harvey 2015).

Henna is a naturally occurring botanical that can be used on hair to achieve a reddish hue. The plant (*Lawsonia inermis*) has been used for more than 6,000 years to tint hair and skin. Henna was popularized in the 1860s by the famous Spanish opera singer, Madame Adelina Patti (1843–1919). In her prime, Patti was well known for her thick auburn hair and earned payment of $5,000 a night in gold. She also inspired legions of fans around the world with her striking good looks, touring from Russia to the United States. The rage for henna created a healthy market for the product to be exported from Turkey to Europe and the United States.

Red hair can prove to be a stigma as well. In medieval Europe, red hair was associated with witchcraft and also as an indicator of potential Jewishness. Many stigmas about the impetuous or violent nature of red-haired people date to this period.

See also: Hair; United Kingdom.

Further Reading

Downing, Sarah Jane. 2012. *Beauty and Cosmetics 1550–1950*. Oxford, England: Shire Publications.

Eupedia. 2016. "The Genetic Causes, Ethnic Origins and History of Red Hair." *Eupedia*. Accessed September 2, 2016. http://www.eupedia.com/genetics/origins_of_red_hair.shtml.

Harvey, Jacky Collis. 2015. *Red: A History of the Redhead*. London: Black Dog & Leventhal.

Killgrove, Kristina. 2015. "DNA Reveals These Red-Haired Chinese Mummies Come From Europe and Asia." *Forbes*. July 18. Accessed September 2, 2016. http://www.forbes.com/sites/kristinakillgrove/2015/07/18/these-red-haired-chinese-mummies-come-from-all-over-eurasia-dna-reveals/#4480d440a423.

Moore, Laoise T., Brian McEvoy, Eleanor Cape, Katharine Simms, and Daniel G. Bradley. 2006. "AY-Chromosome Signature of Hegemony in Gaelic Ireland." *American Journal of Human Genetics* 78, no. 2: 334–38.

Sherrow, Victoria. 2006. *Encyclopedia of Hair: A Cultural History*. Westport, CT: Greenwood Press.

RITUAL CLEANSING (RITUAL PURIFICATION)

Ritual cleansing not only removes unsightly dirt, bodily fluids, or other physical traces of contamination; the act also symbolically purifies and prepares a person's body to engage in sacred activities like worship or prayer. Ritual cleansing is seen in a variety of world faiths, including Buddhism, Christianity, Islam, Hinduism, Shintoism, Baha'i, and Judaism. Many temples, churches, and mosques provide worshipers with basins or other accommodations to ritually mark their presence upon entering the sacred space.

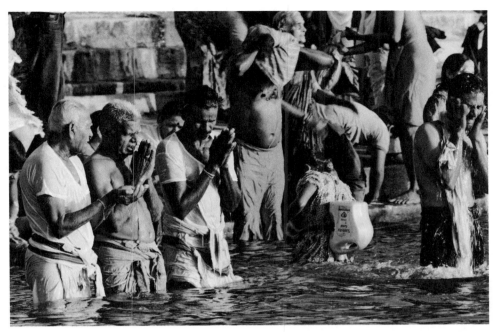

Hindus bathe in the Ganges River in Varanasi, India. Ritual cleansing removes dirt, bodily fluids, and other physical traces of contamination, but it also symbolically purifies and prepares a person's body to engage in sacred activities like worship or prayer. (Hecke01/Dreamstime.com)

Frequently, religious participation requires the observance of ritual ablutions. An ablution is the act of washing oneself or of washing certain parts of one's body, often in a prescribed way and with a specific intentionality. Some ablutions may also be performed by ritual practitioners to cleanse certain sacred objects. Ablutions may be accompanied by prayer, such as in the Islamic observance of **wudu.**

Cleanliness may also be associated closely with morality, as in the aphorism "cleanliness is next to godliness." Biblical exhortations demand ritual purification to deal with bodies soiled by menstruation, childbirth, sexual relations, nocturnal emissions, skin disease, and death. In Hinduism, many cities provide *ghats*, which are staircases built into the side of the Ganges River bank allowing pedestrians access to the water of the sacred river. Hindus are urged to keep their external body and the environment pure, as this attention to purity will exercise a healthy influence on their inner lives as well.

Public bathing in a ritual context may also be seen as a symbol of purification for an individual who is poised to change their social status. Converts and other new members of the faith are often welcomed in the context of baptism. For Jews, the ritual cleansing called *mikvah* must occur in a natural river, spring, or stream or in a special bath that contains rainwater. For those of the Shinto faith, ritual purification (*misogi*) must involve naturally running water, especially a waterfall (Yamakage 2007).

In terms of aesthetics, beauty is often interpreted as that which is clean and pure. Even prior to the germ theory to account for the spread of disease and illness, many civilizations of the ancient world provided citizens with large communal bathing facilities for health and recreation. On a practical level, ritual cleansing can assist the body in preventing potentially health-threatening infections or illnesses.

In recent years, a new movement has raised awareness in the **United States** on the part of health seekers to "eat clean" and to also initiate regular "detoxes" or "cleanses" of their bodies to eliminate, reduce, or shed all of the chemicals that have been ingested over the course of a lifetime. The movement, which is often paired with exercise programs, promotes a "getting back to basics" approach, with few or no processed or packaged foods. Advocates for the movement argue that the results of a "clean" diet not only include **weight** loss, but also improved energy levels and more radiant, luminous **skin**, **hair**, and eyes. Advocates also suggest that these changes to the way a person approaches eating can have long-term effects that reduce susceptibility to certain diseases and can prolong life (Valpone 2016).

See also: Bathing and Showering; Hair; United States; Weight; Wudu.

Further Reading

Shields, Mary E. 1998. "Multiple Exposures: Body Rhetoric and Gender Characterization in Ezekiel 16." *Journal of Feminist Studies in Religion* 14, no. 1: 5–18.

Valpone, Amie. 2016. *Eating Clean: The 21-Day Plan to Detox, Fight Inflammation, and Reset Your Body*. Boston: Houghton, Mifflin, Harcourt.

Yamakage, Motohisa. 2007. *The Essence of Shinto: Japan's Spiritual Heart*. New York: Kodansha International.

SALONS

A salon is an establishment where a hairdresser, beautician, or technician conducts business associated with the beauty industry. In general, salons can be divided into "hair salons" and "beauty salons," though many establishments combine services to offer a wide array of spa-like treatments, including **hair removal**, **manicures** and **pedicures**, **tanning**, facials, and massage. Because of their foothold in the business of beauty, many consider salons to be "recession proof," because of evidence that beauty spending actually increases in times of economic distress (Trainer 2016).

Sociological studies of salons concentrate on how knowledge about beauty and taste may circulate among people of many nationalities, social **classes**, and social groups to create a certain standard of beauty that is widely shared and considered to be attractive (Ossman 2002, 57). These techniques, practices, and ideas about new forms of beauty have the power to transform the relationships between people and even have the power to affect the ways that people think about themselves.

Another important aspect of the salon experience is that it places choice at the center of beauty, power, and the economy. Building upon a metaphor that equates beauty with freedom, Ossman argues that salons "open a space where we can produce airy bodies with quick limbs that move with ease over vast expanses" (2010, 29). Salons also create a space where clients find it thera-

> "Natural beauty takes at least two hours in front of a mirror."
> —PAMELA ANDERSON

peutic, like to be pampered, like the luxury, or need the social contact. Stylists and those who work in salons are extremely attuned to detailed knowledge of women's beauty-specific cognitive maps because they get to know their patrons well, through intimate discussions, and over the course of many years (Getz and Klein 1994). Patrons come to salons in part due to appearance anxiety coupled with a sense of dependence upon the hairdresser (Ibid.) Hairdressers may assist with this sense through creating an anonymous friendship and the illusion of loving.

Whereas doctors repair the physical body, a stylist is repairing the perpetually unstable capacity of the patron to create a coherent presentation of the self. A salon is place to go to get "fixed" or to get "done," and the patron places herself in a position where she negotiates with a stylist what her presented self will be like. She gives the stylist a tremendous amount of interpersonal power to construct an essential feature of her identity (Getz and Klein 1994, 135). Despite the relatively impersonal, utilitarian, and temporally infrequent visits to the salon, many patrons report a sense of intimate caring and loving within the salon that reassures the patron that she is worthy or cared about. Such a perception of intimacy and connection must take into account the significance of touching, which is often only found in primary relationships, but must exist by definition in the relationship between a patron and a stylist.

Kang's ethnographic study of Korean women immigrants in New York City documents nail salons as a rich empirical site to examine the concept of "body labor" and to look at the intersections between gender, migration, race relations, and the emotional and embodied dimensions of service work (2010, 3). Immigrant women who work in American nail salons shared their stories with Kang to illustrate the ways that racial ideologies propel thousands of Asian immigrant women into beauty work that both conceals and reproduces racial inequalities and underscores the expansion of the global service economy under the veneer of women's supposedly common investment in beauty and beauty practices (Kang 2010, 5). Clients include white middle-class women and working-class African American women who often have different expectations of pampering and extra perks, like hand massages during their manicure. In Kang's study, African American clients were less likely to expect or demand pampering than their white counterparts, focusing their experiences instead on more elaborate aesthetic nail designs, which they co-created with their nail technicians (2010, 167). Recently, a coalition of labor rights organizers successfully mobilized and represented nail salon workers against salon owners to oppose exposure to toxic chemicals, low wages, and a lack of overtime pay combined with irregular meal and break times and a lack of accommodation for child care issues within the workplace.

Immigrant African women entrepreneurs who open braiding salons in large cities face similar issues to those studied by Kang. Hair braiding salons are sites where undocumented African workers often put in long, physically demanding hours creating elaborate hairstyles for African American women who are positioned differently in the global political economy (Mbakwe 2016). These salons represent a point between the formal and the informal economy that governs much beauty work around the world. Because cash is the preferred form of currency, many braiders are not paid an hourly wage, but only a portion of a flat fee for an involved task that may take up to a day to perform. The lack of regulation and social networking that accompanies word-of-mouth advertising for braiding salons disadvantages young immigrant women who work in the field who may not know the language and who have no recourse for intervention when they are asked to work excruciatingly long hours. On the other hand, official regulation for the salons also threatens to close down some businesses because of excessive needs for what some view as punitive and unnecessary training, licensing, and paperwork.

See also: Barbershop; Class; Hair; Hair Removal; Manicure; Pedicure; Tanning.

Further Reading

Getz, J. Greg, and Hanne K. Klein. 1994. "The Frosting of the American Woman: Self-esteem Construction and Social Control in the Hair Salon." In: *Ideals of Feminine Beauty: Philosophical, Social and Cultural Dimensions*, edited by Karen A. Callaghan, 125–46. Westport, CT: Greenwood Press.

Kang, Miliann. 2010. *The Managed Hand: Race, Gender, and the Body in Beauty Service Work.* Berkeley, CA: University of California Press.

Lawson, Helene. 1999. "Working on Hair." *Qualitative Sociology* 22, no. 3: 235–57.

Mbakwe, Christiana A. 2016. "The Hidden World of Harlem's African Braiders." *Okay Africa* Accessed October 1, 2016. http://www.okayafrica.com/culture-2/african-hair-braiders -harlem.

Ossman, Susan. 2002. *Three Faces of Beauty: Casablanca, Paris, Cairo.* Durham, NC: Duke University Press.

Trainer, David. 2016. "Sally Beauty Holdings Sitting Pretty in Recession Resistant Cosmetics Business." *Forbes.* May 20. Accessed October 1, 2016. http://www.forbes.com/sites /greatspeculations/2016/05/20/sally-beauty-holdings-sitting-pretty-in-recession -resistant-cosmetics-business/#5d49904f3ad6.

SCARIFICATION

Scarification, sometimes called "cicatrization," is similar to tattooing in that it creates a permanent mark in the skin in a desired shape or design. Deliberate scars that convey literal or symbolic meanings to both the person being scarred and their social community can be achieved through a variety of techniques. The most common technique is "cutting," in which skin is cut carefully with a sharp tool such as a scalpel or knife into a desired pattern with the intent to leave a visible, raised scar after the wounds heal. In "branding," a heated piece of metal is applied to the skin in such a way as to leave a pattern within the burn marks. Another technique for scarring is called "packing," in which a raised scar is created by inserting material into the cut in order to form keloids within the skin as it heals. Laser branding, also called electrosurgical branding, is a newer technique that allows an artist to cut and cauterize the skin using a tool much like a welder would use. Each of these techniques involves physical pain and is irreversible. It should also be noted that there are physical risks to the practice, such as bacterial infection and other potentially serious complications.

Though scars are often considered beautiful, they also signify something more meaningful to members of the culture. This painful procedure is often performed as a rite of passage marking the transition from childhood to adulthood in parts of Africa and Oceania, although the practice is increasingly being adopted by "neotribal" Westerners. Scars are usually more prominently visible on darker-skinned people than are tattoos.

A number of ethnic groups across West Africa practice scarification. In the historic Benin Kingdom, keloid scars, referred to as "beauty berries" by Sir Richard Burton who visited Benin City in the late 19th century, were placed on women over each eyebrow. Called *iwu*, scars were also strategically cut into thighs, calves, cheeks, between the breasts, in the small of the back, and on the shoulders to enhance attractiveness. "As part of the cultural geography of the body, *iwu* mapped out ethnic terrain and transformed the self, inscribed male and female personhood, denoted stratification by pedigree, and delineated selected occupational roles" (Nevandomsky and Aisien 1995, 68).

For the Tiv people of Nigeria, scarification is part of a beauty regimen that involves oiling the skin, dressing beautifully, chipping the teeth, and incising the skin with

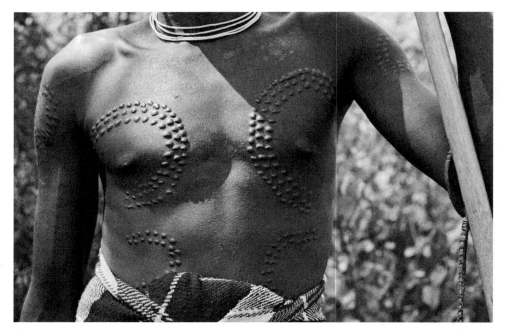

A Mursi man with scarred chest, Omo valley, Ethiopia. Sometimes called "cicatrization," scarification creates permanent marks in the skin in a desired shape or design. Scars may be considered beautiful, but they also signify something more meaningful to members of the culture. (Veleknez/Dreamstime.com)

geometrical scars (Bohannan 1956). The effect of the scars, made with a sharpened nail or a razor, may be emphasized by rubbing camwood or charcoal into the wound as it heals. Women frequently bear scars on both their backs and their stomachs in patterns that are considered both beautiful and sexy. It is also believed that certain scarification patterns promote fertility and indicate the ability of a woman to manage the pain necessary for bearing children. Facial scars are also considered attractive to the Tiv. Typically, a sharpened twig of the *Uapaca guineensis* tree is used to preview the scarification pattern. Skin pricked with this twig bears a mark for two to three months. Efforts are made to find the most flattering patterns to emphasize the best points of a face before the design is made more permanent through cutting. For example, prominent cheeks may be made more prominent by doubling the shadows cast upon them through raised scars. A nose may be made to appear longer or shorter through a deep mark. The ultimate goal of Tiv scarification is to increase the attractiveness of an individual, and the process may take decades. As men and women age through their life course, they include additional patterns upon their faces and bodies. They believe that the pain they endure in the process contributes to the beauty (Bohannon 1956, 130).

Historically, among the Igbo, similar techniques for scarring were reported. Distinct facial tattoos signified noble status, place in the birth order, and a connection with the celestial world (Jeffreys 1951). In other parts of Nigeria, the legacy of facial scarring, especially of Yoruba women, took on renewed importance during the tumultuous years of colonialism to denote identity and social status. Tattoos and scars came to connote ethnic identity because the images inscribed into the skin had geopolitical specificity and significance (Ojo 2008). In some parts of Yorubaland, marks held by certain elite families signified wealth, beauty, and class status, and the phrase *aláílówó ko 'là* ("he who has no money to procure marks") was used as a pejorative for someone considered poor. Facial tattoos are usually inherited by children through their father, though children may be given their mother's facial stripes under certain circumstances (Orie 2011).

Scarification practices are also noted in some East African tribal groups, including the Karo and Nyangatom of southern Ethiopia. Among the Oromo of Ethiopia, women typically enhance their beauty with colorful beads, headbands, tattoos, and scars, called *haaxixa*. "Scars are usually incised with a sharp thorn or razor that lacerate the first few layers of skin above the eyebrow, along the bridge of the nose, and on the cheeks that heal in a recessive dell" (Klemm 2009, 61). The scars are strategically placed at the onset of puberty in order to enhance the features considered beautiful. This enhancement is emphasized sometimes with the application of dots of nail polish, meant to draw the eye and harness visual attention.

For the Baluyia of Western Kenya, "the body arts were an especially important aspect of artistic expression, consisting of clothing, accessories, jewelry, scarification, and painting" (Burt 1982, 68). Baluyia women traditionally wore an apron with a tail made of strings twisted from banana fibers and as much **jewelry** as they could afford, including strings of beads, metal ornaments, and cowrie-studded leather straps as headbands, earrings, necklaces, pendants, armlets, wristlets, rings, waistbands, leglets, and anklets. Additionally, their mostly naked bodies were scarred and painted with clay pigments. Scars were created by lifting the skin with a thorn and using a razor to cut a lozenge-shaped welt in patterns that radiated outward from the navel. Scarification was considered a prerequisite to marriage and was considered a marker of sexual availability: the tenderness required to handle healing skin was thought to add to sensitivity during lovemaking.

Scarification is also commonly practiced in Oceania. Men of the Tanga of New Ireland in Melanesia wear elaborate facial tattoos and often scar areas of their chest between the nipples and the outer part of their upper arms. Young men begin the lifelong process of scarring, which is accomplished with a razor-sharp piece of bamboo or an obsidian blade and then rubbed with lime, causing them to heal as scars raised about three-eighths of an inch above the rest of their skin (Bell 1949). These extremely painful scars are either done by a friend or self-inflicted. Scars may also be used as a way of initiating a member into a dancing or singing group.

In the Sepik region of Papua New Guinea, the chest, back, and buttocks of a young male initiate are sliced by an elder with the sharpened edge of a bamboo blade in order to create a distinctive pattern reminiscent of crocodile skin. The resulting scars are thought to represent the teeth marks of a crocodile that has been swallowed, and thus mastered, by the young man during the ceremony (Guynup 2004).

Today, many adherents to the aesthetics of the "modern primitive" or "neotribalism" movement seek scarification as a way of marking their flesh. Just as the painful practice of scarification is used to demonstrate mastery or a lack of fear necessary for a rite of passage, many Westerners who practice these forms of **body modification** argue that the physical discomfort and health risks that the process entails allow them to experience a kind of intensity that is often missing in their daily lives. Along with tattooing, some argue for more rigorous legislation to prevent minors from engaging in this distinctive and irreversible practice (Oultram 2009).

See also: Body Modification; Jewelry; Tattoos.

Further Reading

Bohannan, Paul. 1956. "Beauty and Scarification among the Tiv." *Man* 56: 117–21.

Bell, Frank L. S. 1949. "Tattooing and Scarification in Tanga." *Man* 49: 29–31.

Burt, Eugene. 1982. "Eroticism in Baluyia Body Arts." *African Arts* 15, no. 2: 68–69.

Guynup, Sharon. 2004. "Scarification: Ancient Body Art Leaving New Mark." *National Geographic*. Accessed July 15, 2016. http://news.nationalgeographic.com/news/2004/07/0728_040728_tvtabooscars.html.

Jeffreys, Mervyn David Waldegrave. 1951. "The Winged Solar Disk or Ibo ItΣI Facial Scarification." *Africa* 21, no. 4: 93–111.

Klemm, Peri M. 2009. "Oromo Fashion: Three Contemporary Body Art Practices among Afran Qallo Women." *African Arts* 42, no. 1: 54–63.

Ojo, Olatunji. 2008. "Beyond Diversity: Women, Scarification, and Yoruba Identity." *History in Africa* 35: 347–74.

Orie, Olanike Ola. 2011. "The Structure and Function of Yoruba Facial Scarification." *Anthropological Linguistics* 53, no. 1: 15–33.

Oultram, Stuart. 2009. "All Hail the New Flesh: Some Thoughts on Scarification, Children and Adults." *Journal of Medical Ethics* 35, no. 10: 607–10.

Nevandomsky, Joseph, and Ekhaguosa Aisien. 1995. "The Clothing of Political Identity: Costume and Scarification in the Benin Kingdom." *African Arts* 28, no. 1: 62–73.

Pitts, Victoria. 2003. *In the Flesh: The Cultural Politics of Body Modification*. New York, Palgrave Macmillan.

SEXY

The word "sexy" is an adjective used to describe people who are highly attractive and sexually appealing. What the specifics of that characterization and opinion are, however, can vary. The elements of what makes a person "sexy" are linked often to elements of physical appearance—eyes, legs, rear end, or hair—but can also be associated with elements of fashion and dress or personality features such as confidence or intelligence (Barnes and Williams 2011).

The rise of the idea of being "sexy," according to philosophers like Michel Foucault, came from a rejection in the West of earlier attempts to manage, discipline, and regulate the body. According to Foucault, by the 1960s in many cultures, capitalism and the structure of capitalist society had shifted away from a Victorian effort to hide and control sexuality and more toward a celebration of sex, moving from coercion (tamping down sexual ideas) to provocation (hoping to stimulate sexual reactions) (Rutherford 2007).

By the 21st century, scholars were talking about an "eroticization" of the world, where more and more elements of popular culture and marketing were about being "sexy." Arguments for this shift include the explosion in popularity of pornography, the increasing appearance of naked skin in advertising, and the success of Viagra and other treatments for male impotence (Rutherford 2007).

This emphasis on being sexy in the current century has also increasingly extended to children, with some expressing alarm about how young bodies are sexualized more and more. Both boys and girls suffer "age compression" in this area as their bodies are eroticized through costumes and clothing while at the same time being bombarded with sexually provocative advertisements and images (Levin and Kilbourne 2009).

Part of the reason that this trend sparks concern is in the roots of the concept of being "sexy." The connotation of the word "sexy" is different from "beautiful" in the way it points to a person's sexual desirability—the way others view an individual as an aspirational sexual partner, not just for procreation, but also for enjoyment.

Perhaps because of this, some link the concept of "sexy" to being physically fit and ready to engage in sex. Physical acts of sex are centered in the body, and the body's ability to react, with blood flow to the appropriate organs and the sensitivity that the blood flow brings, increase sexual energy and satisfaction. Studies have found that every 10 percent of weight lost through exercise in an overweight person resulted in significant improvements in all areas of a person's sex life (Mallet 2009. This type of idea of what is "sexy"—as an ideal of bodily perfection in a classical sense—is supported by scholars who note that bodies that are smooth, symmetrical, and flawless, "ordered and processed by fitness," are often the "sexiest" and most erotic images (Rutherford 2007).

Another element of bodily attraction is scent. Pheromones, naturally occurring substances that the body secretes, send airborne messages about availability to members of the opposite sex, triggering an attraction response. Smell is a key attractor for both men and women (Powell 2006). In one study, 89 percent of men said that a woman's scent would boost her attractiveness, and 60 percent said that it is often the key reason they pursue a woman (Cosmopolitan 2002). Conversely, women are equally attracted by a man's scent, especially that produced by the male pheromone androsterol, the scent found in fresh sweat (Fox 2016).

Some researchers believe that men's and women's preferences in scent and their perception of some scents as "sexy" is actually a biological adaptation that leads individuals to pick people who are genetically best suited to be a mate and produce the healthiest children. Women think that men whose immune systems match best with their own are the sexiest, and females can even identify by smell those men whose bodies are most symmetrical (Naked Science 2016)

Scientists who study the biological and "animal" nature of sexual attraction also argue that intelligence and kindness are seen as attractive across cultures and around the world. Both intelligence and kindness are signs of good genetics and the ability to provide for and care for the partner and offspring. Contentious and difficult people may have more sexual partners (perhaps because of the elements of risk and excitement described later), but agreeable and intelligent people have more long-term relationships (Barker 2014).

In this, sexiness can be understood as being as much mental as it is physical. One proponent of confidence and self-acceptance as the keys to being sexy, beyond a physical appearance that conforms to social norms of thinness, is fashion model Stella Ellis, a successful professional who has walked the runway for major European fashion designers. In her memoir, which doubles as a beauty manual on being "sexy," Ellis seeks to convince women to embrace their bodies, with curves or without, as a way to achieve the approval and admiration of others and build their own confidence. Ellis' work suggests both clothing that emphasizes curves, which evolutionary psychologists argue are tied to sexual attraction, and also to dress "up" in a way that communicates success and a high level of self-care (Ellis 2010).

Ellis is not alone in identifying nonphysical attributes as "sexy." Humor is sexy to both sexes. Women prefer men who will make them laugh, whereas men prefer women who will laugh at their jokes. Exchanging personal information is also "sexy" for both genders. Feeling emotionally intimate and close is seen as attractive. But being perceived as "hard to get" is another element seen as sexy for both genders. This feeling that the other person is very desirable to many people, and therefore hard to catch, is particularly sexy when that person then gives some indication that he or she might be specifically interested in you (Barker 2014).

The feeling of excitement and pursuit, especially for men, can create the image of the woman as sexier. Elements of fear and risk in the context of meeting a mate make other individuals more attractive and can heighten sexual attraction (Naked Science 2016).

See also: Airbrushing; Disciplinary Practices/Disciplinary Power; Perfumes and Scented Oils; Symmetry; Weight.

Further Reading

Barker, Eric. 2014. "Science of Sexy." Accessed September 29, 2016. http://time.com/2859728/science-of-sexy-5-things-that-can-make-you-irresistible/.

Barnes, Bronwyn, and Nakisha Williams. 2011. "We Asked . . . What's the Secret to Being Sexy?" *InStyle* 18, no. 2: 62.

Cosmopolitan. 2002. "The Sexy Power of Your Scent." *Cosmopolitan* 233, no. 4: 232.

Ellis, Stella. 2010. *Size Sexy: How to Look Good, Feel Good, and Be Happy—At Any Size*. New York: F+P Media.

Fox, Kate 2016. "The Smell Report." Accessed September 29, 2016. http://www.sirc.org/publik/smell_attract.html.

Levin, Diane E., and Jean Kilbourne. 2009. *So Sexy So Soon*. New York, Ballantine.

Mallett, Tracey. 2009. *Sexy in 6: Sculpt Your Body with the 6 Minute Quick-blast Workout*. New York: Da Capo Press.

Naked Science. 2016. "Naked Science: What's Sexy." Accessed September 29, 2016. http://channel.nationalgeographic.com/videos/whats-sexy.

Powell, Helena Frith. 2006. *Be Incredibly Sexy: 52 Brilliant Ideas for Sizzling Sensuality*. Oxford, England: Infinite Ideas.

Rutherford, Paul. 2007. *A World Made Sexy: Freud to Madonna*. Toronto: University of Toronto Press.

SHAPEWEAR. *See* Corsets, Shapewear, and Waist Trainers.

SHAVING. *See* Hair Removal.

SHEA BUTTER

Shea butter is an important ingredient in a variety of cosmetics and skin care products, especially those that promise improved skin elasticity and collagen production. Shea butter is made from the nuts and seeds of the shea tree (also called by the French name, *karité*, and scientifically classified as *Butyrospermum parkii*), which grows throughout the mixed climate savannah/sahel region of nineteen African countries. The country with the highest shea butter production today is Burkina Faso (Moudio 2013). These trees represent an important resource for the community: maximum productivity of the tree is reached after fifty years, and they remain fully productive for more than a century. The trees reach a maximum growth of ten to fifteen meters and do not even begin to flower until they are at least twenty years old. The tree appears in oral tradition, being the source of an ointment used on the legs of Sundiata Keita, ruler of the Mali Empire, in childhood. Legend suggests that Mande kings climbed the shea tree as part of their coronation celebration and as a symbol of royal power. Arabic written records from the 13th century confirm that shea butter was traded as far south as the Volta River in Ghana for products from the coast, including fish and salt (Carney and Elias 2006). Archaeological evidence shows evidence of shea butter production in Mali dating to the 14th century (Neuman, Kahlheber, and Uebel 1998). The global trade in shea nuts goes back to ancient **Egypt**, where it was in high demand to protect skin and hair from the hot sun, and continued to be heavily traded to the Middle East and European markets throughout the Middle Ages. Scottish explorer Mungo Park, who visited West Africa in the mid-1800s, commented on the importance of shea butter in daily lives and mapped the extent of the shea tree's habitat.

Traditionally, shea nuts were eaten by West African peoples during the annual rainy season, also known as the hungry season, as it represents the part of the year just before ground crops had ripened. Shea nuts provide a valuable source of dietary fat and are associated with health, well-being, and vitality. The creamy butter, which can remain as a solid in temperatures up to 120 degrees Fahrenheit when prepared properly, is also used as a topical medicine. Shea products are used by West African healers as anti-inflammatory ointments and as an insect repellent (Goreja 2004). Shea nuts are also used locally in cooking, soap making, lamp oil, and as gifts between women (Greig 2006). Refined shea butter can also be used as part of a hair care regimen in order to add control and sheen to dry hair. Shea butter was also rubbed into the skin on a regular basis to keep the skin soft, supple, and "bright." Shea butter is also used commercially as a substitute for cocoa butter and added to low- to mid-priced chocolates. For this reason, the price of shea is often tied to volatile global commodity market prices, rising and falling with the relative value of cocoa.

Since the 1990s, shea butter has been gaining importance as a profiled ingredient in cosmetic and skin care products (Elias and Saussey 2013). Significantly, shea butter is one of the few agricultural crops that is solely managed and processed by West African women (Carney and Elias 2006). The "fair trade" label matters to conscientious consumers who are the target audience of these campaigns. Shea butter marketing campaigns are often paired with gender equality and sustainable development objectives. High-profile Western cosmetics companies like The Body Shop or L'Occitane are willing to pay higher prices for quality oil produced by African women, and female Western consumers at the other end of the "ethical sourcing" commodity chain are eager to be linked to African women producers. Women's labor and expertise are essential to the management of the crop, and over time, women's culturally based agroforestry traditions have established the tree species outside its traditional range because of the preference for the taste of foods cooked in shea butter (Carney and Elias 2006, 247) and their reliance on the product to smooth and brighten their skin.

Processing the nuts is a time-consuming process that frequently involves the kin-based labor of related women of all ages. These women spend an average of ten hours transforming ten kilograms of shea nuts into about one kilogram of butter, with additional time necessary to collect the nuts, firewood, and water used in the production process (Chalfin 2004). Labor is shared. First, the fruit pulp is eaten and the kernels are either buried to prevent germination or set in the sun to dry for five to ten days. Alternatively, the nuts may be roasted in a kiln over a constant wood fire, if available.

The next phase of production involves the removal of the nut's outer shell, and the vigorous use of a stone, a wooden mallet, or a roller to release the kernels and press the oil. The kernels are roasted in a pot over a fire, which accelerates the coagulation of the oil within the kernel. The warm kernels are pounded manually in a mortar with a pestle into a paste the same consistency as peanut butter. Women often perform this labor on their knees by grinding the paste across a flat rock with a stone roller. Water is gradually added to the coarse paste, and the mixture is kneaded and washed many times to achieve the desired consistency and color. The solid fat is then melted and boiled, skimmed and decanted, and left for a few days to cool into a solid. The final product is rolled into fist-sized balls, to be stored for up to two years or sold in the local market.

Other factors also add to the costly nature of the product. One source estimates that it takes between 8 and 10 kilograms of firewood to produce 1 kilogram of shea butter, and women can spend three to five hours a day collecting water during the dry season. In recent years, mechanized equipment has become available to minimize the requirement for additional firewood and raise the yield of oil gained from the nuts. However, the introduction of new technologies into traditional household processes often weakens women's control of production by displacing the need for the specialized knowledge and labor.

The American Shea Butter Institute is a bio-tech institute that began in 2001 to provide consumer and industry education on shea butter and to stimulate the global shea butter value chain. The institute Web site explains that shea butter is distinct from other seed oils in that it can have up to 17 percent more nonsaponifiable oil than other seed oils. This quality is important for two reasons: first, the nonsaponifiable oil does not turn into soap when combined with an alkali, but creates a barrier on the skin that helps to retain moisture, and second, this oil contains valuable phytonutrients and vitamins that promote healing by stimulating the production of collagen. In addition to moisturizing skin, shea butter can be used for a variety of functions, including dry skin, skin rash, peeling skin, blemishes or wrinkles, itching skin, sunburn, small skin wounds, stretch marks, insect bites, frostbite, muscle fatigue, skin allergies, eczema, and dermatitis. The collagen-stimulating properties of refined shea butter also make it an attractive ingredient in expensive anti-**aging** serums. The institute also created a classification system to rank the quality of products from Class A to Class F.

See also: Egypt; Hair.

Further Reading

American Shea Butter Institute. 2016. "Shea Institute." Accessed April 15, 2016. http://www
     .sheainstitute.com.
Carney, Judith, and Marlène Elias. 2006. "Revealing Gendered Landscapes: Indigenous
     Female Knowledge and Agroforestry of African Shea." *Canadian Journal of African Studies* 40, no. 2: 235–66.
Chalfin, Brenda. 2004. *Shea Butter Republic: State Power, Global Markets, and the Making of
     an Indigenous Commodity*. New York: Routledge.
Elias, Marlène, and Judith Carney. 2007. "African Shea Butter: A Feminized Subsidy from
     Nature." *Africa* 77, no. 1: 37–62.
Elias, Marlène, and Magalie Saussey. 2013. " 'Unveiling the Gift that Keeps Giving': Para-
     doxical Narratives of Fair Trade Shea Butter." *Sociologia Ruralis* 53, no. 2: 158–79.
Goreja, W. G. 2004. *Shea Butter: The Nourishing Properties of Africa's Best-Kept Natural Beauty
     Secret*. New York: Amazing Herbs Press.
Greig, Delaney. 2006. "Shea Butter: Connecting Rural Burkinabè Women to International
     Markets through Fair Trade." *Development in Practice* 16, no. 5: 465–75.
Moudio, Rebecca. 2013. "Shea Butter Nourishes." *African Renewal*. August. Accessed Octo-
     ber 12, 2016. http://www.un.org/africarenewal/magazine/august-2013/shea-butter
     -nourishes-opportunities-african-women.
Neuman, Katharina, Stefanie Kahlheber, and Dirk Uebel. 1998. "Remains of Woody Plants
     from Saouga, a Medieval West African Village." *Vegetation History and Archaeobotany* 7,
     no. 2: 57–77.

SKIN BLEACHING. *See* Skin Whitening.

SKIN TONE

One of the universal, or near-universal, elements of beauty identified by evolutionary psychologists and anthropologists is skin color (Etcoff 2000). Whether because skin color is a sign of youth, health, class, status, or sexual interest, the color and tone of skin are among the most common elements of social beauty norms. In many cultures and at many times through history, lighter skin has been preferred, especially for women. In other moments, however, skin color and tone that communicate genetic and physical health through finding the "medium" of the color spectrum is the desired color. Whether in bleaching or tanning skin, the universal agreement is that skin color is important to beauty norms around the world.

Many cultures prefer lighter skin on women and darker skin on men. From Japan to Europe, this standard may be explained by the preference for women to appear more youthful and more delicate, less like they work outside or have spent years in the sun (Etcoff 2000). Youth is a signal to potential mates of fertility and child-bearing capability, and the highlighting of women's weakness or delicacy makes clear the gender difference between male and female. This differentiation, the clear visual clues as to who is male and who is female, is also a universal beauty preference. Humans like to be able to tell the gender of a person based on their appearance, whether in clothing or hair length (Etcoff 2000).

Men of any racial group tend to have darker skin than women in the same group, and this difference is preferred by most women. Women might find a light-skinned man "beautiful," but often also identify him as "too feminine," and therefore not the preferred sexual partner. Darker-skinned men, however, are more likely to be described by women as "attractive," in the sense that they are attracted to him as a potential mate. Psychologists theorize that women prefer the darker skin that indicates more age and capability to work outside as signs that a man is energetic, masculine, and can be depended on to both provide and protect the family (Etcoff 2000).

Due in part to the pervasive influence of colonial history and the global imposition of notions of power and value that privilege a Euro-descended background, in many cultures "whiteness" has become symbolically associated with not just beauty, but modernity and civilization. More than just a denomination of skin color, the idea of "whiteness" can be understood as shorthand for decency, intelligence, attractiveness, wealth, and high social status because of the association with the conquering powers (Charles 2011). In many parts of Asia, lighter skin is also a sign of indoor work or leisure and can be a signal of the moral and intellectual worth of a person. Light skin means a higher caste or social class, an intellectual job, or family wealth that precludes manual labor. For these reasons, in many parts of the world, skin bleaching through a variety of products and practices is a relatively common phenomenon. In Africa, Asia, and the Caribbean, skin-bleaching or skin-whitening products are used routinely (Dlova et al. 2015).

Ochronosis

The global preference for whiter, lighter skin means that many people use skin-lightening products that contain the chemical hydroquinone, which works by impeding the body's ability to produce melanin, the pigment responsible for skin's color. Regular application of hydroquinone means less melanin and lighter skin in some users. Regular and long-term application of the chemical on the skin, however, can also ironically damage it, making the color irregular and making the skin darker, causing dermatitis and exogenous ochronosis—a condition in which large bluish-black patches appear on the treated areas. Some areas of Africa, such as South Africa, have seen the condition of ochronosis reach epidemic proportions because of the widespread and chronic use of hydroquinone by South African women.

The preferences for women of lighter skin color in dating and marriage is a world-wide phenomenon that has been demonstrated as gaining steam in many areas in the 21st century. In India, where light skin for women drives a huge skin-lightening product market, online dating and matchmaking services allow men to filter their results to leave out darker-skinned women (Jha-Nambiar 2008). In the United States, light-skinned African American women continue to be considered more attractive than their darker-skinned compatriots by potential mates (Chien Ju 2004). And in the Caribbean, being married to or partnered with a "browning," or light-skinned, woman is a symbol of status and success for Jamaican men (Hope 2006).

This widespread and well-documented preference for lighter-skinned women, then, might seem to run contrary to the common practices of tanning in lighter-skinned European and North American cultures. Similar to the association of light skin with higher class in Asian cultures, tanning became popular in the United States as a sign of affluence, wealth, and leisure in the 1920s. The association of tanned skin with exercise, health, and the ability to travel to tropical locales has persisted into the 21st century (Hemrich et al. 2014). These preferences in Europe and North America for tanned skin mean that both men and women engage in tanning practices, whether outside, in tanning beds, or using cosmetics, activities analogous to the skin-bleaching practices of other areas of the world.

One possible explanation for the dual movements toward tanning and bleaching may be found in the concept of the "average" as a global beauty preference. Multiple studies have found that humans, from Oceania to the Americas, prefer faces and bodies that are seen as not "too" anything. Not too dark or too light, not too tall or too short, not too fat or too thin. The average in studies is consistently rated as more attractive than any exaggerated feature (Adams 2006). Evolutionary psychologists theorize that this type of preference is linked to the perceived health of the individual. People who demonstrate genetic diversity through mixing are less susceptible to disease and less likely to be carrying predispositions to genetic ailments. In terms of skin color, then, this demonstration of mixing, and therefore preference, is sometimes called the "mixed race, pretty face" theory (Etcoff 2000).

This preference for genetic diversity may explain the skin tone of the contestants in a global beauty pageant such as Miss Universe. Contestants who come from populations with darker skin are often selected for their lighter version of their nation's coloring. Contestants who come from populations with lighter skin engage in tanning to become darker. All are seeking the average, medium skin that communicates a "pretty face."

See also: The Caribbean; China; India; Skin Whitening; Tanning.

Further Reading

Adams, William Lee. 2006. "Mixed Race, Pretty Face?" January 1. Accessed July 28, 2016. https://www.psychologytoday.com/articles/200601/mixed-race-pretty-face.

Charles, Christopher A. D. 2011. "Skin Bleaching and the Prestige Complexion of Sexual Attraction." *Sexuality & Culture* 15, no. 4: 375–90.

Chien Ju, Huang. 2004. "Skin Colors, Self Perceptions, Racial Identities, and Preference of Mate Selection of African Americans." *Conference Papers—American Sociological Association* 1–20.

Dlova, Ncoza C., Saja H. Hamed, Joyce Mahlako Tsoka-Gwegweni, and Anneke Grobler. 2015. "Skin Lightening Practices: An Epidemiological Study of South African Women of African and Indian Ancestries." *British Journal of Dermatology* 173: 2–9.

Etcoff, Nancy. 2000. *Survival of the Prettiest: The Science of Beauty.* New York: Anchor.

Hemrich, Ashley, Laura Pawlow, Andrew Pomerantz, and Dan Segrist. 2014. "Current Versus Ideal Skin Tones and Tanning Behaviors in Caucasian College Women." *Journal of American College Health* 62, no. 8: 588–91.

Hope, Donna. 2006. *Inna Di Dancehall: Popular Culture and the Politics of Identity in Jamaica.* Mona, Jamaica: University of the West Indies Press.

Jha-Nambiar, Sonora. 2008. "Looking for Love in All the White Places: A Study of Skin-Color Preferences on Indian Matrimonial and Mate-Seeking Web Sites." *Conference Papers—International Communication Association* 1–31.

SKIN WHITENING

The cosmetic practice of seeking lighter, whiter skin through the application of lotions, creams, and other treatments is a widespread practice across the world and among both men and women. From Asia to Latin America and the United States, people of both sexes seek whiter skin for a variety of reasons, but always with the belief that the lighter appearance will make them more attractive. This practice, as with many types of beauty work, is not a new innovation, but has its roots in many nations, in centuries past.

The ancient Greeks used a skin-whitening cream filled with lead, and in the Europe of the 1600s and 1700s, for example, aristocrats also used a lead oxide powder to lighten their skin before peeling it off with mercury-based masks (Mapes 2008). Historically, in both China and Japan, people drank potions made with ground pearls and applied lotions made with mercury to whiten skin. Cosmetics, such as thick powders, were also applied to the face to give a whiter appearance (Bray 2002). Lead, mercury, and arsenic, though toxic, have been used continually throughout history and across the globe in the pursuit of whiter skin.

In the 21st century, worldwide, there are a dizzying array of products produced and marketed that claim to whiten skin, and the market for skin lightening keeps growing. In 2011, the World Health Organization reported that 61 percent of all skin care products sold in India were skin-lightening creams. The number of consumers for the products was equally high in Africa: in Nigeria 77 percent of women polled reported using skin lighteners, and numbers were similarly high in many Asian nations such as Malaysia and South Korea (World Health Organization 2011).

With the demand for the products growing, the number of brands and choices increases. Many of these products continue, however, to contain chemicals and compounds that have been proven to be dangerous to the user's health. Mercury is still a commonly used ingredient because of its effectiveness. Mercury inhibits the production of melanin, which causes skin pigmentation and effectively produces whiter skin. Mercury-based soaps are popular as skin-lightening tools in Africa, and mercury is found in many Asian skin-lightening creams (Nakano Glenn 2008). Although mercury does effectively lighten the skin, it also carries with it a whole list

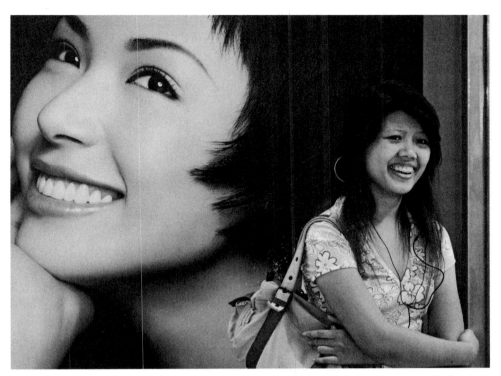

A shopper looks on while seated near a large advertisement for light skin in Bangkok, Thailand. With rising incomes, more and more Asians are turning to products to lighten their skin color, and cosmetics companies are cashing in. (AP Photo/Sakchai Lalit)

of dangers, from kidney damage to depression, anxiety, and psychosis. Mercury can also, ironically, cause skin damage such as rashes, discoloration, and scarring (World Health Organization 2011).

Mercury soaps are not, however, the only choice for skin whitening. Some skin-whitening creams contain botanical elements such as soy, arbutin, or kojic acid. These botanicals, although safer than mercury, are not generally as effective. The most effective agent put in creams and treatments used by physicians is hydroquinone, an organic compound. Again, although this ingredient is believed to be safer than mercury, which has well-proven damaging effects, hydroquinone has shown some cancer-causing effects and is only available by prescription in the United States (Stoppler 2006). Another method used by cosmetic surgeons for skin lightening is a series of intense pulsed light treatments, in which a laser is used to lighten skin (Schlessinger 2008). In August 2016, the Food and Drugs Authority of Ghana banned the sale of all cosmetic products containing hydroquinone (Voice 2016).

So what drives the desire for whiter skin? Why run these great risks? The answer to that question can vary according to region and the individual who is engaged in skin-whitening practice. For some, lighter skin automatically carries the connotation of wealth and a higher social class. For others, light skin symbolizes an attractive fragility and delicacy. In each case, however, light skin is associated with beauty.

The European correlation between white skin and high status is the root of the term "blue bloods," an idea that true nobility's skin was translucent enough to see their veins. In China, there is a saying that "one whiteness can cover three kinds of ugliness." In China, having light skin is synonymous with elegance and nobility, and the term often used to describe the ideal skin tone is "white jade" (Leong 2006). This connection between the lightness of skin and the high social position of the person with that skin was equally true in China as well as other parts of Asia, such as Korea and Japan, where it was assumed that only peasants needed to work outside, and therefore had darker skin (Leong 2006).

The historical prejudices and assumptions about the correlation between lighter skin and higher monetary and social worth continue into the 21st century. Multiple studies undertaken by sociologists and anthropologists have revealed the way in which skin color and tone significantly affects people's ability to get a job or find a mate. In nations such as Venezuela, Brazil, and the United States, research shows how many people find others with a darker skin to be less intelligent, trustworthy, and attractive (Nakano Glenn 2008). It is undeniable that some associate lighter skin with the Caucasian appearance and the power, privilege, and prestige that is often associated with the European and American presence and lifestyle. In South Africa, for example, the colorist ideologies brought by colonists and continued into the 20th century emphasized the correlation between darker skin, primitiveness, uncleanliness, and poverty (Nakano Glenn 2008).

Some researchers, however, maintain that this racially based colorist prejudice is not the only reason for people to pursue lighter skin. Scholars in Indonesia, for example, have proposed that the drive for whiter skin in that nation is the pursuit of a "transnational" ideal of beauty that does not signal just a Caucasian racial heritage, but rather a "cosmopolitan," internationally recognized, and embraced beauty ideal that symbolizes the ability to move from one local, national, or regional context to another easily and be seen as beautiful in each (Saraswati 2010). In this argument, the beauty ideal of lighter skin is tied to the universal embrace of lightness correlating with beauty.

See also: Brazil; Chemical Peels; China; Greece; India; South Korea.

Further Reading

Bray, Marianne. 2002. "Skin Deep: Dying to Be White." Accessed November 21, 2015. http://edition.cnn.com/2002/WORLD/asiapcf/east/05/13/asia.whitening.

Leong, Solomon. 2006. "Who's the Fairest of Them All? Television Ads for Skin-Whitening Cosmetics in Hong Kong." *Asian Ethnicity* 7, no. 2: 167–81.

Mapes, Diane. 2008. "Suffering for Beauty Has Ancient Roots." November 11. Accessed November 21, 2015. http://www.nbcnews.com/id/22546056/ns/health/t/suffering-beauty-has-ancient-roots/#.VlDQ0r9cjVI.

Nakano Glenn, Evelyn. 2008. "Yearning for Lightness: Transnational Circuits in the Marketing and Consumption of Skin Lighteners." *Gender and Society* 22, no. 3: 281–302.

Saraswati, L. Ayu. 2010. "Cosmopolitan Whiteness: The Effects and Affects of Skin-Whitening Advertisements in a Transnational Women's Magazine in Indonesia." *Meridians: Feminism, Race, Transnationalism* 10, no. 2: 15–41.

Schlessinger, Joel. 2008. "Ask the Doctors." *Cosmetic Surgery Times* 11: 14.

Stoppler, Melissa. 2006. "FDA Proposes Hydroquinone Ban." Accessed November 21, 2015. http://www.medicinenet.com/script/main/art.asp?articlekey=64167.

The Voice. 2016. "Ghana to Ban Sale of Skin Bleaching Products." *Jamaica-Gleaner.* Accessed June 16, 2016. http://jamaica-gleaner.com/article/world-news/20160531/ghana-ban-sale-skin-bleaching-products.

World Health Organization. 2011. "Mercury in Skin Lightening Products." Accessed November 21, 2015. http://www.who.int/ipcs/assessment/public_health/mercury_flyer.pdf.

SOCIAL CONSTRUCTION OF BEAUTY

What is considered beautiful can change dramatically according to historical circumstances, geographical distribution, and social interactions between people. The notion of beauty, and of the body itself, changes according to a variety of social and cultural factors. For this reason, many social scientists and gender scholars take the view that beauty is socially constructed; that is, the differences between individuals that make one more beautiful and the other less beautiful are not actually based in some biologically quantifiable reality or "truth." Rather, subtle social meanings that are derived from extensive individual and collective experiences come to shape and influence what a culture thinks of as "beautiful" or "ugly." Social construction also refers to the social practice of perceiving and defining people as beautiful and how these practices come to fit our social beliefs, continually reinforcing the standards of beauty within the social group. Social constructions of beauty eventually come to be accepted as the "normal standard" or as the "natural standard." These standards may be very durable, lasting for generations, or they may be suddenly and unexpectedly influenced by new technologies, new influences, or new experiences.

Although the social notions of beauty accepted by any given culture might be widely agreed upon, it is, of course, the individual who experiences the lived reality of beauty (or its lack thereof). Psychologists can observe the ways in which the biological factors that influence beauty can alter the experiences of an individual, either through continual praise and reaffirmation because the individual conforms to or exceeds a cultural standard of beauty, or through discouragement and self-loathing when the individual does not measure up to what might be culturally expected as a minimal standard of beauty. Frequently, those suffering from **eating disorders** and **body dysmorphic disorders** can relate to the profound dissatisfaction and misery created by seemingly arbitrary, socially constructed standards of beauty. Those considered ugly or **obese** may be relegated by the group or by themselves to marginal social positions and deprived of opportunities to thrive in their own culture.

> "It is amazing how complete is the delusion that beauty is goodness."
>
> —LEO TOLSTOY

People may also choose to ignore or resist norms of physical appearance, though there may be social consequences for going bald, refusing to dye one's hair, or for having small breasts. **Gender**, of course, also plays a role in the stigma of not measuring up to standards of beauty dictated by a culture. Experiences, opportunities, and burdens are differentially available to males and to females because of social views about maleness and femaleness (Kramer 2011, 5). The consequences for a woman who does not conform to the arbitrary social construction of beauty might be significantly harsher than for those of a man.

The social construction of beauty can also be sensitive to differences in age, race, and social **class**. Multiracial feminism, especially that which is informed by an intersectional approach, observes that the conditions of peoples' lives are influenced by significant divisions based on race, class, and sexuality. Particularly in postindustrial, capitalist cultures, there exist, at any given time, a multiplicity of femininities and masculinities that influence the meanings of one's situated location within a social structure, and in turn, influence the degree to which an individual may have access to resources, influence over the decisions of others, or relative power in a given social situation. "Doing gender," as a kind of **performance**, often involves invoking normative socially constructed standards of beauty that may work in one's favor. For those who are unable to manage these critical performances, other alternatives may be available, or there may be disappointments. For example, Hesse-Biber (2007) documents a rising interest on the part of young, occupationally successful African American and Latina women in urban areas of the eastern United States to be thin. This suggests that the white, middle-class social construction of an ideal body shape is spreading, transforming preexisting social constructions about physical beauty. Intersectional approaches to how beauty is socially constructed yield better insight into the ways in which these ideas spread.

See also: Body Dysmorphic Disorder; Class; Eating Disorders; Feminism; Gender; Obesity; Performance/Performativity.

Further Reading

Hesse-Biber, Sharlene. 2007. *Am I Thin Enough Yet?* New York: Oxford University Press.
Kramer, Laura. 2011. *The Sociology of Gender: A Brief Introduction*, 3rd edition. New York: Oxford University Press.

SOUSA, OSMEL

Venezuelan **pageant** guru, coach, judge, and self-proclaimed "Beauty Czar," Cuban-born Osmel Sousa has huge international influence in the world of beauty and beauty pageants (AP 2009). A controversial figure held in high esteem for his work and also vilified for his notions about beauty, he has dominated the international pageant world for four decades.

Sousa, who emigrated to Venezuela at the age of 13, began his career as an artist and illustrator who specialized in drawing the female form. His breakthrough into the world of international pageants happened when in 1969, he was hired by the Miss Venezuela organization as a pageant gown designer. During this time, Sousa also began secretly advising a few contestants. The success of his prodigies resulted in him being named president of the Miss Venezuela organization in 1981 (Miss Venezuela 2016).

Starting from the belief that natural beauty is a false ideal, Sousa created a boot camp–style training regimen of dieting and plastic surgery. As part of a well-organized nationwide recruiting program, Sousa sought "diamonds in the rough" and molded them to his vision of beauty. "I derive my enjoyment by changing the women for the better," Sousa has been quoted as saying, "otherwise, it would be a bore" (Omestad 2001).

The drive to perfect the female form includes a celebration of plastic surgery as an acceptable type of beauty work. Whereas other nations banned cosmetic surgery, Sousa has always embraced the practice. For Sousa, these procedures are a necessary and reasonable part of the process of molding a beauty queen, say-

Pygmalion

Pygmalion, a Greek figure made famous through the work of the Roman poet Ovid, is a sculptor who carves his vision of the perfect woman out of ivory. Once the statue is completed, Pygmalion is so enamored of his vision of beauty that he falls in love with the statue and loses interest in real women. Pygmalion prays to Aphrodite to make the statue real, a prayer that the goddess answers, turning the statue to life. The idea of a man creating his own vision of perfect beauty in a woman because real women are inadequate is an idea that continues to be relevant through 21st-century culture. Viewing women as both objects and raw material to be molded into the perfect, ideal beauty norm is seen particularly in modern films, such as *My Fair Lady*, *Pretty Woman*, or *Ruby Sparks*.

ing, "If a girl needs a nose job, you get her one. It's an industry so we strive for perfection. We can't settle for mediocrity" (Styles 2014).

Tellingly, Venezuela has had more international beauty queens than any other nation. Sousa's career has led him to train contestants from other nations. In the United States, Sousa is one of the coaches and judges on the Spanish-language program *Nuestra Belleza Latina* [Our Latin Beauty], a hugely popular and long-running reality show on the Univision Network. The program brings in young women from Latin America and Hispanic communities around the United States to be groomed and prepared for careers as models, television hostesses, and actresses. Sousa is likened to Simon Cowell in his severity, scathing criticisms, and insults to contestants.

Sousa remains a controversial figure for many of his views and opinions. The Beauty Czar has been quoted as saying that "inner beauty doesn't exist. That's something that women who aren't pretty invented to justify themselves" (Neuman 2013). He disregards female activists who criticize his attitudes toward women, saying of **feminist** organizations, "Those organizations were created by ugly betties with no hope of a fix! They're all horrendous!" (Styles 2014). The attitude that women are only valuable if they conform to Sousa's vision of beauty is made more troubling by his views on race. Sousa has made deeply troubling comments on the issue of race and beauty. In a 2002 documentary he confided to the interviewer, "Venezuelan black women are not beautiful" (Beauty Obsession 2002).

See also: Feminist; Pageants—Local, National, International; Plastic Surgery; Venezuela.

Further Reading

AP. 2009. "Beauty Guru Osmel Sousa Shapes Miss Universe." September 24. Accessed August 12, 2016. http://www.dawn.com/news/923751/beauty-guru-osmel-sousa-shapes-miss-universe.

Beauty Obsession. 2002. Film. ABC Australia, Journeyman Pictures.

Kearney, Ryan. 2013. "Of Airport Animals and Beauty Pageant Bastards." *New Republic* 244, no. 20: 10–11.

Miss Venezuela. 2016. "Osmel Sousa." Accessed August 12, 2016. http://www.missvenezuela .com/osmel-sousa.

Neuman, William. 2013. "Mannequins Give Shape to a Venezuelan Fantasy." Accessed August 12, 2016. http://www.nytimes.com/2013/11/07/world/americas/mannequins-give -shape-to-venezuelan-fantasy.html?pagewanted=1&_r=4&smid=fb-share.

Nichols, Elizabeth Gackstetter. 2014. "Virgin Venuses: Beauty and Purity for 'Public' Women in Venezuela." In: *Women in Politics and Media: Perspectives from Nations in Transition,* edited by Maria Raicheva-Stover and Elza Ibroscheva. London: Bloomsbury.

Nuestra Belleza Latina. 2016. Accessed August 12, 2016. http://www.univision.com/shows /nuestra-belleza-latina.

Omestad, Thomas. 2001. "In the Land of Mirror, Mirror on the Wall." *U.S. News & World Report* 131, no. 3: 33.

Styles, Ruth. 2014. "'It's Like a Competition for Plastic Surgeons!' The Extreme Beauty Queens of Venezuela Prepared to Spend Thousands on Getting the Perfect Face." February 5. Accessed August 12, 2016. http://www.dailymail.co.uk/femail/article-2552401 /Its-like-competition-plastic-surgeons-The-extreme-beauty-queens-Venezuela-prepared -spend-thousands-getting-perfect-face.html#ixzz4H7jiPZ7U.

SOUTH KOREA

The small Asian nation of South Korea is the nation with perhaps the highest per-capita spending and effort put into beauty work. Both men and women in South Korea are deeply invested in their physical appearances and engage in a wide range of beauty work to achieve their ideal of beauty. Cosmetics, plastic surgery, and other types of activities are extremely common in a nation with full-length mirrors in every subway car.

Cosmetics are one weapon in the South Korean arsenal of beauty. South Korea is a world leader in the development and sale of beauty products, in 2014 exporting more than a billion dollars in cosmetics to international markets worldwide. The products produced in Korea, however, are also widely used by both male and female Koreans. Products such as skin care creams, lipstick, and eyeliner are worn, marketed, and sold by the stars of Korean pop music and by regular Koreans across the nation (Shaeffer 2015).

For both men and women in South Korea, a daily skin care regimen can include the use up to 18 products per day (Hunt 2011). The interest in and work on cosmetics in the nation has led international magazines to proclaim South Korea a "skin-care superpower," where the formulas and skin care technology are more than a decade ahead of anything that Europe or the United States produces (Hunt 2011).

The Korean interest in cosmetics goes beyond simple skin care, however. Colorful and artistic cosmetic products such as eyeliner, blush, and lipstick are also popularly used by men and women. Men, in particular, are much more likely to use cosmetics in South Korea than in other nations. South Korean men are the world's top per-capita consumers of skin care products, buying four times more than the men in the second-place nation of Denmark. In a market in which men spend more than a billion dollars a year on cosmetics, it is not surprising that national and international brands market directly to Korean men. In the 21st century, the products advertised even included a special line of skin care and camouflage-style makeup for those men completing their mandatory military service (Novak 2015).

The specific cultural value placed on beauty work and appearance for men in South Korea has generated a special term for beautiful, well-groomed men, *kkotm-nam*. This term, 꽃미남, in Korean, alternatively spelled *kkonminam* when transliter-ated, roughly means "flower boy" and is often compared to the idea of the metrosexual (Yang 2014). The term refers to those young men who follow the inspiration of K-pop music stars and cultivate a beautiful, more traditionally feminine or "cute" image that puts emphasis someone who smells good, has delicate features, has excellent manners, wears tight-fitting clothing, and has immaculately coiffed hair. This trend, which started in South Korea, has also moved into other parts of Asia, such as China and Japan (Yang 2014).

Cosmetics are not the only big business in South Korea. The International Society of Aesthetic and Plastic Surgeons reported in 2014 that South Korea performed the third most cosmetic procedures of any nation on the planet, only following the United States and Brazil (ISAPS 2015). Given that South Korea's population of 49 million citizens is only a fraction of the populations of the United States and Brazil (320 million and 204 million, respectively), this means that South Korea has the highest rate of plastic surgery, per capita, in the world.

Much of South Korea's history with plastic surgery dates from the Korean war of the 1950s. The American presence in the nation helped change and shape beauty ideals, especially the desirability of Occidental, or Western, eyes. U.S. surgeons based with the military, such as Dr. Ralph Millard, began to do the medical research into the process of eyelid opening and to publish findings on best practices in the field (Haiken 1999). Today, however, South Korea is itself a leader in the training of plastic surgeons and the research and publication of new methods and treatments.

Estimates place the percentage of South Korean women who undergo plastic surgery between 30 and 50 percent, and the number of men who undergo proce-dures between 15 and 20 percent. For many South Koreans, eyelid or nose surgery is a common high school graduation gift (Marx 2015). The ISAPS reported that in 2014, more than 100,000 blepha-roplasties and rhinoplasties were performed in South Korea (ISAPS 2015).

The most popular and famous locale for plastic surgery proce-dures in South Korea is in the capital of Seoul, in an area known

K-pop

K-pop is a highly visual musical form that originated in South Korea. Starting in the 1990s, by 2016 K-pop already had a huge influence in both music and style throughout Asia, Europe, and the United States. K-pop music is a fusion of hip-hop, rock, electronica, and pop music, often performed by groups of beautiful young "flower boys" in boy bands of four or more members. The performance of the music is an integral element of the style, with music videos featuring sharp dance rou-tines and colorful, stylish costumes and makeup for the performers. The K-pop band BigBang, with elabo-rate hairdos, flamboyant makeup, and theatrical cos-tumes, was the first to have a video (Fantastic Baby) reach more than two million views on YouTube.

as the "self-improvement district." This district, in the high-end neighborhood of Gangnam, houses between 400 and 500 different clinics and hospitals in one square mile of the city (Marx 2015).

The clinics in Gangnam offer a wide array of products and services that reflect South Korean norms and ideals of beauty. In addition to eyelid opening surgery and nose jobs that add a defined point to the nose, jawline shaving is a popular procedure. A reflection of the South Korean preference for smaller faces, many South Koreans have bone from their jaws removed through shaving, reduction, and contouring. Sometimes called "v-line surgery," the goal of the procedure is to lessen the roundness of the face and produce a V-shaped jawline (Marx 2015).

See also: Advertising; Eyelid Surgery; Metrosexual; Nose Jobs; Plastic Surgery.

Further Reading

Haiken, Elizabeth. 1999. *Venus Envy: A History of Cosmetic Surgery.* Baltimore: Johns Hopkins University Press.

Hunt, Kenya. 2011. "The New Skincare Superpower." *Marie Claire* (US Edition). May. 18, no. 5: 244.

ISAPS. 2015. "Global Statistics." Accessed November 16, 2015. http://www.isaps.org/Media /Default/global-statistics/2015%20ISAPS%20Results.pdf.

Marx, Patricia. 2015. "About Face: Why Is Seoul the World's Plastic Surgery Capital?" *The New Yorker.* March 23. Accessed November 16, 2015. http://www.newyorker.com /magazine/2015/03/23/about-face.

Novak, Kathy. 2015. "Why South Korea Men Are Buying Tons of Cosmetics." October 4. Accessed November 17, 2015. http://money.cnn.com/2015/10/04/news/south-korea -men-cosmetics.

Shaeffer, Kayleen. 2015. "What You Don't Know About the Rise of Korean Beauty." September 9. Accessed August 16, 2016. http://nymag.com/thecut/2015/09/korean-beauty -and-the-government.html

Yang, Hsing-Chen. 2014. "Flower Boys on Campus: Performing and Practicing Masculinity." *Journal of Gender Studies* 23, no. 4: 391–408.

SUPERMODELS

Models, or men and women who fashion designers use to showcase their clothing, have been used widely since the 19th century. In the 1800s, models wore and helped to sell clothing designs by appearing in publications like magazines and newspapers and at private shows for wealthy clients, in a similar fashion to the work of models today. The phenomenon of the "supermodel," however, is a purely late 20th-century and 21st-century phenomenon.

Originally, the idea of a model was to be a living "clothes hanger," not to be noticed for their own body, but only to display the clothing for sale. Through the vast majority of the 20th century, few, if any, models were known by name and none had the kind of international celebrity that would

"Inner beauty, how we think, how we act, how we see things, is reflected in how you look."

—CAROLINA HERRERA

start being common in the 1990s (Etcoff 2000).

Although a few models, such as the British model Twiggy, did receive some recognition for their work, the supermodel phenomenon is usually traced back only to the 1990s, when British *Vogue* magazine identified five models on its cover as the "Top Models in the World" (Etcoff 2000). The models featured on that cover, Linda Evangelista, Cindy Crawford, Naomi Campbell, Christy Turlington, and Tatjana Patitiz, are often considered the first "super" models.

Each of the women in this list, and the other women who have since been identified as supermodels, conformed to general social norms of weight, height, hair texture, and facial features. Female supermodels for fashion modeling generally are asked to be at least five foot nine inches tall, and slim, with thirty-four or thirty-five-inch hips, twenty-four-inch waist, and thirty-four-inch bust. These measurements are very uncommon and mark models as "special." As an example of the unusual nature of this body type, the average height of a woman in the United States in 2016 was five foot two inches, and the average waist size was thirty-seven inches (CDC 2016). Women who fit the requirements to be a supermodel are "statistical rarities" that combine very lean bodies with curves (Etcoff 2000).

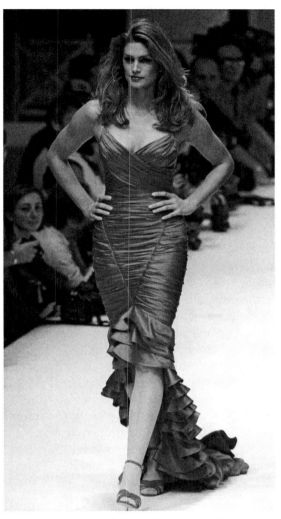

American supermodel Cindy Crawford sports a sleeveless evening dress designed by Herve Leger at a fashion show in Paris, October 18, 1995. (AP Photo/ Remy de la Mauviniere)

The requirements for body shape for female supermodels are just as difficult for the average woman to achieve as the requirements for male supermodels. In the 21st century, the list of supermodels has expanded to encompass men, including Tyson Beckford, Sean O'Pry, and David Gandy. To become supermodels, men generally do not have specific requirements of measurements, but are expected to be tall, lean, and athletic with clearly defined, shredded, muscles and the "Dorito-shaped" body that is a hallmark of progressive muscularity (Hrivnak 2015). Men seeking to become models and supermodels follow the program of adding muscle and stripping away fat, a procedure that requires a very restricted diet and long hours in the weight room (Bailey 2015).

To be a supermodel, a man or woman must certainly conform to social norms of beauty. Some say, however, that reaching true "super" status has less to do specifically with looks and more with name and face recognition: familiar faces help sell products better. Businesses will often pay more for a model whose face is already famous and trusted as an effective selling tool (Times 2015).

The collection of five women featured on the cover of the previously mentioned edition of British *Vogue* in 1990 had their superstardom reinforced and spread by businesses with special appearances on the catwalk for the Italian designer Gianni Versace, in the music video for George Michaels' "Freedom," and in a famous car advertisement (Times 2015). The 1992 advertisement for an economy car called the Vauxhall Corsa became famous not only for the five supermodels who appeared in it, but also for the amount of money each model earned for her participation, reportedly more than $700,000 each (Winter 2013).

It is these very large paydays, combined with the very strict height and weight requirements, that drive much of the controversy and discussion about supermodels. Are they a negative influence on the body image of men and women, leading many to engage in unhealthy dieting, exercise, or surgical practices? The death of Ana Carolina Reston due to anorexia in 2006 is an example of the harmful effects of the restrictive body demands of the industry. Reston, a top model from Brazil, was due to fly to Paris for a photo shoot the day after she died, demonstrating how her literally starved body fit the ideal for the profession (Telegraph 2006).

Some others, however, argue that for young women especially, supermodels represent not sex objects, but success objects that can inspire young women to succeed in business, using "beauty and beauty technologies as another weapon in the Power Girls' arsenal" (Tom 2002). The power, success, and wealth of a supermodel such as the Brazilian Gisele Bündchen, who in 2015 was the world's top paid supermodel, earning $44 million dollars a year through her modeling, fashion lines, and other business ventures. Bündchen earned even more than her pro football player husband, Tom Brady (Pedro 2015). Bündchen, at five foot eleven inches tall, with measurements of 36-24-35, is an example of both the very unusual body type needed to succeed and the success possible in modeling and business for those women with an appropriate body type.

See also: Brazil; Eating Disorders; Height; Progressive Muscularity; United Kingdom; Weight.

Further Reading

Andrade, Pedro. 2015. "The Cost of Being a Male Model." *ABC News*. July 1. Accessed August 16, 2016. https://www.youtube.com/watch?v=f1U66uhY7wM.

Bailey, Mark. 2015. "Ten Body Shaping Secrets from Male Cover Models." *Telegraph UK*. Accessed August 19, 2016. http://www.telegraph.co.uk/men/active/11342141/Ten-body -shaping-secrets-from-male-cover-models.html.

CDC. 2016. "Body Measurements." Accessed August 16, 2016. http://www.cdc.gov/nchs /fastats/body-measurements.htm.

Hrivnak, Filip. 2015. "Where Are All the Male Supermodels?" Accessed August 16, 2016. http://www.vogue.com/13452046/next-male-supermodel-is-coming.

Telegraph. 2006. "Too Skinny Model Dies of Anorexia." Accessed August 16, 2016. *The Daily Telegraph (Sydney)*. November 17. *Newspaper Source*, EBSCOhost.

Times. 2015. "Tears, Tantrums and 10K a Day." *The Sunday Times*. 22, 23, 24, 25. Accessed August 16, 2016. *Newspaper Source*, EBSCOhost.

Tom, Emma 2002. "Supermodels for Modern Girls." Accessed August 16, 2016. *The Australian. Newspaper Source*, EBSCOhost.

Winter, Katie. 2013. "Teenage Kate Moss Makes One of First TV Appearances with Christy Turlington, Linda Evangelista and Naomi Campbell in Vintage Vauxhall Ad." Accessed August 16, 2016. http://www.dailymail.co.uk/femail/article-2383729/Teenage-Kate-Moss-makes-TV-appearances-90s-supermodels-vintage-Vauxhall-ad.html#ixzz4HVR37tZN.

SYMMETRY

Symmetry is understood as an objective equilibrium between two identical forms or two equal sets of formal characteristics (van Damme 1996, 77). Regardless of size, symmetry matters. In order to register attractiveness, a curvy body can have just as much symmetry as a lanky, lean one; round faces can be as symmetrical as square faces. Cultures may have varying standards of the ideal size or shape of a beautiful person, but the notion of symmetry remains the same.

In general, almost all cultures prefer an ideal face and body that appears well proportioned and balanced. Studies show that people who are asked to rank images of other people according to relative attractiveness are most attracted to composite images of faces and bodies that demonstrate symmetry than any single image (Savacool 2009, 9). Artists have known about this principle of idealized symmetry for 2,500 years: the Greek philosopher Euclid provided the first written description of "the golden ratio," a mathematical formula based on the principles of symmetry that finds the ideal distance between two points and lines intersecting as 1:1.618. This key symmetry ratio, known as *phi* in Greek and sometimes referred to as "the Golden Ratio," can be seen in the ancient sculptures of the Parthenon, the dimensions of da Vinci's "Vitruvian Man," and the face of the Mona Lisa, and in contemporary beauty analyses provided online by a company known as "Beauty Analysis," which allows users to superimpose a symmetrical grid known as the "Golden Mask" on top of a photo of their own face (Golden Number 2016). Research also confirms that infants will stare longer at images of people with symmetrical faces than asymmetrical ones and adults prefer symmetrical bodies as well, which they associate positively with physical health and strength (Savacool 2009, 10).

However, studies show that when human replicas (in robotics or computer generations, for example) appear too perfectly symmetrical, the results actually elicit negative emotional feelings of eeriness or revulsion. This phenomenon is known as the "uncanny valley hypothesis" and suggests that the human sense of idealized beauty does not require "perfection," but rather desires some measure of imperfection in order to generate positive feelings of empathy and recognition of personhood. Some researchers suggest that the symmetrical perfection of robots or androids compels viewers to fear their own mortality and triggers deeply rooted psychological defenses for coping with the inevitability of death, including fears of soullessness and the fear of being replaced.

A concept perhaps as important as symmetry to understanding how the human brain evaluates beauty is the related concept of "balance," which is a more subjective and less tangible form of visual equilibrium, often "sensed" and not necessarily quantifiable. The notion of balance is used to designate what is felt to be an equilibrated relationship between two or more nonidentical forms, even though there may be minute differences between the two that could be verifiably measured. Sometimes, balance and symmetry are very closely related—as in the arrangement of **hair** or the placement of earrings or other **jewelry**. Other times, there is more latitude given to the ways in which two objectively asymmetrical features are "balanced" to create a pleasing effect that strikes the viewer as beautiful. Van Damme (1996) gives the example of the ways in which female breasts and buttocks are assessed to create an **hourglass shape**: the figure is not necessarily evaluated by drawing an axis that runs vertically through the female figure, but rather, the viewer may have appreciation for the ways in which the body can create a balanced asymmetry, especially in motion.

Art historians, seeking to establish guidelines for "ethno-aesthetics," have conducted research trying to establish the shared value for the importance of symmetry and balance in creating pleasing pieces of visual art or in assessing what features they designate as most crucial for establishing standards of human beauty. The Dan, Senufo, Tiv, Chokwe, and Turu have no indigenous word for "symmetry," but they are able to describe the concept to summarize the concept of balance in the masks that they make designed to embody the most valued qualities of the human face. In Igbo, the concept of "kwabim" translates as balance, and is important for describing aspects of beauty. Similarly, the Batammaliba word "yala" means evenness or balance, and the Mende term "mbe-ma" refers to a similar concept. The Fang concept of "bipwé" also means balance, not only in visual aesthetics, but also in the concept of moderation (van Damme 1996). Across Africa, moderation is frequently an attribute credited not only to physical balance, but also to moral attractiveness. Careful attention to symmetry designating "beauty" by the viewer is also found in Surinam, the Trobriand Islands, and among a wide variety of Native American peoples.

However, many of these cross-cultural experiments on "ethno-aesthetics" also confirm findings already reported for Western subjects: novelty, complexity, and surprisingness, when presented to the viewer under the right circumstances and in the right quantities, appear to elicit a pleasurable effect that may override the desire for perfect symmetry (van Damme 1996, 65).

See also: Hair; Hourglass Shape; Jewelry.

Further Reading

The Golden Number. 2016. *Phi, The Golden Number*. Accessed March 15, 2016. http://www .goldennumber.net/beauty.

Savacool, Julia. 2009. *The World Has Curves: The Global Quest for the Perfect Body*. New York: Rodale.

Van Damme, Wilfried. 1996. *Beauty in Context: Towards an Anthropological Approach to Aesthetics*. Leiden: EJ Brill.

TANNING

For many generations, porcelain skin untouched by the sun revealed a life of leisure spent indoors. Those who had to work outdoors as laborers or fieldworkers were recognizable by their darker skin. Spanning back to the Greek and Roman empires through the days of Jane Austen, women tried to create pale skin using a variety of **skin whitening** techniques, some of which contained toxins like arsenic that harmed them or even shortened their lives.

Following the Industrial Revolution, the logic about the skin of the worker changed: in an industrial age, low-**class** workers toiled indoors. The average working person's life was now spent living and working under damp, cramped conditions in small rooms in order to avoid the soot and smog of the streets. Ailments like rickets and tuberculosis became commonplace (Wilkinson 2012), and many doctors prescribed sunbathing as a remedy for those who could afford it. Wealthy sufferers in the early 1900s traveled to sunny spots to lie out on chaise lounge chairs and "take the sun" (Palmer 2012).

The French fashion designer Gabriel Bonheur "Coco" Chanel is generally credited with popularizing the tanned skin of the wealthy elites when she took too much sun on a Mediterranean cruise in 1923. In the summer of 1927, *Vogue* **magazine** featured a tanned model on the cover, challenging the well-established precedent of the lily-and-rose complexion as the standard of beauty (Downing 2012, 51). Tanned arms and backs appeared with evening gowns, and formal gloves were abandoned. Sandals became de rigeur for vacationing socialites. With these changes, the Riviera in the south of France rapidly became a "stockingless heaven," according to *Vogue* magazine (Downing 2012).

In addition to popularizing the tan, Coco Chanel is credited with freeing women from the confining cage of the corset in the early 20th century. She popularized a casual, sporty silhouette, which encouraged women's movement and darker skin. Chanel resignified the sun-kissed, bronzed look as a mark of leisure and privilege.

Today, tanned skin is often associated with health and vitality. White Americans, Australians and Europeans believe that tanned skin is a sign of health, and a 2006 study of Australian teenagers found that tanned models were deemed to be more attractive than lighter-skinned models (Palmer 2012).

Tanned skin has also become an important signifier of **masculinity**. Studies find that darker tans are considered healthier for men than for women (Palmer 2012). Male celebrities like Cary Grant actively worked on their tans, and male politicians like Mitt Romney and Donald Trump use spray tan to maintain a healthy glow.

Sun lamps and tanning beds are widely available across the Western world to help light-skinned customers turn their skin a more attractive, darker shade of tan. Warnings from the U.S. Food and Drug Administration caution that tanning lamps may be more dangerous than natural sun because people can use them all year round, not allowing their skin time to heal in between doses of ultraviolet (UV) radiation. Additionally, tanning beds allow a person to expose all of their skin at one time, causing a larger strain on the body's natural ability to heal itself.

Like many beauty practices, tanning also poses some health risks. When skin is exposed to the sun, a natural pigment called melanin is produced to protect the body from UV radiation. Excessive UV exposure causes direct and indirect damage to the skin, causing rapid aging or wrinkling, impairment of the immune system, and increased risk of skin cancers. The rise in skin cancer associated with sun bathing has concerned dermatologists and oncologists. By the 1970s, a wide array of suntan lotions was replaced by sunscreens that used sun protective factor (SPF) technologies to block the harmful rays of the sun.

To avoid excessive UV exposure, many seeking darker skin sought out spray tans. Most spray tan technology applies the same process that makes an apple turn from white to brown when exposed to the air. When applied evenly to the skin using an aerosol spray, the naturally occurring chemical dihydroxyacetone (DHA) changes from a colorless sugar derived from sugar beets to an attractive shade of color when it comes into contact with the oxygen in the air. (Some complain that the DHA color is too orange in hue; another spray tan ingredient called erythrulose can also be used for a more "tan" color. The effects of a spray tan are temporary, as people are constantly shedding the top layer of skin and replacing it with new cells. Spray tans can be applied at home or professionally in order to get even coverage and even specialized shading effects.

Other bronzing agents or temporary dyes may also be used on the skin to create the illusion of tanned skin. However, many of these will rub off with sweat or bathing. Bronzing agents are often added to plant-based moisturizers in order to help the skin absorb the tanning solution more quickly.

Some celebrities decry the fashionable practice of tanning. There are parts of the world today where darkened skin still indicates a lower class status. In **India**, many consumers seek a skin tone known as "wheatish," trying to avoid darker-colored skin that hints at an outdoors lifestyle. In **China**, beachgoers sometimes wear a "face-kini," a balaclava-like mask, in order to shield the skin of their faces from tanning (Palmer 2012).

See also: "Black Is Beautiful Movement," or Black Power; China; Class; India; Magazine; Masculinity; Skin Whitening.

Further Reading

Chaney, Lisa. 2012. *Coco Chanel: An Intimate Life*. New York, Penguin.

Downing, Sarah Jane. 2012. *Beauty and Cosmetics 1550–1950*. Oxford, England: Shire Publications.

Palmer, Brian. 2012. "When Did Tanned Skin Become Fashionable?" *Slate*. October 10. Accessed October 6, 2016. http://www.slate.com/articles/news_and_politics/explainer

/2012/10/romney_s_spray_tan_when_did_white_people_start_deliberately_tanning
_themselves.html.

Wilkinson, Sophie. 2012. "A Short History of Tanning." *The Guardian*. February 19. Accessed
October 6, 2016. https://www.theguardian.com/commentisfree/2012/feb/19/history-of
-tanning.

TATTOOS

The earliest evidence of tattooing is found on the body of a mummy from the Italian-Austrian border. Discovered in 1991, Ötzi the Iceman displayed small tattoos in the shape of dots and crosses on his lower spine, right knee, and ankle joints. Archaeologists speculate that the 61 separate tattoos were added to Ötzi's body about 5,200 years ago, not for beautification but rather as a therapeutic remedy to alleviate joint pain possibly caused by arthritis (South Tyrol Museum of Archaeology 2013).

The word "tattoo" comes from the islander word "tatatau" from British explorer James Cook's expedition to Tahiti in 1769. The first Europeans to tattoo themselves were sailors, but the practice spread quickly upon their return home.

Though tattoos can be a sign of beauty, they are also a mark of stigma. Tattoos can indicate important spiritual ideals, but mainstream religions like Judaism, Christianity, and Islam actively condemned them. The permanence of tattoos was also used at various times in world history as a punishment or indelible identifying marker on the bodies of slaves, convicts, or members of a persecuted group, including concentration camp victims of the Nazis.

Evidence of tattoos appears in the ancient remains of Egypt, Nubia, Thrace, Greece, Japan, Mexico, Greenland, and Polynesia (Lineberry 2007). The first evidence of cosmetic tattoos that were likely designed to be pleasingly decorative comes from ancient **Egypt**. The tattoos, dotted patterns of lines and diamonds, were made by pricking the skin with specially designed wooden tools and then rubbing in a dark pigment that contained a high percentage of soot. Brighter colors were also used. Some women mummies from the era were also tattooed with figures of the dwarf god Bes on the thigh area (Lineberry 2007).

Iron Age burials of the Pazyryk culture in the Altai Mountains, located at the juncture of present-day Siberia, Kazakhstan, Mongolia, and China, display a wide range of human burial mounds where entire horses were sacrificed and buried with the deceased. Horses were important for both the daily lives of these nomadic people and their religious ideology, which included a permeable boundary between human and animal, living and dead, and a rider and her horse. In this cold environment, many of the frozen embalmed mummies found in the tombs still possess enough skin to make out the dramatic features of animal tattoos, including birds, fish, reindeer, ibexes, mountain sheep, felines, and probably most importantly, horses (Argent 2013). The most famous of these mummies is a fifth-century elite woman sometimes sensationally called the "Siberian Ice Maiden," who was unearthed with dozens of tattoos, six horses (saddled and bridled), a three-foot-tall headdress, and a container of marijuana (PBS 1998). Researchers believe that she likely suffered from cancer, exacerbated by a fall from a horse, and the cannabis was used to alleviate her pain in her final hours. Some have called her tattoos "the most complicated and the most beautiful" of those found in the ancient world (Siberian Times 2012).

Tattooing, and body painting in general, can be thought of as a way to differentiate the body of the human from the natural world. For many cultures, visible markings on the body indicate what Turner calls "the social skin," that which identifies a person's achievements or their group membership (Turner 1980).

Tattoos and other body paintings may also distinctively mark social rank and **class**. In his influential memoir written during the 1950s, Lévi-Strauss said of the native Brazilian Guaycuru peoples (also called Kadiwéu or Caduveo), "The nobles bore, quite literally, the 'mark of rank' in the form of pictorial designs—painted or tattooed—on their bodies" (Levi-Strauss 1974, 161). Both men and women wore elaborate tattoos, often augmented with body paint.

Moko facial tattoos are symbolically significant for the Maori people of New Zealand for the ways they represent ancestral lineages. Originally, these tattoos were worn as a sign of status, but today, many Maori men and women wear "moko" as an honorary reflection of their cultural heritage. Moko tattoos are usually done on the head and face, which is considered to be the most sacred part of the body. The Maori also tattoo the lips. A Maori woman with full, blue lips is considered the most beautiful and desirable. Another culture that historically practiced facial tattooing was the Lai Tu Chin tribe of Myanmar (Teicher 2016). Dramatic "spider-web" tattoos were part of coming-of-age ceremonies for young women and were considered marks of beauty. The ink was made from organic ingredients, including soot from cooking lids and plant material. Old women describe the process as lengthy and painful, especially in the eyebrow and eyelid area. Outlawed in the 1960s, the practice of facial tattooing for young women went underground, though it was still practiced by some in remote locations by women who waited for the soldiers to leave. Young women today are no longer receiving the characteristic facial tattoos.

Among the most colorful tattoos found around the world are the incredibly lush **Japanese**

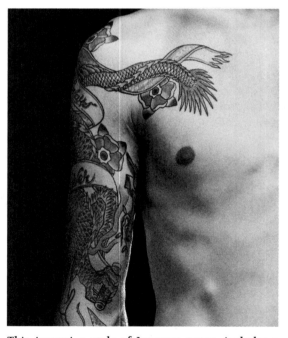

This *irezumi*, a style of Japanese tattoo, includes a dragon, origami crane, and flowers. Tattooing, and body painting in general, is a way to differentiate the body of the human from the natural world. For many cultures, visible markings on the body indicate achievements or social status. (Scott Dumas/Dreamstime.com)

tattoos called "*irezumi*" (also called *bunshin*). The intricacy of *irezumi* was inspired by Edo period woodblock artists (1600–1868), who considered human flesh to be the ultimate canvas and used many wood-blocking tools for transferring designs to bodies, including chisels, gouges, and a unique ink (called Nara ink), which turns blue-green under the skin. Popular *irezumi* designs include elaborately coiled dragons; lavish flowers, fish, and birds; Buddhas and Buddha themes; natural elements, such as bamboo, leaves, and feathers; images of the "Floating World" derived from *ukiyo-e* prints; and hybrid and mythical beasts, usually depicted in action. Another technique is called "*kakushibori*," literally "hidden carving," to "hide" tattoos in discreet body locations where they are unlikely to be seen, like the armpit or inside the thighs. *Kakushibori* also refers to the practice of "hiding" a word within a design, such as weaving the characters (letters) of a word into the scales of a fish or the petals of a flower. *Irezumi* tattoos are done by hand and take a very long time to complete, taking several visits of many hours each to accomplish the outline, coloring, and shading. The technique is reportedly more painful than Western tattoos, which are mostly done by machines. Artist practitioners spend years apprenticing to learn all the various techniques. Some *irezumi* enthusiasts cover their entire bodies in tattoos, called a "body suit," which covers the neck, chest, back, legs, and arms, but always leaves an unlinked space at the center of the body. This style of tattooing inspired Ed Hardy, the widely recognized popularizer of the contemporary American tattoo styles.

Today, tattoos are often adopted by individuals as "body projects" designed as conscious and long-term strategies to alter the body as a way of rejecting cultural norms or to mark specific aspects of their personal journey (Pitts 2003). Tattoos are chosen to emphasize personal agency and to celebrate the various forms of body modification and individual sources of suffering and pleasure. Tattoos as a form of intentional **body modification** may also mark membership in a counterculture community.

See also: Body Modification; Class; Egypt; Japan; Moko Tattoos.

Further Reading

Argent, Gala. 2013. "Inked: Human-Horse Apprenticeship, Tattoos and Time in the Pazyryk World." *Society and Animals* 21:178–93.

Levi-Strauss, Claude. 1974. *Tristes Tropiques*. New York: Atheneum.

Lineberry, Caitlin. 2007. "Tattoos: The Ancient and Mysterious History." *Smithsonian*. January 1. Accessed October 13, 2015. http://www.smithsonianmag.com/history/tattoos-144 038580/?no-ist.

PBS. 1998. "Ice Mummies: Siberian Ice Maiden." *NOVA*. November 24. Accessed October 13, 2015. http://www.pbs.org/wgbh/nova/transcripts/2517siberian.html.

Pitts, Victoria. 2003. *In the Flesh: The Cultural Politics of Body Modification*. New York: Palgrave Macmillan.

The Siberian Times. 2012. "Siberian Princess Reveals Her 2500 Year Old Tattoos." *The Siberian Times*. August 14. Accessed October 13, 2015. http://siberiantimes.com/culture /others/features/siberian-princess-reveals-her-2500-year-old-tattoos.

South Tyrol Museum of Archaeology. 2013. "Ötzi the Iceman." Accessed July 22, 2016. http://www.iceman.it/en/oetzi-the-iceman.

Teicher, Jordan G. 2016. "The Dwindling Facial Tattoo Tradition of Myanmar's Lai Tu Chin Tribe." *Slate*. July 17. Accessed October 11, 2016. http://www.slate.com/blogs/behold /2016/07/17/dylan_goldby_photographs_the_tattooed_women_of_myanmar_s_lai_tu _chin_in.html.

Turner, Terence. 1980. "The Social Skin." In: *Not Work Alone: A Cross-Cultural View of the Activities Superfluous to Survival*, edited by Jeremy Cherfas and Roger Lewin, 112–40. London: Temple Smith.

Young, William C. 1994. "The Body Tamed: Tying and Tattooing among the Rashaayda Bedouin." In: *Many Mirrors: Body Images and Social Relations*, edited by Nicole Sault, 58–75. New Brunswick, NJ: Rutgers University Press.

TEETH BLACKENING

In Japan, glossy black surfaces, like those that appear to be lacquered, are considered beautiful. During the Meiji era (1868–1912), teeth were commonly dyed black for festivals, wedding ceremonies, and funerals in order to achieve a pleasing black look that was considered more beautiful than white teeth. Black teeth were most common among married women and signified sexual maturity. The dye for the procedure was historically made by dissolving iron filings into vinegar and then combining this solution with tannins such as may be found in tea or sake. To improve the taste of the bitter drink, cinnamon, cloves, and anise could be added to it. The illusion of darkened teeth allowed one to present a wide smile without showing the teeth, which may have been damaged from decay. In any case, the dye was applied daily and said to actually prevent tooth decay. The practice was banned by the Japanese government in 1870 as part of nationalist efforts to "modernize" the country. In 1873, the empress began to promote a **teeth whitening** campaign.

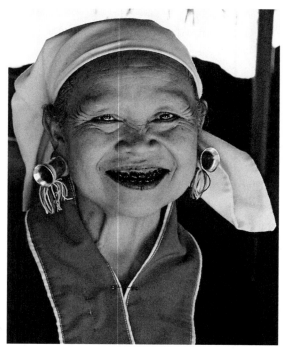

A Lahu woman in rural Thailand smiles, showing black teeth caused by chewing herbs. It is possible that the practice originated to protect teeth from cavities. (Guido Vrola/Shutterstock)

The practice of blackening teeth, *ohaguro*, has been practiced intermittently by Japanese aristocracy or by certain people with particular professions during previous historical eras. For example, throughout the Heian period (794–1185), samurai and pages working in large temples dyed their teeth. During the Sengoku period (1467–1603), daughters of military commanders would blacken their teeth as part of a coming-of-age ritual.

After the Edo period, only male aristocracy dyed their teeth due to the odor and the labor required to complete the process. The exception to this rule was **geisha**, who frequently blackened their teeth in order to make their whitened skin appear more luminous. With such bright white skin, many geisha feared that their teeth would appear yellowish in comparison.

Historically, the people of Vietnam also colored their teeth. A French survey conducted in 1938 found that 80 percent of rural Vietnamese living in the hills practiced teeth blackening, likely in an effort to protect the teeth from cavities and to distance themselves from demons and wild animals that were known to have gleaming white teeth (Nguyen 2011). Teeth are blackened in part as the result of frequent chewing of betel nut, a mild stimulant that grows on local trees. However, people also "paint" their teeth. Traditionally, among the Si La, a Tibeto-Burmese–speaking group that lives in the hills, men paint their teeth red using a resin that is obtained from the secretions of a tiny aphid-like insect that sucks the sap of a host tree (Nguyen 2011). Si La women prefer to paint their teeth black using a paste-like concoction of burned coconut husk combined with nail filings, which is then adhered to the teeth and allowed to soak into the enamel. Alternatively, black dye may be made by diluting resin in a combination of lemon juice and rice alcohol, along with shavings of iron or copper, which yield a blue-black "paint" that can be applied to the teeth. The practice is no longer widely observed by young people of the region. Similar practices of teeth blackening were also practiced by several ethnic minority groups in neighboring Laos, Thailand, and China, including the Hani, the Katu, the Blang, the Dai, the Hmoob, the Jino, the Lahu, and the Yao. Many members of these groups continue to chew betel nut regularly, which stains the teeth.

In the past, the practice of teeth blackening was also observed in some parts of India as part of a life cycle event indicating the onset of sexual maturity. Not only the teeth but also the gums are dyed a darker shade with a mixture of iron and copper sulfate, tannins, and other agents to create a solution called missī, thought to be used once by Fatima, the daughter of the Mohammed. The act of blackening teeth in India is considered to have sexual overtones and is most commonly practiced by prostitutes. Evidence of teeth blackening can also be found in western Amazonia and Madagascar (Zumbroich 2012).

Teeth blackening may also include selective blackening of one or more teeth to achieve a particular effect. Similarly, in some cultures, removal of teeth to modify the smile is also considered a form of teeth blackening. In north central Australia, for example, once an Arunta or Kaitish boy reached maturity, ritual tooth extraction of two upper teeth was observed as a rite of passage (Spencer and Gillen 1899). For the pastoralist Dinka of Sudan, four to six of the lower teeth are removed for both boys and girls as a rite of initiation and sign of beauty (Pitt Rivers Museum 2011).

Teeth blackening and the removal of teeth are distinct practices that differ from the celebration of a naturally occurring or cosmetically created **tooth gap**. In some West African societies, bright, white, shiny teeth are key to beauty, but a prominent tooth gap between the two front teeth with a small display of pink skin is often considered the optimal beauty for a smile in both men and women, but especially for women. Some speculate that at least historically, the gap between teeth was considered attractive for the Mende people of West Africa because it furthered the punning interplay between the mouth and the genitals common to the society (Boone 1986, 100). The opening between the teeth suggests the opening between a woman's legs, and a girl with open teeth would have been considered a more passionate lover (Ibid.).

See also: Dental Hygiene and Cosmetic Dentistry; Teeth Whitening.

Further Reading

Boone, Sylvia Arden. 1986. *Radiance from the Waters*. New Haven, CT: Yale University Press.

Nguyen, Lanh. 2011. "Tooth Blackening: The Forgotten Tradition." *Travel Dudes*. December 12. Accessed July 1, 2016. http://www.traveldudes.org/travel-tips/tooth-blackening -forgotten-tradition/14811.

The Pitt Rivers Museum, University of Oxford. 2011. "Body Art: Shaped Teeth." Accessed July 1, 2016. http://web.prm.ox.ac.uk/bodyarts/index.php/permanent-body-arts/resha ping-and-piercing/158-african-lip-plugs.html.

Spencer, Baldwin, and Francis James Gillen. 1899. *The Native Tribes of North Central Australia*. Sacred-texts.com. Accessed September 15, 2016. http://www.sacred-texts.com/aus /ntca/ntca14.htm.

Zumbroich, Thomas J. 2011. "'Teeth as Black as a Bumblebee's Wings': The Ethnobotany of Teeth Blackening in Southeast Asia." *Ethnobotany Research and Applications* 7: 381–98.

Zumbroich, Thomas J. 2012. "Don't Show Your Molars to Strangers: Expressions of Teeth Blackening in Madagascar." *Ethnobotany Research and Applications* 10: 523–39.

Zumbroich, Thomas J. 2015. "The Missing-Stained Finger-tip of the Fair—A Cultural History of Teeth and Gum Blackening in South Asia." *eJournal of Indian Medicine* 8: 1–32.

Zumbroich, Thomas J., and Brian Stross. 2013. "Cutting Old Life into New: Teeth Blackening in Western Amazonia." *Anthropos* 108: 53–75.

TOOTH CHIPPING (TEETH CHISELING, TEETH MODIFICATION, TOOTH SHARPENING)

The practice of tooth modification can be seen historically in a number of different regions around the world. Depending on the style the culture prefers, teeth can be filed flat or exaggerated into sharp points. Tooth modification is potentially painful and dangerous, as the removal of enamel can expose the nerve inside the tooth and allow bacteria to infect the pulp within the tooth. Pain, discomfort, and swelling would likely require a tooth that was not properly prepared to be extracted. In some cultures, specific teeth are also deliberately removed in order to enhance beauty, a process called ablation. For added beauty, in some parts of the world, teeth may also be intentionally stained either on the tooth itself or in the surrounding soft tissue (called a gingival tattoo).

In Africa, the cliff-dwelling Dogon people of Mali are one group that historically filed their teeth into sharp points. The goal was to create teeth that looked like a loom to evoke the sense that speech that passed through the mouth wove into a tapestry of reality (Pitt Rivers Museum 2011). On the other side of the African continent, the Makonde people of southern Tanzania also practiced teeth filing and chipping into sharp points to mark individuals who had undergone rites of passage and were accepted adult members of the group.

The Basongo Menos people of present-day Democratic Republic of Congo also covered their faces in **tattoos** and filed their teeth into sharp points, a practice commented upon derisively by European colonialists who went to the region seeking rubber in the late 19th century. Also known as the "Zappo Zap," this group's larger name derives from Belgian speculation that they practiced cannibalism and were named for "*ba*" (the people), "*songa*" (to file), and "*meno*" (teeth) (Phipps 2002, 137). In an upsetting example of the racist politics comprising anthropology and "evolutionary science" of the day, Ota Benga (1883–1916) was a young Congolese boy who was "imported" to the United States for display at the St. Louis World's Fair in Missouri in 1904 in part because of his dramatically sharpened front teeth. He was later exhibited at the Bronx Zoo where he was forced to share quarters with an orangutan before being released to live in a church-sponsored orphanage in Virginia. Sadly, Benga took his own life in 1916 (Newkirk 2015).

A number of Indonesian cultures also have traditionally practiced teeth chiseling. Sometimes, teeth were chiseled in order to emphasize humanity. In Bali, teeth are thought to represent anger, jealousy, fear, and other negative emotions. Pointed teeth were culturally associated with monsters and witches. People were encouraged to file their teeth flat to discourage any potential associations with evil intentions.

However, in other parts of Indonesia, teeth were deliberately chiseled to enhance a dramatic, otherworldly effect. The Mentawai people of Sumatra are a seminomadic foraging group who practice animism. Their faith connects them deeply on an individual and communal level to their rainforest environment. Traditionally, both men and women used a chisel to file their teeth to increase their beauty and to draw totemic connections to the animal world in which they lived. Members of the group also practiced **tattooing** with a needle, hammered with a piece of wood by a shaman to create a geometrically pleasing design that mimicked the look of a rainforest animal or bird.

Central Americans also historically practiced teeth modification. Ceramic figurines from the Remojadas style (BCE 100 to 800 CE) of the Veracruz region demonstrate sharpened incisors. In addition to filing their teeth to pleasing shapes with stone abraders, the ancient Maya used hardened bone drills, aided by water and abrasive sand (or powdered quartz), to carve into the enamel of teeth in order to set stones in the smile. Mayans filled the resulting cavities in the exposed teeth with colorful stones like jade, obsidian, pyrite, hematite, mother-of-pearl, or turquoise in order to enhance beauty and prestige. Practitioners had to be careful not to drill too deeply into teeth to avoid exposure of the pulp and potentially dangerous infections; it was also possible that the inlay protected the teeth from decay. Stones were then held in place with pressure or cement made of organic materials. Partial to the semidivine properties of certain semiprecious stones, especially jade, these tooth ornaments sat within prominent front teeth of both men and women for a more dramatic smile during the Classic era (250–900 CE). By the Postclassic era (900–1500 CE), archaeologists estimate that about 60 percent of the population was engaging in some form of dental modification (Williams and White 2009).

South American Indians of the Amazon Valley are also known to file their central incisors to sharp points in imitation of the piranha fish who occupied the river. Sharpened teeth may have been considered a mark of beauty and ferocity.

See also: Dental Hygiene and Cosmetic Dentistry; Maya; Tattoos.

Further Reading

Newkirk, Pamela. 2015. *Spectacle: The Astonishing Life of Ota Benga*. New York: Harper Collins.

Phipps, William E. 2002. *William Sheppard: Congo's African American Livingstone*. Westminster, England: John Knox Press.

The Pitt Rivers Museum, University of Oxford. 2011. "Body Art: Shaped Teeth." Accessed July 1 2016. http://web.prm.ox.ac.uk/bodyarts/index.php/permanent-body-arts/resh aping-and-piercing/164-shaped-teeth.html.

Soule, Jean-Philippe. 2004. "The Mentawai: Shamans of the Siberut Jungle" [Web site]. Accessed July 31, 2016. http://www.nativeplanet.org/indigenous/cultures/indonesia /mentawai/mentawai.shtml.

Williams, Jocelyn S., and Christine D. White. 2009. "Dental Modification in the Postclassic Population of Lamanai, Belize." *Ancient Mesoamerica* 17, no. 1: 139–51.

TUAREG

Sometimes referred to as the "aristocrats of the Sahara," the distinctive-looking Tuareg people and their challenging pastoralist lifestyle in the stark desert environment inspire an appreciation of their long-lived civilization since medieval times, when it thrived in an economy that relied on camel-laden caravans to trade gold, perfume, salt, and spices across the Sahara Desert.

Traditionally, the head (*eghef*) was considered the source for intelligence, and the **hair** was considered an outer manifestation of a person's intellect. Women maintain luxuriant and intricately braided hair, as unkempt hair is considered a sign of madness. Local plants, including the crushed leaves of black benniseed (*talekkodt*) or the white raisin tree (*deje*), are used to produce shampoos to keep the hair clean and free of lice. Sometimes camel urine is used as a hair tonic to prevent dandruff or to lighten the color of the hair. Some women also make a nourishing **pomade** of dark sand and animal fat to coat the hair before braiding it into an elaborate hairstyle.

Though most Tuareg today are Muslim, women typically do not veil or observe *hijab* (Rasmussen 2013). Attractive women are expected to be heavy, with limited bodily mobility as they practice "light" tasks close to home (Ibid.). Women receive the tents that make up the mobile living compounds as part of their dowry; they decorate the insides of the tents with lush rugs and textiles. The Tuareg practice bilateral descent, which means that women can inherit from both their mothers and their fathers. They enjoy relatively high status relative to many other pastoralist and Muslim societies.

Tuareg women also use cosmetics and makeup to emphasize their features. They line their eyes with powdered kohl stone, which also serves to reduce glare in the desert sun. They use both moistened and powdered *tahijjart*, a fruit from the gum tree, as a shimmery eye shadow. Desert date oil (*taboraght*) may also be used as a skin moisturizer. The oil also acts as a medicine against skin irritations. Another

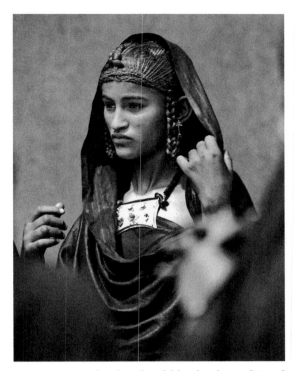

Tuareg woman, hands colored blue by the traditional indigo dye in her clothes, performs a dance in Timbuktu, Mali. (AP Photo/Ben Curtis)

oil, pressed from seeds of low, scrubby trees, may also be used as a skin moisturizer or to soothe skin that has been exposed to the sun. Women use henna (sometimes called *mehendi*, referred to as *anhalla* by the Tuareg) to tint their hands and feet with designs.

Aromatic fragrances are highly valued by the Tuareg, believed to carry protective properties. *Adaras*, a resin of the African myrrh tree, is burned in low braziers within the tents of the women. The heady fragrance also serves to keep bugs away. Women crush the flowers of tropical evergreen trees (*Mitragyna inermis*) and the bark of the shittah tree (*Acacia seya*) into another type of incense that is especially favored by pregnant women.

In terms of jewelry, the Tuareg shun gold, preferring silver. Their jewelry also incorporates cowrie shells (emblematic of fertility) and carnelian (for protection against loss of blood). Triangular or circular pendants are thought to ward off the evil eye, and four-branched crosses made of silver are also popular as symbols of scattering evil and danger to the four winds. The most famous Tuareg jewelry is known as the *khomissar,* a stylized hand to keep harm at bay (Winkel and Winkel 2006).

Today, Tuareg people are challenged by more than just their ecosystem, with their loss of autonomy after incorporation of their nomadic way of life into the sedentary nation-states of Mali, Niger, Algeria, and Libya (Rasmussen 2013). Additionally, armed conflicts for independence, as well as the incursions of Islamists into their region, have compromised their ability to practice their traditional culture.

See also: Hair; Pomade.

Further Reading

Beholding Beauty. 2016. "Five Beauty Rituals from the Saharan Aristocrats." Accessed October 1, 2016. http://www.beholdingbeauty.com/tuareg-women-five-beauty-rituals-from-the -saharan-aristocrats.

Rasmussen, Susan. 2013. "Do Tents and Herds Still Matter? Pastoral Nomadism and Gender among the Tuareg of Mali and Niger." In: *Gender in Cross-Cultural Perspective,* edited by Caroline Brettell and Carolyn Sargent, 139–47. New York: Routledge.

Winkel, Bertie, and Dos Winkel. 2006. *Vanishing Beauty.* Amsterdam: Prestel.

U

UNITED KINGDOM

During the Middle Ages, extravagant displays of beauty were widely discouraged by women in European cultures due to morality restrictions imposed by the church. Beauty could be considered a gift from God, but it was considered wrong for a woman to openly acknowledge or enjoy her beauty because it was widely believed that the devil might tempt her to be vain, enticing men into immorality. Women were discouraged from wearing cosmetics or revealing clothing. However, long, luxurious hair was an acceptable medium for beauty: Lady Godiva famously rode naked in protest of high taxes wearing only her long hair. As the Crusades began, the chivalric code allowed men and women to channel their inner feelings more openly, giving rise to songs and poetry extolling the beauty of one's beloved (Downing 2012). Women removed their **eyebrows** through vigorous plucking to leave their faces delicate, vulnerable, and pious. To highlight a high, elegant forehead, women also **removed their hair** by plucking their natural hairline up to the top of the head and away from the borders of the face to create an elongated oval. The effect was then emphasized by a stiff white headdress, with only a hint of color on the cheeks and lips (Downing 2012).

It was a common Tudor belief in the 16th century that witches had some kind of ugliness or deformity. As the daughter of Anne Boleyn, the second wife of the infamous Henry VIII who was suspected of witchcraft, Queen Elizabeth I made a point of cultivating beauty. She wore huge, richly jeweled gowns to inspire a larger-than-life presence and used heavy cosmetics to disguise smallpox scars on her face. Like many wealthy women of the era, Elizabeth whitened her complexion with ceruse, a concoction of finely ground white lead powder mixed with vinegar. The white-as-milk ideal visage of the day set off a clear, high aristocratic forehead that was meant to be kept blemish free by avoiding the sun. One of the most innovative beauty treatments of the era was a kind of chemical peel using eggs, vinegar, turpentine, sugar-candy, camphor, rock alum, quicksilver, lemon juice, tartarum, and white onion mixed into a paste, applied liberally at night, and allowed to dry. One surgeon's notes remark that burns could result (Downing 2012). Less expensive (and less toxic) treatments could also be made using ground alabaster or starch mixed with perfume. Critics charged that ceruse smelled unpleasant up close and could cause headaches, swollen eyes, receding gums, hair loss, and tremors.

Elizabethan women also wore rouge made from a white lead base dyed with red crystalline mercuric sulfide, madder, cochineal, vermilion, or alkanet root. Rouge was applied to highlight the cheeks and intensify the bone structure of the face. Women in the Tudor era also wore color on their lips, using a "pencil" made of

Windsor Beauties

Charles II of England earned the title "The Merry Monarch" when he came to the throne during the Restoration Era after more than a decade of austere, Puritanical rule. His court was characterized by hedonism that included a bevy of attractive women, many of whom were his mistresses. During the 1660s, court artist Peter Lely painted three-quarter-length portraits of ten of the most beautiful women of the court. These women (who looked remarkably similar to each other with tightly curled hair, sleepy bedroom eyes, and dramatically low necklines) came to be known as the Windsor Beauties. The most notorious and well-known of these beauties was the scandalous Barbara Villiers, who had at least five children with Charles II and fueled court gossip until she was replaced by a younger favorite, Louise de Kérouaille.

ground alabaster mixed with a coloring agent, usually alkanet (from the plant *Alkanna tinctoria*) or dye from the East Indian brazil tree, formed into a stick and dried in the sun. The cosmetics on the face were then "fixed" with a glaze made of egg white, which added a porcelain shine and gave the cosmetics more durability (Downing 2012).

Elizabethans also emulated the Roman goddess Venus, who reputedly had a single beauty spot, one small mark of darkness to highlight her perfect complexion. "Patches," or beauty spots, began to appear in the late 16th century and reached their height in the 17th century. Beauty spots could be made of black silk or velvet and were glued to key areas of the painted face to highlight beauty. Each "patch" position had a specific name: "the coquette" was situated near the smile, the "passionate" was placed at the side of the eye, and the "gallant" was positioned in the center of the cheek much as a dimple. Some women wore patches strategically to camouflage moles or smallpox scars. Although the "dot" was the classic shape, stars and crescent moons became popular, and ladies became so addicted to patches that satirists of the age mocked women who applied them too liberally (Downing 2012).

The Puritans abhorred cosmetics, believing such vain usage to be even more heinous a crime than committing adultery. The Puritans strongly believed that Eve's biblical role in the original sin symbolized women's inherent moral weakness. It was essential that women not be exposed to temptations of vanity or frivolity, as they were more susceptible to sin than men, although they did have the potential to be more disciplined than men when they applied themselves to the task of moral living. Women were expected to marry in order to have children. Courtship practices were very strict, and the weddings themselves were very simple and stark. Women were expected to dress modestly, covering their hair and their arms. Women who were found guilty of attempting to seduce men through "harlotry" or imprudent applications of their feminine wiles could be stripped to the waist and publicly humiliated. Sometimes, "immodest" women could be whipped in front of the church congregation.

The porcelain perfection of artificially whitened faces, called *à l'Anglaise*, eventually lost favor on both sides of the Channel during the Revolutionary era. An emerging passion for nature and the countryside brought in simpler styles for hair and cosmetics. The stiff and towering **hair** arrangements of the previous era were replaced by looser chignons with cascades of ringlets (Downing 2012). Thick white makeup was replaced with lighter powders made from talc and rouge made from organic ingredients of vegetables, sandalwood, brazil wood, and saffron. The Romantic era inspired young women to achieve a dark, slightly glazed look by dropping belladonna into their eyes to dilate their pupils into poetic, dark pools. (Such treatment could also cause blindness.) The term "dandy" originated to describe a particular aesthetic style for young men during the British Regency period (1790–1840). The style of the day had political overtones, as many young people supported the French Revolution and its message of democratic access. Eschewing the powdered wigs and breeches with tights of the previous era, this generation of men dressed more simply, preferring starched white shirts, expertly fitted suits, and simple boots polished to a high shine (Sherrow 2006).

Into the Victorian period, pressure remained on women to appear beautiful and youthful without any hint of artifice. Expensive beauty treatments in lush packaging, such as "Magnetic Rock Dew Water of Sahara for Removing Wrinkles," appeared for wealthy women able to pay £2 2s for a bottle (twice the weekly wages for a working-class family). Many of these potions were dubious or fraudulent. By the end of the 19th century, some women were beginning to work in department stores and offices or attending university. In 1878, Mary Haweis, a vicar's wife and member of the Dress Reform Society, published *The Art of Beauty*. She argued that it was not wicked or immoral for a woman to make an effort to be beautiful; rather, such efforts were in perfect keeping with the cultural standards of good taste (Downing 2012). Makeup began to be seen as a barometer of emancipation, worn by the new generation of women eager to undertake legitimate careers and engage the world on their own terms.

Throughout the mid-century war years, when cosmetics could be hard to find, British women were still encouraged to look good in an effort to keep the spirits high in the fight against the Nazis. An advertisement for cosmetics read, "No lipstick—yours or anyone else's—will win the war. But it symbolizes why we're fighting" (Lawrence 2015). Conventional wisdom agreed that Hitler abhorred makeup as un-Aryan (Lawrence 20115), so British women rationed their bright red **lipstick** and black mascara. To fill the gap, they also made a lip stain out of beetroot and "mascara" out of boot polish (Lawrence 2015).

During the so-called "Swinging Sixties," London was the headquarters of the international cultural scene that drove new trends in music, dance, and "mod" beauty fashions. Designer Mary Quant introduced the mini skirt, which went on to revolutionize women's wardrobes, and Twiggy became a global superstar as the model who most closely embodied the youthful look of the era.

In 1981, Prince Charles introduced the world to his fiancée, the young Diana Spencer. Her wedding dress, with giant sleeves and acres of fussy lace, became emblematic of the 1980s. Her hairstyle was quickly emulated around the world, as was her impeccable fashion sense. Princess Diana eventually became an international icon, her grace and personal appeal instantly recognizable, especially through her humanitarian efforts. Her effortless style continued to attract the attention of the world until her tragic and untimely death in an automobile accident in 1997.

Diana's son, William, proposed to Kate Middleton while on vacation in Kenya in 2010, and the two married the following year. Since that time, Middleton (now known as the Duchess of Cambridge) has become a powerful force in setting standards of international fashion and beauty trends around the world. For example, the £14 "George" coral-colored skinny jeans she wore to play field hockey in 2012 experienced an 88 percent increase in sales after she was photographed in them, prompting the media to dub her influence "the Kate effect" (Rawi 2012). When the Duchess of Cambridge wore a dress by the maternity brand Seraphine in an official portrait with Prince George, the company's sales bumped by more than 50 percent in forty-eight hours (Poulter 2015). Middleton's sister, Pippa, has also drawn admirers. Following the Royal Wedding in 2011, many commentators discussed "Pippa's **bum**" (Rankin 2016).

See also: Butts and Booty; Eyebrows; Hair; Hair Removal.

Further Reading

Downing, Sarah Jane. 2012. *Beauty and Cosmetics 1550–1950.* Oxford, England: Shire Press.

Lawrence, Sandra. 2015. "Beetroot and Boot Polish: How Britain's Women Faced World War 2 Without Make-up." *Telegraph,* March 3. Accessed October 1, 2016. http://www .telegraph.co.uk/women/womens-life/11393852/Beauty-in-World-War-2-How-Britains -women-stayed-glamorous.html.

Poulter, Sean. 2015. "The Kate Effect Could Double Maternity Brand's Turnover." *The Daily Mail.* April 20. Accessed October 1, 2016. http://www.dailymail.co.uk/news/article -3047988/The-Kate-effect-Sales-favourite-maternity-label-double-fans-camp-outside -hospital-ready-royal-arrival.html.

Rankin, Seija. 2016. "In Honor of Pippa Middleton's Engagement, Let's Look Back at the Most Ridiculous Headlines from the last Royal Wedding." *E! Online News.* Accessed October 1, 2016. http://www.eonline.com/news/781022/in-honor-of-pippa-middleton-s -engagement-let-s-look-back-at-the-most-ridiculous-headlines-from-the-last-royal -wedding.

Rawi, Maysa. 2012. "The Kate Effect Soars Again." *The Daily Mail.* March 16. Accessed October 1, 2016. www.dailymail.co.uk/femail/article-2116038/The-Kate-effect-strikes-Sales -coral-coloured-jeans-soar-Duchess-wore-pair-play-hockey.html.

Sandbrook, Dominic. 2006. *White Heat: A History of Britain in the Swinging Sixties.* New York: Little, Brown.

Sherrow, Victoria. 2006. *Encyclopedia of Hair: A Cultural History.* Westport, CT: Greenwood Press.

UNITED STATES

The United States is a relatively young nation founded mainly by Puritan Christians seeking religious freedom in the 17th century. These immigrants, and their attitudes toward physical appearance, bodies, modesty, and vanity, still underlie many issues regarding beauty in the United States today.

For the Puritans, the conduct, appearance, and behavior of each member of society was an integral part of the moral worth of the group. If one member of the Puritan community sinned, it was understood to be a stain on the community as a whole and a threat to the spiritual health of all. The Puritans believed that punishment might ensue from individual sin, and the community might become the victim of God's wrath for not policing the group as a whole (Vaughan 1997). For this reason, both customs and laws were very specific in regulating the personal behavior of individual citizens in Puritan communities, including those related to physical appearance.

Many laws in the 17th-century colonies were aimed at preventing the sin of pride and vanity. Specific regulations were drafted that made clear how much finery in the way of jewelry, lace, or linen could be worn. Indeed, clothing that contained any silver or gold thread, silk or lace was outlawed. Embroidery, needlework decoration, hatbands, and other decorations were similarly against the law in the Puritan colonies. Many hairstyles were outlawed for both men and women, being considered dangerously vain. These included long hair for men and hair visible outside the cap of women (Vaughan 1997).

For the Puritans, committing the sin of vanity risked punishment for all from God, and these laws were enacted to stop behaviors that were "prejudicial to the common good" (Vaughan 1997, 180). Individuals, their needs, and desires were, in this way, less important than the whole community, and each individual was taught to draw less attention to themselves, and especially their appearance, as they sought to perfect their inner self for the benefit of the whole. This type of thinking, of the way in which we dress in the United States having a direct effect on the moral worth of the whole community, is still visible in laws and rules such as school dress codes, which restrict what students can wear for the stated reason that individuals who draw attention through their appearance are distracting to others in the community, damaging their educational experience.

In the 21st century, the diverse and complex society that is the current United States still struggles with the tensions between a human desire to be appealing to others and the puritanical heritage that cautions us all against vanity and individual preference. These debates are particularly visible in the field of plastic surgery, where both practitioners and patients, still holding on to Puritan assumptions about vanity and self-indulgence, must negotiate a fine line between having a procedure to fix a "deformity" or for simple "vanity." This has meant, for many, "if the aim was to look better, the surgery was unacceptable. If the goal was to be less conspicuous, the procedure was permissible. The problem was where the line should be drawn and who was to draw it" (Feldman 2004).

Much of this debate in the United States revolves around a double narrative that each citizen learns as they grow up. On the one hand, Americans learn that they shouldn't "judge a book by its cover" and that "real beauty is on the inside," messages that fit with the Puritan concept of spiritual rather than external and physical worth. However, at the same time that Americans are surrounded by books and movies with that message of "it's who you are on the inside that counts," they are also faced with a never-ending barrage of advertisements, television programs, competitions, and decisions in life that emphasize how important physical appearance is. For every children's book that teaches about inner beauty, there are four reality shows looking for the next Top Model or showcasing the beauty and beauty work of celebrities like the Kardashians.

The focus on celebrities and their appearance then reveals another key element of U.S. beauty culture, the way that American society conflates appearance with success. For men especially, attractiveness is tied directly to displays of status and success. Many studies show a preference among women for men with more resources and higher income. If this is the preference for women, it is what men in the United States will set out to achieve (Etcoff 2000). In studies of men in the United States, anthropologists have shown how men specifically acquire and wear items such as expensive designer shoes and watches—those types of accessories specifically prohibited by the Puritans—as visual symbols of their wealth and achievement (Masi de Casanova 2015).

For women in 21st-century America, the fine line between the Puritan ideal of inner, natural beauty and the drive to conform to beauty norms that expect ever whiter skin, more voluminous hair, and shapelier bodies creates daily negotiations of expectations. Study after study demonstrates that women are rewarded for conforming as closely as possible to the social norms of beauty, and cultivating beauty costs money and takes work (Etcoff 2000). Women, like men, receive specific benefits for their appearance in both professional and personal success, and therefore it is logical that they seek to pay attention to beauty and beauty work. Cosmetics, hair products, jewelry, clothing, exercise, dieting, and plastic surgery are all reasonable methods to achieving a beautiful appearance and therefore a better job, higher salary, and more desirable mate.

There continues, however, to be widespread criticism of those women who are "too obviously" engaging in beauty work in a way that reminds us of the public shaming methods of the Puritans. Returning to the famous 21st-century American beauty Kim Kardashian, we can see how these two lines of rhetoric converge and compete in the United States. On the one hand, Kardashian is open and clear about the beauty work that she engages in, writing extensively about dieting, exercise, plastic surgery, and other beauty work to her huge following on social media (French 2016). The appetite for Kardashian's thoughts and experiences on beauty work, as well as for the photos of the beautiful results of that work, has garnered her millions of followers and made her a multimillionaire who can garner $300,000 for a single appearance (Ingram 2016).

Despite Kardashian's personal, professional, and financial success at working the expectations and norms of beauty, however, she is also constantly criticized.

America's (and the Worlds') Next Top Model

The reality television program *America's Next Top Model*, hosted and produced by American supermodel Tyra Banks, was a televised competition that ran for twenty-two seasons through 2015. The show gathered ten or more aspiring models and put them through a series of makeovers, trainings, and competitions before selecting a winner. The program offered two coaches and a series of lessons and photo shoots that were then judged by Banks and a panel who critiqued the contestants' progress. Although the show was criticized for the body-shaming comments of the judges and the fact that the contest never succeeded in creating a true "supermodel," it was hugely popular worldwide during its run. The program aired in 170 nations across the planet, and twelve nations, from Australia, to Poland, to Hong Kong, aired their own, nationally produced versions of the competition.

Those who fault the celebrity for her openness about her beauty work and her body often return to the types of puritanically based arguments about inner beauty being more important or the need for modesty and lack of pride and vanity (Saul 2016). Many often also call out the celebrity for her focus on her own appearance, her continuous use of "selfie" images to promote her own appearance, and her unabashed appreciation of her own form. As one art critic notes, this spawns "knee-jerk criticisms of crassness, shallow opportunism, and surface-only illusion" (Saltz and Wallace-Wells 2015).

See also: Hair; Jewelry; Plastic Surgery; Vanity.

Further Reading

Etcoff, Nancy. 2000. *Survival of the Prettiest: The Science of Beauty*. New York: Anchor.

Feldman, Ellen. 2004. "Before & After." *American Heritage* 55, no. 1: 60.

Ingram, Mathew. 2016. "Why Kim Kardashian Is Almost as Smart as Donald Trump About Social Media." Accessed August 23, 2016. http://fortune.com/2016/07/18/kardashian-donald-trump.

Masi de Casanova, Erynn. 2015 *Buttoned Up: Clothing, Conformity and White Collar Masculinity*. Ithaca, NY: Cornell University Press.

Saltz, Jerry, and David Wallace-Wells. 2015. "Jerry Saltz: How and Why We Started Taking Kim Kardashian Seriously (and What She Teaches Us About the State of Criticism)." May 20. Accessed August 23, 2016. http://www.vulture.com/2015/05/saltz-how-kim-kardashian-became-important.html.

Saul, Heather. 2016. "Kim Kardashian-West Answers Criticism from Bette Midler, Piers Morgan and Chloe Moretz over Nude Selfie." March 8. Accessed August 23, 2016. http://www.independent.co.uk/news/people/kim-kardashian-west-answers-criticism-from-piers-morgan-bette-midler-and-chloe-moretz-over-naked-a6918461.html.

Vaughan, Alden T. 1997. *The Puritan Tradition in America, 1620–1730*. Hanover, NH: UPNE.

V

VANITY

Vanity, a complex philosophical, ethical, and religious idea, is, at heart, a description of the human desire for and delight in the good opinion of others (Reed 2012). Each of us is driven in greater or lesser degrees by a need to look good in the eyes of other people. We want to fit in, get along, and be seen as successful.

In specific terms of beauty, this means that we seek to follow social norms of appearance, show that we know what the rules are, and succeed in achieving the highest possible opinion of other people when they look at us. We want others to view us as healthy, wealthy, and attractive. As with other elements of the topic of beauty, this means that human vanity is both a potential virtue and a potential vice. On the one hand, to seek what will make us and our families successful is a positive drive. On the other, to spend too much time and attention courting and obsessing about the opinion of others is a potentially negative habit.

When defining vanity as a concept, there are often two agreed-upon elements: a focus on outward appearance and beauty, and a focus on personal achievement. Both of these two elements incorporate a positive, and sometimes elevated, view of an individual's own appearance and success (Netemeyer, Burton, and Lichtenstein 1995).

Those who might argue that vanity has a positive place in human interactions include the 18th-century moral philosopher David Hume. Hume argued that vanity is a mediator that drives one person to pay attention to the needs, emotions, and opinions of others (Hume 2000). This, for Hume, is the combination of self-interested passion and sympathy. A person displaying vanity is gaining pleasure from another person's pleasure and favorable opinion, but is also seeking to avoid the pain of the discomfort of another person's unfavorable opinion (Reed 2012). This concern and sympathy for others (even in the service of self-interest) can make society run more smoothly.

When we act in a vain manner, we are tacitly paying attention to what others think and feel. It may be true that we are doing so to feel better about ourselves, yet the way we choose to do that is by making others feel comfortable, happy, and pleased. When, for example, a man chooses to wear an expensive watch, he is displaying his success and wealth through his appearance, which makes him feel good, as he knows it will be admired by his friends and his wife or potential mate. Those friends then also feel good to be associated with a successful person and that he has chosen to hang out with them. This is a similar example of a woman having breast enhancement both for the purpose of feeling good about herself and to be admired by more men who appreciate and enjoy looking at the larger breasts.

In agreement then with thinkers like Hume, the Venezuelan designer Carolina Herrera has stated that attention to beauty is a key to the successful interaction of people and that in order to "show sensitivity and respect for the people who surround us, wanting to please and not offend," we must pay close and careful attention to our appearance (Herrera 2012).

Although attention to appearance as a way to make others feel comfortable and pleased can be seen as positive, there are ways in which vanity can be negative. For example, a person choosing to seek excessively the good opinion of others to the point where the actions that the individual is taking as an act of vanity can go too far, and as a result, cause discomfort or pain in others. Returning to the previous examples, the conspicuous display of wealth can be seen as negatively vain if it is so exaggerated that it causes others to feel less important, less successful, or is seen to ignore the pain of the poor.

Celebrities on reality television are often accused of this type of vanity. Plastic surgery, although a recognized avenue to causing pleasure for others, can, if undertaken too often, produce an appearance that actually makes others uncomfortable, as some celebrities have also done. Spending what seem to be excessive amounts on things like air-conditioned dog houses or golden toilets is another type of expression of economic vanity that turns others off.

Vanity leads us all to make personal and consumer choices designed to enhance our physical appearance in a drive to achieve more. The money that we spend on diets and diet programs, cosmetics, clothing, jewelry, and plastic surgery are all driven by our desire to look better and have others hold us in higher esteem, and these can be successful (Etcoff 2000). These practices also, however, have potentially negative results. Both dieting and surgery, if undertaken too radically, can cause health problems and the bad opinion of others. Excessive spending on clothing or jewelry can lead to financial problems (Netemeyer et al. 1995).

The journalist Junius Henry Brown observed in the late 19th century that vanity, if understood as self-love, can be a positive force, but only if held privately and in secret. For Browne, "to have it [vanity] in full force, and yet to hide it adroitly is one of the finest of fine secular arts" (Browne 1891). This is the task faced by most of us working in society, to love ourselves and care about the opinion and comfort of others without being seen to pay too much attention to our appearance and personal beauty.

This is the tension in modern international culture in the 21st century as it was in the 19th. Makeup that looks "natural" and not too obvious is commended and in some cultures necessary to success. Makeup that is obvious and very bright is considered vain. In media, on the Internet, and in conversations, many cultures recommend the "good work" of beauty practices as a way for each of us to take care of ourselves, often relating procedures like facials, dieting, or manicures to healthy self-love and upkeep. However, "a face that's a bit too tight, boobs a bit too big, lips a bit too plump—"bad work"—and you're cast as sad, vain, phony" (Stein, Steinmetz, and Borowiec 2015).

See also: Jewelry; Makeup and Cosmetics; Plastic Surgery.

Further Reading

Browne, Junius Henri. 1891. "The Value of Vanity." *The North American Review* 153, no. 418: 379–81.

Etcoff, Nancy. 2000. *Survival of the Prettiest: The Science of Beauty.* New York: Anchor.

Herrera, Carolina. 2012. "Presentación." In: *100% Chic: Como vestir bien y lograr un éxito seguro,* edited by Titina Penzini, 3. Caracas, Venezuela: Ediciones B.

Hume, David. 1739 (2000). *Treatise of Human Nature,* edited by David Fate and Mary J. Norton. Oxford, England: Oxford University Press

Netemeyer, Richard G., Scot Burton, and Donald R. Lichtenstein. 1995. "Trait Aspects of Vanity: Measurement and Relevance to Consumer Behavior." *Journal of Consumer Research* 21, no. 4: 612–26.

Reed, Philip A. 2012. "The Alliance of Virtue and Vanity in Hume's Moral Theory." *Pacific Philosophical Quarterly* 93, no. 4: 595–614.

Stein, Joel, Katy Steinmetz, and Steven Borowiec. 2015. "Nip. Tuck. Or Else (cover story)." *Time* 185, no. 24: 40.

VENEZUELA

The South American nation of Venezuela is well known for its natural beauty, thousands of varieties of orchids, the world's tallest waterfall, and the most successful string of beauty pageant contestants in the history of the world. Beauty and beauty work are not only a central part of Venezuelan culture, they are a competitive enterprise in the nation. Men and women alike in Venezuela see the achievement of an ideal of beauty as a path to personal and professional success.

In the history of international beauty pageants, Miss Venezuela has won more titles than any other nation. Miss Venezuela has won the Miss Universe pageant seven times, the Miss International pageant seven times, and the Miss World pageant six times (Miss Venezuela 2015). When, in 2009, one Miss Venezuela/Miss Universe crowned a compatriot for the first time as the new Miss Universe, the organization was awarded a citation in the Guinness Book of World Records as the only nation to have achieved that feat.

The success of the nation in international pageants is a reflection of the emphasis that Venezuelan culture as a whole places on beauty for both men and women. At the beginning of the 21st century, a consumer poll of 30 nations revealed Venezuela to be the "vainest" country of all, with 65 percent of Venezuelan women and 47 percent of men admitting that they think about their looks "all the time" (Rother 2000). In an instructive anecdote, the infamous Venezuelan terrorist Carlos the Jackal, responsible for planning and executing the attacks on the Israeli athletes at the Munich Olympics, was finally caught and arrested in the Sudan after his plastic surgeons turned him in. French and Sudanese officials waited until he was anesthetized for a liposuction procedure to reduce the size of his belly before arresting him (Haiken 1999).

This concern is a reflection of the importance of appearance as a signal of family status, high social class, self-control, and good manners. Looking good, for many Venezuelans, is a way of communicating both high standards and respect for others. In Venezuela, both men and women seek to project the image of being "*arreglado,*" a word that means, simultaneously, "made up," "put together," "fixed," and "managed."

When one looks put together, many Venezuelans believe, one projects the image of hard work, self-discipline, and moral strength that makes a person attractive both to potential romantic partners and employers (Nichols 2016). As the hugely successful Venezuelan designer Carolina Herrera notes, the most important accessory a person can own is a good mirror so that one can be sure to "show sensitivity and respect for the people who surround us, wanting to please and not offend" through our appearance (Herrera 2012).

In the pursuit of the "fixed up" ideal, many Venezuelans turn to fashion and beauty experts such as Herrera and the designer Titina Penzini. Penzini, the author of a series of extremely successful beauty manuals under the title *100% Chic: How to Dress Well and Achieve Assured Success*, emphasizes the importance of appearance as a reflection of inner worth. It is through maintaining a correctly turned-out and controlled appearance, then, that Venezuelan women can achieve success, according to Penzini, who declares that "there is nothing more powerful than the image of a woman who is impeccably dressed and turned out for the occasion, with the correct wardrobe, make-up and accessories" (Penzini 2012).

Penzini has written three volumes of her manual, one for women, one for men, and one for children. This last, especially, is an indication of the way in which Venezuelans emphasize the importance of appearance to children as they grow up and learn to participate in society. It is logical, then, for parents of children to seek training in beauty and appearance for their offspring and for adults to additionally continue to seek avenues to achieving both beauty and ensured success.

The beauty pageant system helps provide Venezuelans with both a set of schools and opportunities to compete designed to ensure that their children can participate effectively in society by their appearance. Beauty pageants are held everywhere, from preschools to prisons, and each academic department at a university typically has its own beauty queen. It is not surprising, then, how many Venezuelans send their children to beauty academies, starting as young as age 4. Venezuelan parents are convinced that success in the area of beauty will translate into success in life (Grainger 2012).

In a typical pageant and beauty school, young people, especially girls, learn a range of skills, from how to walk and hold a wine glass elegantly, to the proper application of makeup. In a fashion similar to the U.S. tradition of finishing schools, young women also learn how to make polite conversation and project self-confidence. What's more, professional skills are also part of the training, including training in networking and public speaking (Grainger 2012).

This list of subjects and skills is very similar to those taught at the national training academy for Miss Venezuela contestants, where aspirants receive similar, if more intensive, training. It is likely for this reason that so many Miss Venezuela contestants have gone on to become television journalists, models, actresses, and politicians, reinforcing the public's perception of beauty training and work as a path to success (Nichols 2014).

Many of the skills and techniques taught both at children's academies and the Miss Venezuela house focus on self-discipline and careful body management. Hair and skin care, diet, and exercise are all taught as both paths to beauty and indicators of a person's work ethic and self-control (Nichols 2016). Another related practice is the prevalence of plastic surgery for those seeking beauty. Osmel Sousa, the director of the Miss Venezuela pageant, is open in his view that plastic surgery is just one tool for perfecting the female image, and this openness to cosmetic intervention is mirrored in the wider community where a popular *quinceañera* (fifteenth birthday) gift is a breast enlargement or nose job (Grainger 2012).

It is worth noting that in Venezuela, all of these interests and values are nearly equally true for men as well as women. Especially in the 21st century, beauty pageants are increasingly popular for men, who see the pageants as an equally valid avenue to success in journalism, politics, acting, or modeling. With the same training, and the same willingness to undergo such plastic surgery procedures as nose jobs, ear tucks, chin implants, and operations designed to define stomach muscles, men in Venezuela show their acceptance of the conflation of beauty and success (Grainger 2011).

See also: Hair; Pageants—International, National, and Local Contests; Plastic Surgery.

Further Reading

Gackstetter, Elizabeth. 2016. *No Such Thing as Inner Beauty: Dress, Cosmetics and Success in Venezuela 1850–2015.* New York: Rowman and Littlefield.

Grainger, Sarah. 2011. "Venezuela's Young Men Eye Beauty Contest Success." May 8. Accessed November 19, 2015. http://www.bbc.com/news/world-latin-america-13264460.

Grainger, Sarah. 2012. "Inside a Venezuelan School for Child Beauty Queens." September 3. Accessed November 19, 2015. http://www.bbc.com/news/magazine-19373488.

Haiken, Elizabeth. 1999. *Venus Envy: A History of Cosmetic Surgery.* Baltimore: Johns Hopkins University Press.

Herrera, Carolina. 2012. "Presentación." In: *100% Chic: Como vestir bien y lograr un éxito seguro*, edited by Titina Penzini, vol. 3. Caracas, Venezuela: Ediciones B.

Miss Venezuela. 2015. "Organización Miss Venezuela." Accessed November 19, 2015. www.missvenezuela.com.

Nichols, Elizabeth Gackstetter. 2014. "Virgin Venuses: Beauty and Purity for 'Public' Women in Venezuela." In: *Women, in Politics and Media: Perspectives from Nations in Transition*, edited by Maria Raicheva-Stover and Elza Ibroscheva. London: Bloomsbury.

Nichols, Elizabeth. 2016. *Beauty, Virtue, Power and Success in Venezuela 1850–2015.* New York: Lexington.

Penzini, Titina. 2012. *100% Chic: Como vestir bien y lograr un éxito seguro.* Caracas, Venezuela: Ediciones B.

Rother, Larry. 2000. "Who Is Vainest of All? Venezuela." Accessed November 19, 2015. http://www.nytimes.com/2000/08/13/world/who-is-vainest-of-all-venezuela.html.

WALKER, MADAME C. J.

Madame Walker was among the first black women to develop, market, and advertise hair care products for African American women. By 1910, she was the first self-made woman millionaire and the first black millionaire in the United States. Walker's entrepreneurial strategy emphasized career opportunities for black women within the beauty industry and set the stage for other black women to start their own companies.

The woman who became known as Madame Walker was born in 1867 as Sarah Breedlove in Delta, Louisiana, just after the Emancipation Proclamation was signed, ending an era of slavery. She was orphaned at age seven and suffered a difficult childhood: married at the early age of 14, widowed by the age of 20. Three of her brothers worked as barbers in a St. Louis barbershop, and Breedlove moved there to work as a washerwoman.

When the World's Fair came to St. Louis in 1904, Sarah Breedlove worked as an apprentice to Annie Turnbo Malone, who made shampoos, creams, pomades, and ointments for hair. Initially working on a commission basis, Breedlove's success allowed her to travel to Denver, Colorado, where she met her second husband, Charles J. Walker. Within a short time, she developed a treatment system for hair loss that she called the "Walker system." The Walker system included a shampoo, a pomade to encourage hair growth, vigorous brushing, and the application of iron straightening combs. The system was promoted as specifically directed toward the special health needs of black women. She sold her homemade remedies directly to black women and recruited a large number of loyal saleswomen, called "beauty culturalists," who sold her products door to door. In 2010, she moved her headquarters to Indianapolis and expanded her sought-after line to include close to twenty hair and skin products. The Madame C. J. Walker Manufacturing Company employed 3,000 women who dressed in a uniform of white shirts, black skirts, and black satchels making house calls. The business expanded to include mail order and international distribution in Cuba, Jamaica, Haiti, Panama, and Costa Rica.

One of Madame Walker's most important contributions was her improvement to the design of the straightening comb, also known as a hot comb. Walker widened the teeth of the hot comb to minimize tangling of coarse, curly hair. After slavery ended, many members of the black community considered hot combs to be controversial because they seemed to promote a "white" ideal of beauty. An important part of Walker's tremendously successful marketing strategy relied on using biblical passages to celebrate the virtues of black women's hair. She invested in a heavy

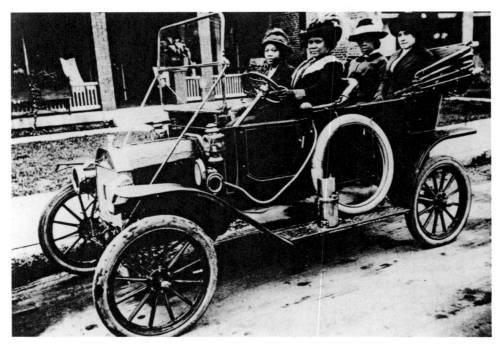

Madam C. J. Walker (driving) was among the first self-made female millionaires in America, representing a rising wave of black women advancing in public life as blacks surged to the cities in the early 20th century. (New York Public Library)

advertising campaign and emphasized that her products could offer black women a healthy, effective way to grow their hair without feeling inferior. Madame Walker advertised her trademark "Walker system" as an advantage for black women's beauty and economic independence. Made of metal, the hot comb is heated and used to straighten moderate or coarse hair from the roots and to create a smoother hair texture. When done properly, the use of hot combs is less damaging to hair than the use of chemical straightening products.

Walker's Manhattan townhouse became a salon for well-known luminaries of the Harlem Renaissance. Toward the end of her life, Madame Walker funded scholarships for women and at Tuskegee Institute and donated large sums of money to the NAACP and other civil rights groups. She died in 1919 at the age of fifty-one from complications due to hypertension.

See also: Barbershop; "Black Is Beautiful Movement," or Black Power; Hair; Salon.

Further Reading

Colman, Penny. 1994. *Madam C. J. Walker: Building a Business Empire*. Minneapolis: Millbrook Press.

History. 1991. "Madame C. J. Walker." Accessed November 21, 2015. http://www.history.com/topics/black-history/madame-c-j-walker.

PBS. 2004. "Sarah Breedlove Walker. They Made America. Accessed November 21, 2015. http://www.pbs.org/wgbh/theymadeamerica/whomade/walker_hi.html.

Wingfield, Adia Harvey. 2008. *Doing Business with Beauty; Black Women, Hair Salons, and the Racial Enclave Economy*. Lanham, MD: Rowman & Littlefield.

WEIGHT

At five foot nine and weighing just under 200 pounds, American men today are about two inches taller and fifty pounds heavier than they were one hundred years ago. During the Civil War, the average American man was an average five feet seven inches tall and weighed about 147 pounds. People in many parts of the world today are notably healthier—and larger—than in eras past. Researchers believe that children's health in very early life is the key to this leap in body size. During the Industrial Revolution, for example, childhood undernourishment weakened and stunted the growth of children, and some historians estimate that at least one in six young adults was dangerously underweight (Sandbeck 2010).

In Europe and much of the Western world, a robust male belly was seen as a sign of bourgeois prestige and vigor, and overweight females of the working class were admired for their additional work capacity and perceived fertility (Vigarello 2015).

In the late 1980s, evolutionary researchers Peter Brown and Melvin Konner (1987) used data compiled by anthropologists in the Human Relations Area File (HRAF) to propose that the physical qualities of plumpness and a moderate degree of fatness were valued in most preindustrial cultures because of fat's adaptive value during times of resource scarcity. Fatter people would be those who were most able to maximize the resources of their environment to create the illusion of abundance, and heavier people would be best equipped to deal with "lean" years when food was hard to come by. The HRAF files, maintained at Yale University, document the findings of over 850 anthropological studies going back to the early 1900s. According to Brown and Konner's analysis of cultures around the world, 81 percent of the societies surveyed preferred plump or moderately fat women, and 90 percent of societies surveyed admired women with large or fat hips and legs. From this analysis, Brown and Konner argued women who carried extra weight would be regarded as beautiful by populations who faced regular resource scarcity, usually due to the climate, and there existed corresponding cultural features to reward women who were able to achieve and maintain higher weights, including the ability to marry more successful mates and have more offspring. In these cultures, thinness would be associated with illness, and extra weight would suggest good health. However, Brown and Konner are quick to point out that true **obesity** is rare outside the Western world. According to medical sources, obesity can cause significant health problems, including elevated rates of diabetes, heart disease, and some cancers. They also point out that women accumulate more subcutaneous fat than men do. In some cultures, such as those that practice **wife-fattening**, this fatness may be actively cultivated, especially among elites.

In the 1990s, another group of researchers revisited the findings of Brown and Konner (1987) using additional ethnographic data. Their findings (Anderson et al. 1992) did not indicate that resource scarcity was necessarily a factor in finding heavier weights in women attractive. Rather, they suggest that two key factors determined societies that valued fatness in women: climate and male dominance. A later study by Ember et al. (2005) agreed that cultures that placed a high value on males being aggressive, strong, and sexually potent (sometimes referred to as "machismo") is highly correlated with cultures that value heavier women.

Before 1890, plumpness was also considered attractive and quite fashionable in Euro-American culture (Stearns 1997). Women were encouraged to eat heartily during frequent pregnancies. They padded their clothes to appear more voluptuous. Mature men and women were supposed to weigh more than their younger counterparts, and those who did not were looked on with suspicion or were suspected to be ill (Ibid.). Western concerns with weight control and reduction emerged at the turn of the 20th century, when social ideals of wellness shifted to an emphasis on appetite restraint and the new science of nutrition. In a society characterized by overabundance, the appearance of success may be less dependent on the sheer accumulation of wealth and more connected to the ability to control and manage the labor and resources of others (Bordo 1993, 192). By 1911, life insurance companies identified large body size as a risk to survival and worked to compile tables of standard weights (de Garine and Pollock 1995). Weight-reducing diets proliferated. Slender bodies began to be seen as more controlled. Those who were unable to discipline their bodies to the new standards were measured as deficient in their ability to rise to the challenge, and the subsequent use of shame and ridicule emerged to stigmatize heavy men and women (Stearns 1997, 21).

As anyone who has flipped through a fashion magazine can attest, large size is not correlated with beauty in the contemporary world. Fashion trends and stylistic conventions are one area where heavier bodies are excluded, even raising emotional feelings of disgust and revulsion. Excess body weight has come to be seen as a reflection of personal inadequacy, laziness, and a lack of will. The moral requirement to diet depends on a culture of abundance that assumes a person can make the personal choice to diet a viable option in pursuit of a body with the size and shape that marks personal, internal order and as a symbol of the emotional, moral, or spiritual state of the individual (Bordo 1993, 192–93). Since the 1920s, the prevailing trends of feminine beauty in the United States have preferred a thinner ideal, with a spike in some slightly larger bodies during the postwar years like the curvy **Marilyn Monroe hourglass** figure coveted in the 1950s. Speaking for the aesthetic that governed women's bodies in the 1930s, Wallis Simpson, the American-born divorcée who married the former King Edward VIII of England to become the Duchess of Windsor, is rumored to have famously said, "You can never be too rich or too thin" (Anderson et al. 1992). The alarming rise in eating disorders among young women has raised awareness of the potentially harmful effects of unrealistic beauty standards.

Undeniably, symbolic and material rewards exist for those who are most able to conform to exacting standards of beauty. In Western cultures, young women are taught to "police" their own weight in order to adhere to the appropriate idea of "femininity." They do this through continual self-surveillance and self-correction. In his influential essay "The Eye of Power," French theorist Michel Foucault wrote, "There is no need for arms, physical violence, material constraints. Just a gaze. An inspecting gaze, a gaze which each individual under its weight will end by interiorizing to the point that he is his own overseer, each individual thus exercising this surveillance over, and against himself" (1977, 155). Some writers have also argued that female hunger as a proxy for female sexual desire is especially problematized and discouraged by patriarchal cultures during periods of disruption in established gender relations and in the relative economic position of women. The so-called "consuming woman" (Dijkstra 1986) prompts a shift in cultural standards of femininity, insisting upon a more manageable, sylphlike female body (more similar to an adolescent or boy than a fully developed adult woman) in response to male anxiety over women's desires which might potentially go unfulfilled. In such times, whereas women's bodies are encouraged to decrease in size and weight, male bodies are exhorted to gain weight through muscle development. Advertisements for **body-building** products and services may feature well-muscled men, nearly nude, who are large but fat free. There is some evidence, however, that the standards of attractiveness in women's weight may vary according to social location within the dominant culture. The results of several studies indicate that African American men have a preference for a larger ideal female body type than other groups in the United States and that consideration of other factors influence what is considered to be "beautiful" (Bailey 2008, 33).

See also: Bodybuilding; Eating Disorders; Hourglass Shape; Monroe, Marilyn; Obesity; Wife Fattening.

Further Reading

Anderson, Judith L., Charles Bates Crawford, Joanne Nadeau, and Tracy Lindberg. 1992. "Was the Duchess of Windsor Right? A Cross-Cultural Review of the Socioecology of Ideal Female Body Shape." *Ethnology and Sociobiology* 13: 197–227.

Bailey, Eric J. 2008. *Black America, Body Beautiful: How the African American Image is Changing Fashion, Fitness, and Other Industries*. Westport, CT: Praeger.

Bordo, Susan. 1993. *Unbearable Weight: Feminism, Western Culture, and the Body*. Berkeley, CA: University of California Press.

Brown, Peter J., and Melvin Konner. 1987. "An Anthropological Perspective on Obesity." *Annals of the New York Academy of Sciences* 499: 29–46.

de Garine, Igor, and Nancy J. Pollock. 1995. *Social Aspects of Obesity*. Amsterdam, Netherlands: Gordon and Breach Publishers.

Dijkstra, Bram. 1986. *Idols of Perversity: Fantasies of Female Evil in Fin-de-Siècle Culture*. New York: Oxford University Press.

Ember, Carol R., Melvin Ember, Andrey Korotayev, and Victor de Muck. 2005. "Valuing Thinness and Fatness in Women: Reevaluating the Effect of Resource Scarcity." *Evolution and Human Behavior* 26: 257–70.

Foucault, Michel. 1977. "The Eye of Power," In: *Power/Knowledge: Selected Interviews and Other Writings 1972–1977*, 146–165, translated and edited by Colin Gordon. New York: Pantheon.

Gilman, Sander. 2008. *Fat: A Cultural History of Obesity*. New York: Polity Press.

Human Relations Area File. 2016. "Explaining Human Culture." Accessed June 28, 2016. http://hraf.yale.edu/ehc.

Sandbeck, Ellen. 2010. *Green Barbarians: How to Live Bravely on Your Home Planet*. New York, Scribner.

Stearns, Peter N. 1997. *Fat History: Bodies and Beauty in the Modern West*. New York: New York University Press.

Vigarello, Georges. 2015. *The Metamorphoses of Fat: A History of Obesity,* translated by C. Jon Delogu. New York: Columbia University Press.

WIFE FATTENING

Around the world and through time, a robust or full-figured woman is frequently associated with fertility and abundance. In Fiji, "you've gained weight" is traditionally considered to be a favorable compliment. Whereas most Western women spend some amount of their time "watching their weight" with an eye toward decreasing their size, there are examples of women in other parts of the world and at different times who had the opposite desire for their girth.

Archaeologists point to the profusion of "Venus figurines" found across Europe to indicate that as early as the Paleolithic era, human artists were drawn to full-bodied women as the standard of feminine beauty. The most famous of these figures was uncovered in 1908 in Austria, known as the "Venus of Willendorf." Measuring about four and a half inches in height, it was portable and could have been easily carried. The unusual anatomical structure of these figurines, labeled as a "lozenge composition," feature a faceless, often downturned head; arms that either disappear under the breasts or cross over them; a thin upper torso with voluminous, pendulous breasts; large fatty buttocks and/or thighs; a prominent, possibly pregnant abdomen, sometimes featuring a large elliptical navel; and bent, unnaturally short legs that taper to small feet (McCoid and McDermott 1996). McCoid and McDermott hypothesized that the figurines may have been self-portraits made by women themselves to celebrate the beautiful, fertile capacities of a pregnant female body.

The Sirionó people of eastern Bolivia historically fished, hunted, and gathered wild plants. Later, after colonialism, the Sirionó also farmed maize, sweet potatoes, and cassava. They lived in a rich ecosystem where food was abundant. Traditionally, this group was matrilifocal, determining both descent and residency along the maternal line. This means that after marriage, a new couple goes to live in the household of the bride's mother. Women were encouraged to become fat to attract male partners. In 1946, anthropologist A. R. Holberg wrote, "Besides being young, a desirable sex partner—especially a woman—should also be fat. She should have big hips, good sized but firm **breasts**, and a deposit of fat on her sexual organs" (Holmberg, quoted in Ember et al. 2005, 260).

Nauru, an island in the South Pacific visited by Captain Cook, is frequently cited as a place where people's extraordinary body size impresses visitors. More recently, epidemiologists have associated the population of the island with high rates of diabetes and glucose intolerance (Pollock 1995). Residents of the island engage in deliberate fattening activities aimed at changing the body shape of individuals. Fattening processes are also closely associated with two other linked standards of beauty: lightening skin color during extended periods of seclusion resulting from a lack of exposure to the sun and increasing body size in order to improve upon the symbolic value of the fat body deemed beautiful by Nauruans.

Fattening practices on Nauru were historically directed primarily at young women of rank at the time of the first menses. A feast lasting for three days joined members of the group together to celebrate the coming of age of a young woman. Following the celebration, the girl was forbidden to work, secluded for up to six months, and served large amounts of whatever food was available. Often, food was donated by members of the extended matrilineal kin network as a tribute and gift to her mother's family. Anthropologists argue that this period of extended dependency created ties of reciprocity that bound communities together more tightly.

The Naruans also practiced fattening during pregnancy. During this time, a woman was not allowed to work and observed strict food taboos, relying on the help of relatives and friends to bring her large amounts of food to eat. During a woman's pregnancy, her husband was also forbidden to work and was similarly fed by neighbors, relatives, and friends, though he was not expected to observe a period of seclusion. Fat is a sign of beauty, and the entire group joined together to overfeed members engaged in the work of managing fertility. Fattening customs of the island have been disrupted by processes of globalization, which shifted the economic focus of the island communities from fishing and farming to phosphate mining and imported foods. Today, changes in diet, especially the high rates of sugar in imported foods, have created a number of health problems that did not exist when fattening was conducted based on a traditional diet.

Fattening is also practiced among the Annang of Nigeria, where people value a "woman of substance" (Brink 1995). The Annang celebrate the opportunity to "fatten up" girls before marriage in order to make them "fat and beautiful." Undergoing such a period of **weight** gain requires the girls to be secluded and to avoid physical work. A girl who is fattening may also have a smaller child to run errands for her, and she is encouraged to eat whenever she wants. The typical Annang diet is composed of primarily cassava (or manioc, called *garri*), a complex carbohydrate with low vitamin and mineral content. This root staple is prepared by adding it to boiling water to form a thick paste, which is then augmented with a thick vegetable sauce. Yams may also be substituted for garri, as is boiled rice when available. Other foods include eggs, dried and fresh fish, chicken, goat, bananas, plantains, and other fruit, when available. Foods may be fried in palm oil, which is derived from the lush forests that surround the Annang villages.

Dieticians estimate that 89 percent of the Annang diet is derived from "starchy" foods (cassava, bananas, plantain), whereas only 11 percent is derived from protein food (Brink 1995, 76). There is almost no animal fat in the daily diet, and the average daily caloric intake is estimated to be about 1,500 to 2,500 calories per day. Given the level of activity required from the horticulturalist lifestyle of the Annang, it would be very difficult to regularly gain and maintain weight on this amount of calories. Medical anthropologists point to the relationship between the degree of body fat and the onset of menarche in West African and Pacific girls (MacCormack 1982). Usually, between 20 and 22 percent body fat is recognized as the minimum requirement for a girl to be considered fertile. A number of studies conducted in Sweden, France, Belgium, Switzerland, and the United States have raised concerns that the age of puberty is starting younger in girls due to the dramatic changes in nutrition, body weight, and body fat linked to higher rates of **obesity** in recent generations (Chalabi 2013).

Annang culturally prescribed fattening practices, then, must specifically designate and redirect fairly scarce resources to marriageable girls (*mbobo*) in order to allow them to gain weight. The reason for investing such resources into a girl has to do with local ideology and the highly valued belief that a fattened daughter will make a more acceptable bride and mother. The Annang value fattening as part of a traditional system associated with marriage and the custom of bride price, which creates young wives who are viewed as fertile and able to conceive and lactate to create the next generation. The fattening room is a specific, designated place in the compound, usually a barricaded portion of the mother's house in order to seclude the girl from view. During this time, a girl is taught "womanly arts," including how to please her husband, care for children, and maintain a household. She remains naked so that others may observe the successful progress of her fattening. The Annang believe that part of the purpose of fattening is to round the hips of the girl in order to improve her ability to conceive, carry, bear, and feed her child (Brink 1995). The belief is that fattening creates broader hips, which are a requirement for providing a large enough birth canal to limit complications during pregnancy and delivery. The fattening room fulfills the purpose of making the girl beautiful and socially desirable: she shows that her family was able to produce such a fine fat girl in order to become a good wife and mother who will add value to the community.

The Annang also observe shorter periods of fattening for those women of the group who have fallen ill to a variety of ailments. For people who suffer from extreme headaches, protracted thinness, sleeplessness, and infertility, a local diviner or fortune teller may prescribe a period of seclusion and fattening, much like the time spent by marriageable girls.

Tuareg and Moorish peoples of West Africa were historically noted as groups that appreciated a heavier body as a component of idealized female beauty. Among the contemporary desert-dwelling Azagwah Arab people of Niger, girls are often force-fed to accelerate the process of sexual maturity and thus allow the girls to be married and become mothers of the next generation. Female corpulence in the region is celebrated in conversation, song, and ritual. Stretch marks, especially on the undersides of the arms, are one indication of high beauty. One traditional song celebrates the beauty of a beloved who had "stretch marks from her waist to her knee." Another song brags delightedly about a local beauty sporting "three luscious folds" at her stomach (Popenoe 2004, 44).

Women who attain this beautiful bodily ideal of heavy upper arms and breasts with rolls of fat at the waist and a protruding backside over heavy thighs (*zeyn*) typically come from more affluent families who can afford the additional expense of feeding and are able to spare the labor of elite women. Fattened women do not move around very much in order to conserve their hard-won fat stores. They run their households with the assistance of servants from a cross-legged position of respect, seated on mats on the ground. Rather than marking the life course in number of years, the Azawagh Arabs carefully watch the bodies of their daughters for signs of maturation, which indicate their marriageability. With the loss of the first two baby teeth, fattening begins and a girl's hair is braided for the first time. When pubic hair begins to be visible, girls trade in childish clothing for an adult woman's *hawli* (a loose, sari-like dress). When a girl begins menstruating, she is expected to fast during the Muslim holy month of Ramadan.

Like many cultures around the world and through history, the Azagwah Arabs believe in a humoral system of pathology, which means that their ideas about wellness and the body reside in maintaining "balance," which requires individuals to either eat or avoid certain foods and practices in order to keep them healthy. Foods, plants, medicines, diseases, and physical acts are all considered in this balance, usually categorized according to relative "temperature": there are foods and practices thought to be "cool" and those that are considered to be "hot." To begin the process of force feeding (*le-bluf*), which yields the desirable fatness for girls after they have lost their first baby teeth, the caretakers in their lives limit the amount of mobility of the girls. They are usually confined to a tent near their mother and switched from their childhood diet of milky porridge to a regimen of dryish couscous, swallowed down with large amounts of water. Couscous and other dry foods are thought to be "cooler" and curb the dangerous possibility of too much "heat" (also interpreted as sexuality) accumulating in the bodies of the young girls. Girls usually willingly undergo the act of increased eating, but girls may also be forced, through words or more extreme physical means, to continue eating, to eat more, to eat faster, and to remain still. The process of fattening takes many years and is considered "work." Girls are encouraged to cram full the entire cavity of their mouths with each bite, swallowing as quickly as possible and following each bite with large gulps of water. Fattening is thought of as a process of sexualizing the body to the male viewer while diminishing the sexual desires of the girl herself. Throughout their fattening period, girls are fed diets that are high in carbohydrates coming from millet or sorghum, taken with water or milk. The ideal food should either be watery in consistency or taken with a lot of water so that it will disperse properly within the limbs and not accrete at any one spot within the body. A variety of recipes are used to combine millet flour and milk into meals of different consistencies, but not very many flavors. This bland diet lacks fruit or vegetables, and girls who are busy with the task of fattening often avoid taking meals with other members of their families for fear that other foods may "melt" the fat they work so hard to accumulate.

Anthropologist Rebecca Popenoe, who lived among Azagwah Arabs for several years in a small village called Tassara in Niger, suggests that these desert people inhabit their world in a particularly active way, often in the face of great scarcity and limited food choices and the beauty of fattening "feeds" the creation of appropriate sexual desire. The beauty ideal described to her by informants, which is so different from the hourglass aesthetic adhered to in mainstream contemporary United States, relies on deeply felt and interconnected cultural logics about what men and women are, how desire works, and a socially perceived nature of the human body. For these people, female fatness represents an aesthetic of "softness, pliability, stillness," which is seen in direct opposition to the masculine standard of male beauty that privileges "hardness, uprightness, mobility" (Popenoe 2004, 191). These two starkly oppositional views of gendered beauty underscore the cultural ethic of gender complementarity present in the society. The Azagwah Arabs understand the heaviness of the female body to be a symbolic and literal kind of affective labor, which ties the woman's body to the earth in a harmonious way that is pleasing to the people of the society and reinforces aspects of gender identity.

Of course, gender must also be factored into considerations of how heaviness might yield a more attractive body to some cultural viewers. There is evidence that the sons of Nigerian Igbo nobility were traditionally sequestered for some time following their rites of passage into adulthood and left to eat and fatten (Jeffreys 1951, 97). Collective male fattening sessions, called *guru*, are highly valued among the Massa of Northern Cameroon (de Garine 1995). As pastoralists, the Massa live in close proximity to their cattle all year long. Skinny men are considered to be sickly or weak. Young men of the group spend a good deal of their time training and grooming themselves in order to appear beautiful (*naana*), and they take advantage of ceremonies at certain times of the year to demonstrate their physical fitness and skill in dancing, singing, and wrestling. Throughout the year, young men who are able to afford it consume high amounts of proteins and carbohydrates, mostly as cow's milk mixed with a thick sorghum porridge, up to about 7,500 calories per day, in order to maintain a weight that makes them about fifteen pounds heavier than other men in the group. During intense periods of overfeeding necessary for optimal fattening, the men can raise their overall body weight by up to forty-five pounds, which is concentrated mostly in a protruding belly and **buttocks**, deemed beautiful by the aesthetic standards of the Massa.

See also: Body Modification; Breasts; Butts and Booty; Obesity; Weight.

Further Reading

Brink, Pamela J. 1995. "Fertility and Fat: The Annang Fattening Room." In: *Social Aspects of Obesity*, edited by Igor de Garine and Nancy J. Pollock, 71–85. Amsterdam: Gordon and Breach Publishers.

Chalabi, Mona. 2013. "Why Is Puberty Starting Younger?" *The Guardian*. November 4. Accessed February 2, 2016. https://www.theguardian.com/politics/2013/nov/04/why-is-puberty-starting-younger-precocious.

De Garine, Igor. 1995. "Sociocultural Aspects of the Male Fattening Sessions among the Massa of Northern Cameroon." In: *Social Aspects of Obesity*, edited by Igor de Garine and Nancy J. Pollock, 45–70. Amsterdam: Gordon and Breach Publishers.

Ellis, Albert, and Albert Albernal, editors. 2013. *The Encyclopedia of Sexual Behaviour*, vol. 1. New York: Elsevier.

Ember, Carol R., Melvin Ember, Andrey Korotayev, and Victor de Munck. 2005. Valuing Thinness or Fatness in Women: Reevaluating the Effect of Resource Scarcity." *Evolution and Human Behavior* 26: 257–70.

Goode, Erica. 1999. "Study Finds TV Alters Fiji Girls' View of Body." *New York Times*. May 20. Accessed October 11, 2016. http://www.nytimes.com/1999/05/20/world/study-finds-tv-alters-fiji-girls-view-of-body.html.

Holmberg, Allan R. 1946. "*The Sirionó: A Study of the Effect of Hunger Frustration on the Culture of a Semi-Nomadic Bolivian Indian Society*." PhD dissertation. New Haven, CT: Yale University.

Jeffreys, Mervyn David Waldegrave. 1951. "The Winged Solar Disk or Ibo ItΣi Facial Scarification." *Africa* 21, no. 4: 93–111.

MacCormack, Carole. 1982. "Ritual Fattening and Female Fertility." In: *Folk Medicine and Health Culture: Role of Folk Medicine in Modern Health Care*, edited by T. Vaskilampi and Carole MacCormack, 27–28. Proceedings of the Nordic Research Symposium, August, Department of Community Health: University of Kuopio, Finland.

McCoid, Catherine Hidge, and LeRoy D. McDermott. 1996. "Toward Decolonizing Gender: Female Vision in the Upper Paleolithic. *American Anthropologist* 98, no. 2: 319–26.

Pollock, Nancy J. 1995. "Social Fattening Patterns in the Pacific—the Positive Side of Obesity. A Nauru Case Study." In: *Social Aspects of Obesity*, edited by Igor de Garine and Nancy J. Pollock, 87–109. Amsterdam: Gordon and Breach Publishers.

Popenoe, Rebecca. 2004. *Feeding Desire: Fatness, Beauty, and Sexuality Among a Saharan People*. London: Routledge.

Tauzin, Aline. 1986. "*La Femme partagées: contrôle et déplacement de la sexualité feminine en Mauritanie*." In: *Côté Femmes: approches ethnologiques*. Paris: Editions L'Harmattan.

WODAABE FULANI (NIGER)

The Wodaabe Fulani are a nomadic, pastoralist people who live in Niger, West Africa. They are probably best known for their highly photographed annual Gerewol (aka Geerewol, Guérewol; also known in French as *le Cure Salée*) gathering, which is sometimes referred to as a "male beauty contest." This annual gathering places the most handsome men from each lineage in competition with each other to determine which man is the most beautiful and desirable. The masculine power and vitality associated with Wodaabe male beauty are expressed in the dance performances. Men emphasize the physical difficulties of the dance, which demands both strength and endurance from participants.

The Gerewol dance is just one part of a seven-day ceremony uniting the two lineages of the tribe. The colorful dances, called the Ruume and the Yaake, are considered the highlight of the event by outsiders to be "unique and colorful" and have been featured in many documentaries and print advertisements of the popular media. One of the main purposes of the annual gathering is to sanction the initiation of men into adulthood. Men who have reached the age of 36 wear leather aprons and circlets of grass on their head. They bow and are ceremonially blessed by elders. Following this ceremony, the other events of the gathering begin, and the newly initiated men are considered old enough to become heads of households. The newly mature men ride their camels, adorned in expensive leather goods, around the women in order to show them off.

Each day of the gathering, participants engage in a variety of ceremonies and dances. Typically, life for the Wodaabe involves strict gender segregation, which means that men and women do not interact socially. However, on the first night of the event, men and women perform the Ruume, or "welcome dance," together to end the rainy season. For this occasion, men color their faces yellow, the color of magic, and wear colorful beads (Roy 2007). The lead singer paints his face a bright shade of red and leads the assembled group in songs of praise of beauty. They songs include descriptions of long, beautiful arms and legs, soft lips, and the large, round eyes of the beloved. Beautiful men are considered to be those who are tall, with long limbs, white eyes, and white teeth.

The Yaake dance takes place over the course of many days. It is a competition dance, and only the most attractive men of each lineage are invited to participate. Men publicly prepare their bodies for the dance by smearing red clay mixed with butter to their bodies. Crowds can gather around a man as he deliberately applies his makeup and costuming, which is usually thought out long before the day of the event. These men go to great expense in order to create a winning look to woo women during the dance. The secrets of their preparation can be jealously guarded. Some men even admit to mixing elements of "love magic" that they obtain from local healers or holy men into the potions they use to create their final look (Roy 2007). The red clay is mined near Joss in neighboring Nigeria; it represents an expense that must be laid out for participation in the event. The red color is meant to represent the violence of war (Roy 2007). Additional **makeup** is applied to the face in order to highlight and accent lightly colored skin and to make the face look longer, narrower, and more vertical. Men apply blackening agent, used like **lipstick** and eyeliner, to their lips and eyes. The black color used to be made by burning the blood of camels, but today, the black color comes from the burned insides of batteries. Men are aware that these ingredients are toxic, and they are careful not to ingest them. To complete the face, the nose is considered the most important feature. It is shaded and highlighted using makeup to appear longer and thinner. A small white line or dot is sometimes applied to the tip of the nose to make it appear more prominent. Men usually wear long leather aprons and long strands of colorful beads to perform the dance. A sleeveless tunic or brightly colored belt may also be worn. The dancers wear specially wrapped cloth and ropes of beads replete with tall ostrich feathers on their heads as headdresses. They also wear metal bracelets with metal rings around their ankles in order to keep time with the music. It is important for men to appear beautiful and charming, possessed of *tobdu*, translated best as "**sex appeal**." The "semifinalists of the dance, those who make it through the first few days of competition, often have a second outfit that they will wear, exchanging ostrich feathers for more dramatic horse tails or sheep tails.

Throughout the ceremony, both during and following the dance, the emphasis of the performance is on sexuality. Men expect to seduce the sexually eligible women with their cosmetics, clothing, dance moves, and facial expressions. Dancing performances are repetitive, hypnotic, and rely heavily on percussive choral traditions and swaying line dances, where the men link arms, rising and falling on their toes, and using expressive facial contortions and eye rolls to attract the attention of marriageable

Huli Wigman

The many tribal groups of the New Guinea Highlands practice elaborate costuming for rituals and rites of passage. The Huli "Wigman" is so-called because of the large headdress made of the man's own hair, vegetable material, and prestigious bird-of-paradise feathers. Beginning by covering the face with a base of charcoal (a symbol of bravery and virility), men paint their faces bright yellow, edged in white and red, in order to transform into "man-birds." The yellow color comes from a tree known as the "tree of the ancestors." A variety of other colored pigments are rubbed into the beard and used to shade the face in order to intensify the gaze and "sharpen" the beak. Men also pierce their noses with stylized rods of mother-of-pearl, bone, or feather. Just as in the bird hierarchy, female costumes are far less elaborate. Their "plumage" consists of small branches of foliage attached to the small of the back and made to move as if a pendulum by rhythmic swaying of the hips.

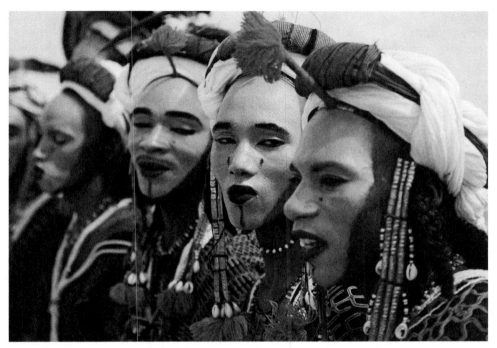

Wodaabe men perform the Yaake dance during Gerewol, an annual courtship festival, Niger. Sometimes referred to as a "male beauty contest," this annual occasion features the most handsome men from each lineage to showcase masculine power and vitality. (Grodza/Dreamstime.com)

women. For this reason, the dance is often interpreted as a "male beauty contest," but it is important to note that the elders actually determine the "winner" of the contest, usually with the assistance of some of the women. Sexual liaisons are inevitable as a result of the event, and lovers may be betrayed or have their hopes dashed. Affairs conducted during the Gerewol may be temporary, or they may be the start of a longer, more permanent relationship. However, at the end of the seven-day event, men who are seeking wives have usually begun the long process of negotiating bride wealth and arranging for marriages to take place within the upcoming year.

Though men may prize the way they look during the performance, it is not always the case that the man who looks the most impressive in his makeup and clothing during the ceremonies is not necessarily viewed as the most handsome without it. In other words, the cosmetics and preparations that prepare the man for the performance are attributed as the source of the beauty.

Of course, culturally appropriate standards exist for women's beauty as well. Wodaabe women are expected to be graceful, proud, and reserved. Adult women frequently present themselves as detached and distant, rarely verbalizing their emotional state. The transformation to womanhood takes place as a series of rites of passage, including **breast binding** to transform the shape of a girl's breasts to those of an adult woman. Adult women also mark their faces with **scarification**. For the most part, women who comport themselves according to this idealized social role can expect to earn the respect of others. Perhaps due in part to the distinctly differentiated gender roles and highly scrutinized level of female behavior in this culture, marital violence may be frequent in this militaristic society that prizes masculinity highly. Other researchers have pointed to the highly significant connection between men and women in managing household economic tasks, including considerations about marriage arrangements for the next generation (Greenough 2012).

See also: Breasts; Breast Binding; Lipstick and Lip Tattoos; Makeup and Cosmetics; Masculinity; Pageants—Indigenous; Scarification; Sexy.

Further Reading

Beckwith, Carol, and Marion van Offelen. 1983. *Nomads of Niger*. New York: Abradale Press.
Greenough, Karen. 2012. "Mobility, Market Exchange and Livelihood Transition: Fulbe Flexibility in Tanout, Niger." *Nomadic Peoples* 16, no. 2: 26–52.
Loftsdóttir, Kristín. 2008. *The Bush Is Sweet: Identity, Power, and Development among WoDaaBe Fulani in Niger*. Uppsala, Sweden: Nordiska Afrikainstitutet.
Loncke, Sandrine. 2015. *Geerewol: Hommes et Musiques*. Accessed October 11, 2016. http://www.ethnomusicologie.fr/wodaabe-loncke/index.html.
Roy, Christopher D. 2007. *Birds of the Wilderness: The Beauty Competition of the Wodaabe People of Niger*. Film. Directed by Christopher D. Roy. New York: CreateSpace.

WRINKLES

An appearance of youth, as evolutionary psychologists tell us, is one of the universally recognized norms of beauty. From Asia to the Americas, young people and young, smooth skin are considered beautiful. It is perhaps for this reason that beauty work to combat wrinkles of the skin has been ongoing for at least three centuries of human history; archeologists have discovered recipes for preventing wrinkles in the medical records of the ancient Egyptians (Etcoff 2000). The appearance of youth is as important for men as it is for women, and both genders seek to prevent, reduce, and eliminate wrinkles.

Smooth skin is particular to youth in all humans. Young people's skin is constantly undergoing change, with new skin cells pushing to the surface every couple of weeks. As skin gets older, this process slows. As we age, our oil glands become less active, and the collagen and elastin—two chemicals that maintain skin's suppleness—begin to break down. This whole process means that skin is drier and less pliable and more apt to wrinkle and sag (Etcoff 2000).

Aging is not the only thing that affects the development of wrinkles in human skin, however. Activities that damage skin as we age can accelerate the process, especially damage from the sun or the toxins of cigarette smoke.

> "Beauty is the first present nature gives to women and the first it takes away."
> —FAY WELDON

Prolonged exposure to the sun quickens and deepens the development of wrinkles, and heavy smokers of cigarettes develop more wrinkles than do nonsmokers (Etcoff 2000).

The drive to rid our faces of the signs of **aging** has led, over the years, to a long history of treatments for wrinkles. In ancient Egypt, in BCE 400 Cleopatra was reported to have bathed in donkey's milk every day, using the alpha-hydroxy agents in the milk to soften and exfoliate long before scientists would identify those compounds (Morrill 2016). Other ancient peoples found similarly intuitive and effective antiwrinkle remedies, such as creams that loosed dirt, oil, and dead skin cells and aged red-wine masks that we now know contained beneficial antioxidants (Morrill 2016).

Other historical treatments for wrinkles, however, have not been supported by modern science. Practices such as the Elizabethan trend of putting slices of raw meat on the face or the ancient Greek practice of using masks made of crocodile dung do not currently have any scientific research to back their effectiveness (Leal 2015).

Some treatments across history have also been not only suspicious in their effectiveness, but dangerous both to the user and to others. In Victorian times, one common antiwrinkle skin treatment for faces was the chemical mercury, which works by corroding and sloughing off large sheets of skin from the face. Mercury is also toxic and can cause a range of neurological conditions (Leal 2016).

Even more chillingly, the 15th-century Hungarian Countess Elizabeth Bathory de Esced (known as the Blood Countess) killed more than 600 peasant girls in order to bathe in their blood to maintain her youth and treat the signs of aging (Sheppard 1995). Although this practice is clearly both horrifying and criminal, the idea of using blood to fight the signs of aging has not diminished over the centuries. In the 21st century, the rise of the "Vampire Facelift," in which a patient's own blood is injected into and then smeared over the face, purports to have scientific validity as a way to fight wrinkles, though most of the scientific community in 2016 remains skeptical (Pesce 2013).

In the 21st century, a range of antiwrinkle treatments have been scientifically proven to remove or reduce the appearance of wrinkles. These treatments generally come in three categories: surgery, injectable substances, and topical or surface creams and treatments.

Surgeries designed to combat the signs of aging include facelift procedures, in which skin is stretched and reattached to smooth out wrinkles, but also less famous surgeries such as barbed suture lifts, forehead lifts, and laser facial resurfacing (ISAPS 2016). The first two of these procedures use different techniques to lift and stretch the skin on a patient's face to smooth out wrinkles, whereas the last uses a carbon dioxide laser to resurface the skin of the face by eliminating several layers (ISAPS 2016).

Another way in which 21st-century patients reduce the appearance of wrinkles is by injecting one of a series of substances into the face and neck, filling in the places where skin has sagged or relaxing the muscles that keep skin puckered. Fillers such as collagen, hyaluronic acid, or calcium hydroxyapatite microspheres are medically accepted substances that can fill in these areas, as can the injection of a patient's own fat from a different part of their body in a treatment called fat transfer (ISAPS 2016).

Finally, there are a wide variety of substances that people can apply to the surface of their skin to remove or reduce wrinkles. Some of these substances are designed to add back in the collagen and elastin lost through aging, plumping up and smoothing lines, and some are designed to take off layers of skin, removing the older skin cells and allowing the younger ones to come to the surface. Examples of the first type of treatment include lotions and creams, which contain plumping ingredients such as collagen, elastin, retinol, or even eggshell membrane (Morill 2016).

The second variety of cream, designed to remove older skin, may contain chemicals such as alpha-hydroxy acids, glycolic acid, pyruvic acid, or tretinoic acid. These creams can be applied at home, with chemicals in lower concentrations, or in a doctor's office with stronger concentrations of the acid being used (Donahue 2013).

See also: Botox; Chemical Peels; Egypt; Facelifts; Greece; Injections; Makeup and Cosmetics; Youth.

Further Reading

Donahue, Kayleigh. 2013. "Anti-aging All Stars." *Redbook* 220, no. 4: 64.

Etcoff, Nancy. 2000. *Survival of the Prettiest: The Science of Beauty.* New York: Anchor.

ISAPS. 2016. "Procedures: Head and Neck." Accessed July 19, 2016. http://www.isaps.org /procedures/laser-facial-resurfacing.

Leal, Samantha. 2015. "The Craziest Things that People Have Done to Try and Stay Young." Accessed July 19, 2016. http://www.marieclaire.com/beauty/news/a14382/anti-aging -beauty-through-history.

Morrill, Hannah. 2016. "Charting: A Brief History of Anti-Aging." April 14. Accessed July 19, 2016. http://www.harpersbazaar.com/beauty/skin-care/a14980/history-of-anti-aging.

Pesce, Nicole Lyn. 2013. "Kim Kardashian's 'Vampire Facelift' Is a Hollywood Hit that Promises Younger, Firmer-Looking Skin." March 12. Accessed July 19, 2016. http://www .nydailynews.com/life-style/health/kim-kardashian-vampire-facelift-bloody-mess -article-1.1285646.

Sheppard, R. Z. 1995. "Gothic Whoopee." *Time* 146, no. 7: 70.

WUDU

To purify oneself through ritual not only beautifies the body, but also prepares an individual to interact with the divine. In Islam, the practice of *wudu* is considered a minor ritual ablution and is performed several times each day. It prepares the faithful for participation in *salat* (prayer). The ritual involves using clean, clear water to purify and clean specified parts of the body in a ritualistic fashion. The act of wudu consists of washing the six organs of wudu: the face and both forearms, the head, and both feet. The process usually begins with an intention (*niyyat*) designed to focus the mind. The next step is washing of the hands. The left hand is used to wash the right hand (all the way up the wrist) three times; then the reverse action is performed. Water is then taken into the mouth and swished to rinse any lingering food, and water is also inhaled into the nostrils to clear the sinuses. Next, the face is washed from the edge of the hair to the chin, beginning with the right side of the face. Then

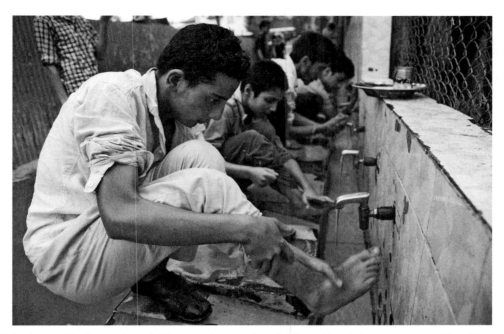

Kashmiri Muslim orphan children perform wudu, ritual washing before prayers and breaking their day-long fast, at the Rahat Manzil Orphanage in Srinagar, Indian-controlled Kashmir, July 6, 2015. Muslims across the world observe the holy fasting month of Ramadan, where they refrain from eating, drinking and smoking from dawn to dusk. (AP Photo/Dar Yasin)

the lower arms are washed from wrist to elbows. Again, the right arm is used to wash the left arm three times, and then the action is reversed. The wet hands are then used to wipe the head from the forehead to the hairline, down the hair, the back of the neck and across the temples, including attention to the insides of the ears. The back of the ear should also be cleaned. Finally, the feet are cleaned to the ankles, using the pinky finger to reach between each of the toes. The action begins on the right foot and then continues to the left foot. The final step of wudu is to raise the right index finger to the sky and recite a brief prayer. The body is now suitably cleansed to perform prayers.

Another ritual ablution, considered a major ablution, is known as *ghusl*. This ablution refers to full body washing and is necessary after sexual intercourse or other sexual acts. The intention of the purification is to remove any unclean elements of daily living, including urination, defecation, or the release of gas. Women are also responsible for daily ritual ablutions and *ghusl*. These differ from the wudu exhortations for men in that there are additional steps to purify the body following monthly periods and postnatal bleeding. In addition to the steps of wudu, water should also be poured over the head three times so that it flows over the entire body. Water is then poured three times over the right shoulder, followed by three dousings over the left shoulder. Private parts should then be washed thoroughly, followed by hand washing.

Mosques and other public spaces throughout the Islamic world provide special facilities for completing wudu ablutions (Philips 2012). These features are often incorporated into the architecture in such a way that they add aesthetic appeal to the space.

See also: Ritual Cleansing.

Further Reading

Al-Islam. 2016. "Ritual and Spiritual Purity: Wudu." Accessed October 11, 2016. https://www.al-islam.org/ritual-and-spiritual-purity-sayyid-muhammad-rizvi/ii-wudu.

Philips, Geradette. 2012. "The Spirituality of Islamic Beauty." *MELINTAS* 28, no. 3: 255–70.

Y

YAEBA (TOOTH CROWDING)

During the Edo period, Japanese etiquette demanded one to cover the mouth submissively while smiling or giggling, possibly because bared teeth may have been interpreted as threatening or aggressive. During this historical period, teeth blackening became common among elites and **geisha** as a way of deemphasizing the animalistic potential of a woman's mouth.

Whereas the U.S. Department of Health and Human Services estimates that Americans spend more than $100 billion on dental improvements every year, the recent Japanese dental trend of *tsuke yaeba* endeavors to make one's smile look less perfect and more uneven by capping the upper canines. Considered "cute" in high-profile pop singers like Matsuda Seiko, proponents believe that the overall "snaggletooth" effect is endearing and sweet. They believe that the imperfection increases the youthfulness of one's appearance and enhances approachability. *Yaeba* translates as "double tooth" from **Japanese** and costs between $200 and $500 per tooth.

Despite the efforts of this practice to produce a more "authentic" and less perfect-looking woman, it is still the case that many women are undergoing the dental procedure in order to appear more appealing to male partners, who still have the ultimate say on what is considered attractive. Some critics point out that the procedure demonstrates inappropriate sexualization of young girls, as a naturally occurring *yaeba* effect is most visible because of delayed baby teeth.

Tooth Gap, or Diastema

A diastema is a space or gap that can occur between any two teeth, but a "tooth gap" (or *dents du bonheur*, "lucky teeth," in French) refers to a space between the two front teeth. Several Western personalities have unique, prominent tooth gaps, including Madonna, Michael Strahan, Anna Paquin, and David Letterman. A tooth gap can also be considered quite beautiful, gracing the smiles of supermodels Lauren Hutton, Alek Wek, and Lindsey Wixson. The French media declared gapped teeth to be fashionable, and *The Wall Street Journal* suggested that they were one of the most coveted attributes for models at New York Fashion Week in 2009. In contemporary Nigeria, a gap in the middle of the front teeth is a sign of sensual beauty. Women with a tiny space between their teeth are often thought to possess a more potent sexual appeal. Gap-tooth smiles are also prized as lucky or signifiers of wealth in other parts of West Africa and the Caribbean. For the Mende people, a pearly white smile, combined with a small amount of flesh showing between the two front teeth, is considered a beauty mark, a point of both attention and admiration. In the past, any woman born without a gap between her two front teeth would have the upper incisors filed in order to open the space.

The *yaeba* trend in Japan was related to the rise of Okinawan-born techno/pop music star Amuro Namie, who was a spokes-model for the Takana Yuri beauty clinic from 1996–1997. Amuro became well known for her light brown hair, worn long, and her youthful, slim figure. Amuro also wore "sassy" outfits that were closely associated with character-istic brick-sized shoes. By the late 1990s, the enormous platform shoes, boots, and sandals she pop-ularized had reached eight- to ten-inch heels and generated sales around $100 million (Miller 2006). Amuro's popularity also launched a national "small face" fad (*mikuro kei*), spurring the rise in sales of dubious face-slimming creams and masks to women across Japan who hoped to make their relatively round faces look more angular. Nota-

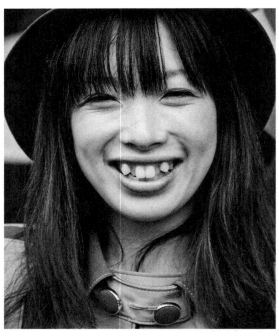

A Japanese woman with *yaeba* teeth. Yaeba, or tooth crowding, is often said to look more appealing, youth-ful, and "authentic" than more conventional repre-sentations of beauty. (Igor Vidyashev/Alamy Stock Photo)

bly, Amuro was described in the media as one of the "hidden uglies" (*basu kakushi*): a woman who does not necessarily embody the most desired, traditional beauty ideals but who is able to transform herself into a style idol through strategic use of fashion and cosmetics (Miller 2006).

In the early 2000s, the big shoes/small faces look made popular by Amuro look-alikes in subcultures of Japan launched more commercial, youth-based beauty trends often referred to as *kogyaru* (an abbreviation of *kōkōsei gyaru*, or high school girls). "Average-looking" amateurs started modeling for edgy fashion magazines. Marketing campaigns began to use images of the *kogyaru* look, characterized by a "school girl" look featuring a miniskirt, bleached hair often worn in pigtails, knee socks scrunched at the ankle, and big shoes with a platform heel. Through media hype, the "girl power" subculture was rendered into a type of "bad-girl" consumer. The *kogyaru* style also evolved into another related youth-based aesthetic called *gan-guro* and favored by hip girls from working-class backgrounds. *Ganguro* emulated the effortless street-wise fashions of the African American "B-Girl" style, sporting processed hair, extreme hair colors, tanned skin, and the use of white or pale makeup around the eyes and on the lips. The style can best be seen in the Japanese female hip-hop artist Hitoe.

All of these "new girl" styles in Japan represent a rejection of cultural proscrip-tions about "proper" female affect and presentation of the self. In the global era, the demure aesthetic of the historic geisha figure is being replaced over and over again by open displays of youth-based independence and challenging attitudes. "The insurrectionary poses that would normally be categorized as rude, whorish, or low-class take on new meanings of hipness when aligned with subcultural fashion and makeup styles" (Miller 2006, 34).

See also: Dental Hygiene and Cosmetic Dentistry; Geisha; Japan.

Further Reading

Considine, Austin. 2011. "A Little Imperfection for that Smile?" *New York Times*. October 21. Accessed October 11, 2016. http://www.nytimes.com/2011/10/23/fashion/in-japan-a -trend-to-make-straight-teeth-crooked-noticed.html?_r=0.

Miller, Laura. 2006. *Beauty Up: Exploring Contemporary Japanese Body Aesthetics*. Berkeley, CA: University of California Press.

Nelson, Sara C. 2013. "Yaeba: Japanese 'Double Tooth' Trend Will Give You a Costly Crooked Smile." *Huffington Post*. February 1. Accessed October 11, 2016. http://www.huffingtonpost .co.uk/2013/02/01/yaeba-japanese-double-tooth-trend-expensive-crooked-smile_n _2596720.html

YOUTH

Many cultures around the world appreciate and promote the qualities of human experience that come with age. Historically, village life was organized around a gerontocratic system of authority, whereby the eldest members of the group were assumed to possess the most wisdom and had the final say on matters facing the group.

The physical qualities of youth are highly prized, especially as markers of vitality and attractiveness. Young faces usually feature large eyes, high cheekbones, and full lips. Youthful bodies are typically supple and firm.

Skin loses the elasticity lent by collagen as it ages, typically resulting in **wrinkles**, crow's feet, drooping eyelids and jawlines, and loose skin around the neck. Skin may become increasingly dry and start to show signs of sun damage. Hair begins to thin, turn grey, or fall out. Additionally, a person's physique shows signs of aging as the metabolism slows and gravity exerts a toll on the body, including sagging breasts or buttocks and redistribution of fat storage, especially around the midsection. Depending upon a variety of lifestyle factors, the average woman gains about sixteen pounds by midlife (Wing et al. 1991).

Especially in the youth-focused United States, people seek to camouflage signs of aging through **cosmetic surgery**, increasingly intense fitness regimens, or expensive creams and lotions intended to "lift" or rejuvenate aging skin. Specific surgeries may include facelifts, injections, or chemical peels or laser resurfacing.

As with many practices dealing with beauty, there is a gendered component to the acceptance of youth and aging. Men are often thought to become more distinguished as they age, making them more attractive to younger women. Though gay men are likely more susceptible to the desire to project a more youthful appearance, many male celebrities have enjoyed longer film careers than their female counterparts as they age into "silver foxes."

Even while those aging within the consumer culture seek to appear younger, there is a parallel effort to make the innocence of youth appear more sexualized, worldly, or adult. Since the highly publicized murder of six-year-old beauty contestant Jon Benet Ramsey in 1997, the idea that even very young children should compete to be named the "most beautiful" has generated discomfort for the ways it promotes a version of perfect childhood innocence within the guise of adult beauty practices, including cosmetics, dyed hair, and sexually suggestive clothing or photographic poses. Child **pageants** and the families of pageant contestants have been featured prominently on several reality television programs.

The use of one's looks as a means of status and power presents profound problems as a basis for one's identity because attractiveness is ephemeral and ultimately unsustainable (Lakoff and Scherr 1984).

See also: Pageants—International, National, and Local Contests; Plastic Surgery; Wrinkles.

Further Reading

Clarke, Laura Hurd, and Meridith Griffin. 2008. "Visible and Invisible Ageing: Beauty Work as Response to Ageism." *Ageing and Society* 28, no. 5: 653–74.

DeWitt, Karen. 1997. "Never Too Young to Be Perfect." *New York Times*. January 12. Accessed October 11, 2016. http://www.nytimes.com/1997/01/12/weekinreview/never-too-young -to-be-perfect.html.

Featherstone, Mike. 1982. "The Body in Consumer Culture." *Theory, Culture, and Society* 1: 18–33.

Giroux, Henry. 1998 "Nymphet Fantasies: Child Beauty Pageants and the Politics of Innocence." *Social Text* 57: 31–53.

Gosselink, Carol A., Deborah L. Cox, Sarissa J. McClure, and Mary L. G. De Jong. 2008. "Ravishing or Ravaged: Women's Relationships with Women in the Context of Aging and Western Beauty Culture." *The International Journal of Aging and Human Development* 66, no. 2: 307–27.

Lakoff, Robin T., and Raquel L. Scherr. 1984. *Face Value: The Politics of Beauty*. Boston: Routledge & Kegan Paul.

Wing, Rena R, Karen A. Matthews, Lewis H. Kuller, Elaine N. Meilahn, and Pam L. Plantinga. 1991. "Weight Gain at the Time of Menopause." *Journal of the American Medical Association Internal Medicine* 151, no. 1: 97–102.

Appendix: Opposing Viewpoints

QUESTION 1
Psychology with a Scalpel: Does Cosmetic Surgery Boost Self-Esteem?

One of the distinct features of cosmetic surgery (sometimes referred to as "plastic" surgery) is that it transforms the face or the body irrevocably. In most cases, there is no way to "undo" the changes made by a practitioner's scalpel. Why might individuals be tempted to make such permanent and irreversible changes to their bodies? What factors motivate a person to wish for such dramatic changes to their appearance? How does one come to value and to prioritize the often painful and costly procedures of plastic surgery?

Some people believe strongly that the physical transformations to one's appearance made possible by medical and technological advances in cosmetic surgery enhance their own personhood, making them more fully into the person that they want to be. Those who seek these surgeries argue that the way a person feels about their own appearance is an integral part of their own wellness and sense of self. Enthusiasts claim that the opportunity to look younger, more attractive, or fitter allows them a wider range of options to create the life they truly desire, and research does show that those who conform more closely to social norms of beauty do have advantages in their personal and professional lives.

Additionally, there are many people who seek cosmetic surgeries to correct disfiguring accidents or birth defects in order to feel "normal." For these individuals, the decision to "go under the knife" is a highly personal one that allows that person to realize a goal about the self.

Typically, there are also those in Western cultures who object to elective cosmetic surgery as evidence of vanity or shallowness. This group, which occasionally includes some feminist activists who reject the rampant objectification of women's appearance in general, argues that those who believe in the individualistic, "empowering" capacity of cosmetic surgery may suffer from potentially dangerous delusions about the overly deterministic primacy of physical appearance and the capriciousness of physical beauty. This perspective argues that such significant changes to one's face or body do nothing to actually enhance the person, but rather, create a false illusion of temporary beauty, which in turn perpetuates unrealistic standards about how people are "supposed" to look.

Beyond issues of morality, vanity, or self-esteem, there are additionally valid concerns about the risks and dangers associated with aesthetic surgery. Any surgical procedure bears risk of side effects, infections, and even death. Surgeries can also fail to achieve the desired goal and may leave a patient feeling worse about their appearance than before. For each person, the risks and potential negative effects must be weighed against what they will gain personally and professionally by altering their appearance.

The following writers share some perspectives on this controversial topic.

RESPONSE 1
Psychology with a Scalpel: Yes, Cosmetic Surgery Boosts Self-Esteem
By Aimee Ross

You know you've thought about it. You have a body part or feature of your appearance that you would change if you could. Everyone does. It's part of the human condition and the psychological desire to feel normal or "fit in." So it makes sense, then, that having plastic surgery—whether reconstructive or cosmetic—to correct or enhance one's appearance also boosts one's self esteem. Statistics, the experts, and most importantly, the patients, all say so.

When it comes to cosmetic surgery, statistics and numbers suggest that perking up an aging body or face is significantly important to people's self-esteem—particularly middle-aged women. According to the American Society of Plastic Surgeons' annual report, cosmetic procedures in the United States in 2015 totaled 15.9 million and cost more than 13 billion dollars, a respective 2 and 4 percent increase since 2014. Women accounted for 92 percent of those having work done, and the largest age group—40- to 54-year-olds—made up almost half (49 percent) of everyone having plastic surgery. The next largest demographic group was ages 55 and over. Breast augmentation, liposuction, rhinoplasty, eyelid surgery, and abdominoplasty (tummy tuck) were the top five surgical cosmetic procedures, and Botox, soft tissue fillers, and chemical peels were the most common minimally invasive procedures. If these numbers (and body parts worked on) aren't convincing enough, the fact that 41 percent of all people having plastic surgery are having multiple procedures done—why not have several things "fixed" while under the knife?—is. In addition, a staggering 47 percent are repeat patients, coming back for more. (It is important to note that an additional 5.8 million reconstructive procedures—for example, tumor removal, scar revision, or hand surgery—were done in 2015, reflecting a different kind of investment in appearance, but they are not included in these numbers.)

The experts are also adamant that cosmetic surgery can boost more than one's self-esteem. Among those dissatisfied with a physical feature, people who actually undergo surgery can experience both psychological and physical benefits (Thorpe, Ahmed, and Steer 2004, 75). According to Honigman, Phillips, and Castle (2004), a "positive change in physical appearance for the patient will lead to an improvement in his psychological well-being, including his self-confidence and self-esteem" (p. 2). Patients hope to align their outward appearance with their body image/inner feelings, and when that happens, their psychosocial functioning increases (Ericksen and Billick 2012, 347), reducing anxiety and increasing social confidence (Honigman, Phillips, and Castle 2004, 5). In turn, all of this can affect a positive attitude, general health, and one's life satisfaction. In particular, Talwar and Puri found that successful scar revisions could dramatically improve a patient's quality of life because they can be psychologically distressing or "an unpleasant reminder of a trauma." Erasing the scar means erasing its memories (Talwar and Puri 2016, 155–156).

Statistics and experts, although significant and credible, don't reflect the actual voice of those who have had or are considering cosmetic surgery—the most important source for evidence of its effects. RealSelf.com, an online community since 2006, claims to be "the largest plastic surgery forum in the world dedicated to sharing what real people say about cosmetic and wellness results for treatments, products, and clinicians." Patients can write reviews, share before and after photos, rate their own results, participate in discussions or Q&As, and generally communicate with others who have had surgery or are thinking about it. In 2014 alone, the site had 51 million visitors (Realself 2016). The top-rated treatments on the site, according to the number of people who reviewed them, are 1. breast augmentation and 2. tummy tuck, both 97 per cent "worth it," and 3. the Brazilian butt lift, 93 per cent "worth it" (Realself 2016). Rhinoplasty, breast reduction, liposuction, scar removal, and eyelid surgery follow, with ratings anywhere from 89–98 percent "worth it" (Realself 2016). One woman from Cincinnati, Ohio, had this to say about her rhinoplasty:

> For years I wondered what it would be like to not be self-conscious about my appearance—in fact, most of my adult life. Finally, at age 55 I decided I'd had enough and to do something about it. While I wish I had had the procedure much sooner, I would advise others that it is never too late to choose to feel good about yourself—to make positive changes. Having the rhinoplasty dramatically improved my self-esteem. I no longer feel self-conscious, I feel more confident—it may sound silly, but this single surgery was a real life changing experience—all for the better! (anonymous, Realself 2016)

Another woman, who reviewed her "mommy makeover" (typically a combination surgery of breast augmentation, tummy tuck, and liposuction), cited an "improved body image after having two children," as well as less back pain since her stomach muscles had been repaired. She went on to say that getting the makeover was "one of the best things" she could do for herself: "If I had to do it over again, I totally would in a heartbeat. I feel so much better about my body. I love my kids but growing a human or two can really take a toll" (Realself 2016). Patients from a retrospective study about cosmetic surgery echoed similar results, particularly in terms of maintaining a youthful or "normal" appearance. One person had upper and lower eyelid fat removed after her rhinoplasty, because "I'm in my early fifties, and now that I've got this joy of not having an awful nose on my face, I felt I deserve a few years left of looking more confident and younger . . . I'm very, very happy with the results" (Thorpe et al. 2004, 82). Yet another person, who had a breast augmentation, said she was happy with results that made her feel more normal: "My breasts . . . don't look false or anything like that and you can't really tell that I've had implants done because I'm in proportion . . . they're just normal, I'm just a normal person now with a normal body" (Thorpe et al. 2004, 85).

Patients can experience negative psychological effects from cosmetic surgery, also. These may include an unchanged self-esteem (Thorpe et al. 2004, 76); depression, social isolation, or even self-destruction; or a loss of identity, or the need for multiple procedures (Honigman et al. 2004, 2). It is important to note, however, that most patients who experience negative psychological effects either already have mental health issues or likely suffer from body dysmorphic disorder, which cosmetic surgery cannot fix, particularly if what the patient wants "fixed" is considered a minimal defect (Ericksen and Billick 2012, 347). Screening patients prior to surgery, as well as offering patients proper presurgical preparation, may help with this. Because the general public has an inflated sense of the benefits of cosmetic surgery along with a minimized sense of risk, having realistic expectations of the results and understanding the risks involved are necessary for patient satisfaction (Ericksen and Billick 2012, 345).

Finally, the cosmetic surgery industry is only getting bigger. No longer is the cost outrageous or the stigma attached embarrassing. In fact, "the trend to seek help from a cosmetic physician is on the rise by more than 200%," and one in five U.S. women aged 18 to 64 are pursuing or plan to pursue plastic surgery (Realself 2016). The reality is that whether reconstructive or cosmetic, invasive or not, surgery of this kind offers hope and the chance for empowerment. When patients can improve their appearance, and thus body image, their self-esteem is boosted, or at the least, they feel "normal" again: a solution that also allows for pursuing a better quality of life.

Further Reading

American Society of Plastic Surgeons. 2015. "2015 Complete Plastic Surgery Statistics Report." Accessed July 22, 2016. https://www.plasticsurgery.org/news/plastic-surgery-statistics.

Ericksen, William, and Stephen Billick. 2012. "Psychiatric Issues in Cosmetic Plastic Surgery." *Psychiatric Quarterly* 83, no. 3: 343–352.

Honigman, Roberta J., Katharine A. Phillips, and David J. Castle. 2004. "A Review of Psychosocial Outcomes for Patients Seeking Cosmetic Surgery." *Plastic and Reconstructive Surgery* 113, no. 4: 1229–237.

Realself. RealSelf, Inc., 2016. Web. Accessed July 22, 2016.

Talwar, Ashutosh, and Neerja Puri. 2016. "A Study on Scar Revision." *Our Dermatology Online* 7, no. 2: 155–59.

Thorpe, S. J., B. Ahmed, and K. Steer. 2004. "Reasons for Undergoing Cosmetic Surgery: A Retrospective Study." *Sexualities, Evolution & Gender* 6, no. 2/3:7 5–96.

Von Soest, T., I. L. Kvalem, and H. E. Roald. 2009. "The Effects of Cosmetic Surgery on Body Image, Self-esteem, and Psychological Problems." *Journal of Plastic, Reconstructive & Aesthetic Surgery* 62, no. 10: 1238–44.

RESPONSE 2
Cosmetic Surgery: Boon or Bane?
By Leah Mueller

Physical appearance is a fluke of nature, as well as the luck of the draw. Some people have the good fortune to possess features that adhere to standardized ideals of beauty. Nature bestows less-than-perfect physical attributes upon others: slightly misshapen noses, protuberant chins, breasts that appear too large or too small. For the most part, folks learn to live with these perceived imperfections. But in a percentage of cases, the individual is so dissatisfied with her or his physical attributes that she or he seeks to alter them through surgical means. The process appears trouble free, yet there are many unseen pitfalls.

Every year, the United States hovers in the top five on worldwide plastic surgery lists. Breast augmentation is a perpetual favorite, totaling 279,143 procedures in 2015, according to the American Society for Plastic Surgeons' own website (American Society for Plastic Surgeons 2015). Liposuction came in a close second during the same year, with doctors performing over 220,000 surgeries.

During liposuction, excess fat deposits are removed from "trouble" spots of the body, such as the upper arms. The physicians then redistribute or discard the extra flesh and reshape the patient's body into a more desirable image. Extra breast padding is usually considered desirable, whereas the same amount of flesh on the upper arms is regarded as a detriment. Through the meticulous rearranging of flesh, doctor and patient seek to sculpt a more ideal physique. For U.S. women, this often translates into large breasts, slender but well-formed biceps, a tiny waist, and a round yet toned posterior.

This sort of body is almost impossible to maintain, especially after the age of 30. The inevitable ravages of time and gravity afflict us all. No one makes it to the grave with the pert body and smooth skin she or he took for granted during youth. This unalterable fact doesn't stop a large percentage of folks from spending a staggering amount of money to combat the passage of time. In 2013 alone, Americans spent the mind-blowing sum of $12 billion on plastic surgery procedures, including less invasive processes like Botox (Patt 2016). Women accounted for over 90 percent of the overall total, accounting for more than 10.3 million procedures.

Though plastic surgery remains most popular among women, a million U.S. men surgically altered their features in 2013. The majority of the procedures revolved around eyelid surgery and male breast reduction. Strangely, though the beauty-enhancing attributes of chest flesh are appreciated on female bodies, they are often shunned and derided on male ones.

The male ideal remains surprisingly similar to that of a Ken doll: muscular washboard abs, powerful legs, chiseled features. Similarly, the ideal female physique resembles Barbie's: an anatomically impossible structure to maintain. In real life, such a body would either topple or snap in half like a matchstick.

Needless to say, this pursuit of perfection puts a huge strain on both genders. Females, in particular, receive massive amounts of societal pressure to conform to conventional beauty standards. Little girls get the message early. They spend hours staring at themselves in the mirror, wondering whether they are good enough for society. Often, they feel inferior and do whatever they can to make themselves appear more attractive to others.

As girls mature, the message continues—looking perfect at all times is of paramount importance, and any deviation from this standard can result in severe castigation. As a result, 1 in 200 American women suffers from anorexia, and 2–3 percent are bulimic (Mirasol 2016). College-aged women's numbers are shockingly high: 10 percent of this group suffers at some point from a clinical eating disorder.

Presumably, if excessive exercise and starvation diets fail to achieve the ideal of perfection, cosmetic alteration is an attractive option. The surgery industry preys ruthlessly upon female insecurity. Their glossy pamphlets and Web sites peddle bliss—as long as women alter their features to conform to strict, yet capricious, standards. Changing beauty standards keep plastic surgeons very busy indeed. A modern woman's reasoning often runs like this: if I feel better with larger breasts/smaller buttocks/a shapelier nose/firmer belly, then what is the harm? Why not write a check for a few thousand dollars and go under the knife?

Apart from the hefty monetary expense and the emotional toll of surgical enhancement aimed to correct a lifetime spent disliking one's body, plastic surgery exacts another price—it's dangerous. Serious side effects include hematoma, deep vein thrombosis, nerve damage, and the risk of severe infection. The actual frequency of severe side effects is unknown. A Google search of "How many cosmetic surgery patients have serious side effects?" brought up a plethora of plastic surgery Web sites, but no real numbers. Though the Web site authors wrote glibly about side effects, they were reticent to disclose the prevalence of those complications—a discovery I found suspicious and troubling.

I was unsurprised to learn that cosmetic surgery often exacts a psychological toll as well. Perhaps the most alarming statistic was the rate of suicide among women who had undergone breast augmentation. In several countries, including Denmark, Finland, and the United States, the number of completed suicides was significantly higher among the surgery population (Sansone and Sansone 2007).

No one knows the reason for the correlation between breast augmentation and suicide, but several theories have been posited. Women who undergo this surgery are more likely to smoke and often have lower educational levels than ones who eschew the procedure. Such women are more likely to believe their bodies are their main social currency. When surgery fails to bring happiness, they become depressed.

Overall, the cosmetic surgery process contains more detriments than benefits. The perceived advantages of a sculpted face and body pale beside the danger of unwanted side effects that can lead to health complications, severe postsurgery depression, and even death. Perhaps more insidiously, the cosmetic surgery industry greedily reinforces the message that physical appearance is the main route to satisfaction.

We often forget the body is a container, and the interior is considerably more important than the exterior. No amount of surgery can bring lasting bliss. That strength and grace have to come from within. Perhaps if we placed more emphasis on self-love, the collective need to sculpt our bodies would disappear like the dinosaur. Meanwhile, cosmetic surgery does more harm than good in our continuing quest for happiness.

Further Reading

American Society of Plastic Surgeons. 2015. "2015 Complete Plastic Surgery Statistics Report." Accessed July 22, 2016. https://www.plasticsurgery.org/news/plastic-surgery-statistics.

Mirasol. 2016. "How Many People Have Eating Disorders?" Accessed November 1, 2016. http://www.mirasol.net/learning-center/eating-disorder-statistics.php.

Patt, Bradley. 2016. "How Much Does America Spend on Plastic Surgery?" Accessed November 1, 2016. http://pattmd.com/cosmetic-surgery-2/much-america-spend-plastic-surgery.

Sansone, Randy A., and Lori A. Sansone. 2007. "Cosmetic Surgery and Psychological Issues." *Psychiatry* 4, no. 12: 65–68.

QUESTION 2
Is Beauty a Biological Imperative or a Cultural Preference?

In 1859, Charles Darwin published his paradigm-smashing book *On the Origin of Species*, hypothesizing that all life on the planet evolves through the mechanism of natural selection. He argued that the individuals of a species who prove to be the most fit and best adapted to their environment are the best able to reproduce, passing on their genetic material to the next generation. However, Darwin's famous theory could still not entirely account for seemingly *mal*adaptive traits of some species, including the dazzling beauty of the colorful peacock. How, Darwin wondered, does the improbably extravagant tail of a flightless bird, which should only attract attention from predators and make the male *more* vulnerable to an early death, enable that very same peacock to reproduce successfully? Darwin speculated that "sexual selection" included a predisposition of the individual to feel arousal for particular individuals most able to display the visible cues to health and reproductive fitness. He suggested that successful mating in some species relied upon the ability of the individual to physically signal to potential mates a degree of desirable genetic fitness, interpreted by many scholars as a way of understanding the evolutionary significance of physical "beauty."

Over the years, biologists and social scientists have waged a battle over the continued significance of "beauty" and the degree to which perceived attractiveness influences, inhibits, or enhances personal development and social interactions. Does our species' sense of what is beautiful come from a universal, biological sense of "nature" that automatically registers pleasure or sexual desire on the body? Or is beauty bound up with a dynamic, cultural aesthetic honed in the ways that members of the group are "nurtured" to perceive attractiveness from childhood, and which may change many times during the course of one's life depending on such variables as experience, personal preference, exposure, and open-mindedness? And how might notions of ideal beauty change with time, space, and history? Scholars working in disciplines ranging from evolutionary biology to neuropsychology to cultural anthropology weigh in regularly on what incentivizes individuals to pursue sexual liaisons, but there is still no clear consensus on "the" determining factor shaping beauty. Psychological research does seem to agree that attractive children and adults are treated more favorably by others within their society, regardless of culture. Researchers defined people as attractive when the raters of that study agreed that they were attractive. But what factors specifically comprise a given cultural sense of beauty seem to be highly idiosyncratic. In fact, in cross-cultural investigations, there are remarkably few similarities in beauty preference that stand out.

The following writers offer more perspectives on this thought-provoking topic.

RESPONSE 1
What Could You Expect from a Nation that Has Won a Total of 22 International Beauty Pageants?
By Zaira Reveron

To Venezuelans, beauty certainly is a cultural preference. In this country, there is a multitude of archetypal beautiful women; on the one hand there is the stereotypical girl that conforms to the qualities required by national and international beauty pageants. On the other hand, there is the ordinary woman who, no matter her skin color, the wideness of her hips, bra size, type of hair, hair style, or height, also considers herself beautiful. Nevertheless, for women the important issue is not just to be beautiful, but to be good looking, attractive, elegant, and independent from an economic point of view. This is so, not just to please her partner, but also to feel wonderful or to compete with other women. In any case, the issue of beauty is important for both women and men, and in general for the whole society.

Venezuela is a tropical country located in the northern part of South America. This nation has won a significant number of beauty pageants at an international level. The first one, Miss World pageant, was won in 1955 in London, United Kingdom; from 1979 to 2013 Venezuela won seven Miss Universe titles and seven Miss International titles from 1985 until 2015, in addition to other international and regional beauty pageants. The international beauty pageants have certainly contributed to create a standard and a stereotype of female beauty. Since then the country has gained fame and experience in selecting capable, competent women who have the qualities to win—it has become a common belief for most people that all Venezuelan women are as beautiful as the pageant queens. In this nation, Rodríguez (2005) pointed out that every single town event, school, sports competition, carnival, etc., no matter whether it is small or big, poor or wealthy, close or far away from the city, is enhanced with the election of the "queen of the event." It has become a tradition, and all the girls wish to win—but to be crowned the "queen," one has to be beautiful, well dressed, elegant, and good looking in general.

An important part of the so-called beauty of the Venezuelan women can be dated back to the miscegenation process, a process that began in 1498 when the Spaniards began to colonize the territory. Next, they brought Africans to work as slaves in the coffee and coconut plantations. The integration process deepened when aboriginal, Spaniards, and Africans mixed among themselves. Following independence from the Spanish empire people from European countries, particularly Italy and Portugal, settled in Venezuela. Also, it is necessary to mention that the country received a large group of Jewish immigrants from different countries, like Germany, Austria, Romania, and Poland. Consequently, this migration from different nations and cultures contributed to strengthen the process of miscegenation already in place since the end of the 15th century. In fact, Castro de Guerra and Suárez (2010) have found in their research that Venezuela "is an amalgam country, a country of mestizos in the blood, the mentality and the culture." In general, Venezuelan people are really proud of being the result of the process of miscegenation and of their intercultural mélange. Indeed, in general people are convinced that this variable plays the most important role in being considered beautiful or good looking. Consequently, a good part of the Venezuelan culture consists of doing as much as possible to be beautiful women or handsome men.

It was common that women worked hard on their physical appearance, but nowadays men are also doing the same. Abreu Xavier (2011) has pointed out that Venezuelans love to look great, standing out as the peacock; for this reason they spend a lot of money on their clothing, shoes, accessories, jewelry, cosmetics, fragrances, hair care, hairdressing, makeup, skin care, etc. It seems that the wish to look great is deeply rooted in the Venezuelans. In fact, many of the women employees working as secretaries, saleswoman, or those who have to interact with the public in general are required to look presentable. Analyzing this topic, Finol (1999) asserts that there is a "technology of beauty," which goes from plastic surgery to jogging and body-building techniques." Furthermore, Venezuelan people, both men and women, in their eagerness to be fashionable have undergone different types of cosmetic surgeries to enhance their attractiveness, including nose jobs, breast and buttocks enhancement, liposuction, Botox to smooth face wrinkles, etc. Knowing that, banks as well as big retail pharmacy chains offer loans to their clients, and private hospitals also offer affordable prices and manageable payment mechanisms for cosmetic surgery, for example, buy one get one free. Hence, it is made easier for those interested to find the means to improve their beauty and attractiveness. In this respect, Cabrices (2007) discusses that in Venezuela the purchasing power of the population, the bank's decision to lend money, has allowed for an enhancement in the coquetry of the people.

Women try to be attractive mainly to satisfy themselves and compete among each other, not so much to please their partner. It is common to hear in informal conversations and at different levels of society that *there aren't ugly women, just badly dressed ones*. In the same way, it is necessary to add that makeup and hair care play an important role in the beauty of Venezuelan people. To illustrate the situation, in El Centro Comercial El Valle, a shopping mall located in the south area of Caracas, a lower-class living area in the capital of the country, there are eighty hairdressing salons plus hundreds of nail salons. In an interview with the owner of one of the hairdressing salons of this shopping mall, he pointed out that the majority of their clients require their services once per week. Moreover, he added that men are regular clients of these hairdressers. Likewise, El Centro Comercial Tolón Fashion Mall, located in Las Mercedes, a business area of Caracas, has two hairdressing salons. In an interview with the manager of one these salons, she asserted that their clients require their services every three days. This means that for Venezuelans, no matter the social class, skin color, or occupation, the issue of strengthening their appearance and presentability is of great significance.

To conclude, it is necessary to say that for Venezuelans beauty is a very important issue; the departure point is the miscegenation. From that point, Venezuelans consider themselves beautiful, not only women but also men. However, if it is not the case, there are different mechanisms and ways to become pretty; that is to say makeup, elegant and fashionable clothes, hairdressing, learning how to walk in a beautiful and decent way, plastic surgery, bodybuilding techniques, etc. Perhaps all of these are based on the stereotypes imposed by the beauty industry, but the fact is that the whole nation is deeply affected by the number of times that Venezuelan candidates have won first place in beauty pageants. Consequently, this fact may affect the view that Venezuelans have about themselves; that is to say if Venezuelan women have won such a number of times, then all Venezuelan women have the self-confidence that they must also be beautiful.

Further Reading

Abreu Xavier, Antonio de. 2011. *La pasion criolla por la fashion.* Caracas, Venezuela: Editorial Alfa

Cabrices, Rafael Osío. 2007. "La pujante industria de los sacerdotes del cuerpo." *Debates IESA.* 12, no. 3: 66–72.

Castro de Guerra, Dinorah, and María M. Suárez. 2010. "About the Mixture Process in Venezuela." *Interciencia* 35, no. 9: 654–58.

Finol, José Enrique. 1999. "Semiotics of the Body: The Myth of Contemporary Beauty." *Opción* 15, no. 28: 101–24.

Rodríguez, Albor. 2005. *Misses de Venezuela: reinas que cautivaron a un país: crónicas reportajes y testimonios del concurso Miss Venezuela,* 56. Caracas: Ediciones El Nacional.

RESPONSE 2
On the Irrelevance of Genetics
By Shara Johnson

Although deep in our human brains, there are clearly biologically and genetically motivated factors that drive our decisions toward mate selection, at this point in our evolution, it's impossible to point to a consistent model of beauty as the desirable trait mates look for in one another. Unlike, for example, peacocks, which universally "agree" that majestic tail feathers are the trait that signals health and reproductive suitability, or the birds of paradise, which all evaluate the same specific mating dance, the factors that motivate people around the globe to pursue sexual liaisons have become far more complex than the attraction to an evolved expression of physical and genetic fitness. In fact, genetic suitability has become largely irrelevant.

One common factor shaping a culture's definition of "beauty" is an individual's wealth or potential to achieve wealth or power. When this is consistently expressed by a physical characteristic within a culture, that becomes bound up in sexual attraction. Often these are maladaptive traits that specifically signal a person is of sufficient status or wealth that they need not toil in the common man's physical labor. Obesity has been regarded as beautiful in several cultures because of its cue that the obese individual has ample resources and represents high status. This physical characteristic isn't biologically evolved to induce sexual desire; the desire can only be learned from a culture that places a high value on material wealth.

Although physical fitness is a driver of evolutionary and sexual-selection theories—survival of the fittest (or more fit)—cultural preference for traits in which physical and reproductive fitness are irrelevant has become the prevalent approach to mate selection in humans. One of the most gruesome examples of culturally shaped beauty was the widespread custom of binding women's feet for centuries throughout large areas of China. Many men found these grotesque, deformed feet extremely attractive, yet they don't even look at all like human feet, but something almost equine. An expression of beauty that is more similar to another species entirely than to humans is difficult to argue as biologically evolved, particularly when it has an inverse relationship to physical fitness and is an illustration of pain and suffering rather than the vim and vigor evolution would typically choose.

Yet the bound feet were a fetish for many men, one might argue, because of the social aspects they implied about the woman. It began with wealthy women who were confined to their courtyards by the excruciating pain that prohibited walking much farther, and then lesser-status citizens wished to emulate the upper class, so it subsequently spread to the peasant class as well, which consigned hundreds of millions of women over the centuries to a lifetime of unspeakable pain. Not only were bound-feet women considered attractive within their societies, conversely, those with unbound feet were considered so brute and unattractive as to be under no consideration for marriage. Once foot binding was outlawed in the early 20th century by the government of the newly established Republic of China and reformists pronounced it a symbol of China's backwardness, the practice ceased and is now felt by most Chinese to be an abomination rather than an arousal of desire. So as the Chinese culture changed, its perception of beauty did as well. The inclination of a man to marry and reproduce with a bound-foot woman changed from very high to almost nil within a few decades.

Evolutionary fitness develops in a long-term process; "cultural fitness" can change quickly and dramatically. A current example of this is the frenzy of young people in Iran getting "nose jobs" to alter their facial physique to more closely resemble that of Western populations. Iranians didn't want this alteration until they were exposed to Westerners and Western culture through a variety of visual media that has recently become accessible to them. For millennia, Iranians have felt aroused by other Iranians; that is, their sense of self-beauty and desirability came from within their culture. The sudden wish to emulate the physical traits of those belonging to the dominant global culture cannot be an evolutionary process, particularly when such dominance has historically shifted and nothing indicates it will not shift again. And when it does, notions of desirability will change with it. Many will wish to emulate the dominate culture, whereas a counterculture will also inevitably evolve to conscientiously defy the social norms and establish a sense of beauty contrary to the majority simply for the sake of being contrary (take, for example, the "Goth" culture in America and how it defines beauty).

In many societies, senses of beauty encompass more than just the natural body, but also involve unnatural body modifications. The list of these examples is endless—lip plugs, body piercings, filing teeth, tattoos, and scarification—most of these are identifiers of culture or tribal affiliation. A person from a tribe known for its body scarification is unlikely to find a person from a tribe known for its enormous lip plugs attractive. Along these lines, what a culture considers beauty can often be synonymous with the prominent representation of the culture as a whole.

One illustration of this is the Himba tribe in southern Africa. Hallmarks of traditional Himba culture include the spreading of red clay all over women's bodies and hair; elaborate, impractical hairstyles; and the removal of several bottom front teeth. Not only are these considered attractive among members of their tribe, but they are the most easily and quickly recognizable banners of their long-held cultural continuity, which the Himba place great importance upon.

Mating with healthy people is incontrovertibly a biological imperative, but what are the traits that portray (or betray) poor health? A Google search on "missing bottom front teeth" displays within the first page of results chat and forum discussions that expose the difficulty of accepting people without teeth as attractive, with subject titles such as, "would you date a person missing teeth?" American culture struggles to find beauty in this. I would argue it's because in America, it's a sign of poor health to have teeth missing. In Himba culture, missing teeth are not indicative of poor health but of voluntary cultural identification. Whatever the practice was originally meant to symbolize or portray is no longer relevant; it's now an established tradition, and that in and itself is what makes the dental alteration perceived as beauty in a culture that values tradition.

In my travels through the world, I have met a bound-foot woman in China, I have seen the numbers of women with bandaged noses in Iran, I've stayed among the Himba in Namibia—I've seen all of these different cultures' ideas of beauty, and yet retain my own apart from all of those. This diversity proves the well-known saying, "Beauty is in the eye of the beholder."

QUESTION 3
The Rise of the Transgendered Beauty Pageant: Is Biology a Fixed Category?

Gendered norms and expectations create pressure on individuals to create gender-appropriate bodies. Most people work hard throughout their lives to conform to the ideal version of their gender according to the scripts of the culture, which may include additional complex standards for fitting in according to social class or racial identity. Beauty work is one way in which citizens shape their bodies to conform to societal gender norms, and both bodybuilding and beauty pageants celebrate and reinforce the idealized image of the masculine and the feminine across the world. Beauty work and beauty pageants are two ways in which community members perform the expectations of their gender, race, and class.

Biological gender, however, is not a universally shared concept. Western society is organized very clearly on a two-gender system that most people attribute to a clear-cut, two-sex biology that is often assumed to be "natural." These categories create a binary axis composed of two distinctly oppositional poles called "male" and "female" and based on the biological category of "sex" at birth (sometimes referred to as cis-gender).

However, many non-Western cultures observe a "third gender," a category of individual who is simultaneously considered to be both and neither gender. From the ritualistic role of the *hijira* of India, to the "manly-hearted" *berdache* of the northern plains Native American groups, to the *muxe* role embraced by the Zapotec people in Oaxaca (Mexico), there are many possibilities in the ethnographic literature that recognize a type of person who is neither male nor female.

"Transgender" is a term used to describe those whose gender identity or gender expression does not conform to social expectations for their birth sex. In the last few decades, there has been a rise in the visibility of transgender identities in Western society through the media and popular culture, prompting widespread discussions about the rights of transgender individuals to public spaces. More and more discussion is emerging about gender fluidity and the possibilities of identities "between" the genders.

The rising visibility of non–gender-conforming spaces in the United States and around the world has lent more attention to the ways in which this community celebrates distinct "looks" important to their unique communities. Across world cultures, people whose biological gender does not reflect their experience of their own gendered self practice a wide variety of beauty work to fashion bodies that more closely reflect the gender identity that they feel.

Transgender pageants like Miss International Queen, then, are one example that showcases the work of those seeking to perform a gender identity and beauty ideal that more closely aligns with their experience of self. This calls us to question what meaning we can find from the experience of the transgender pageant and the beauty work of those who do not fit traditional Western binary norms of gender.

The following writers share insights into this emerging site of beauty production.

RESPONSE 1
Transgender Beauty Pageants: An Imperfect Solution
By Tyler Omichinski and Ashley Cyr

Aesthetics and beauty are ever shifting by definition, evolving and changing to match the expectations of society. It is an unfortunate reality that aesthetics and beauty are still used to determine a great deal in our society, and they are often used to specifically determine who is the "other" in a given social context; this "other" all too often falls outside of the in-group of the aesthetic or the beautiful.

Beauty pageants are a means through which we determine and regulate the definition of beauty, and therefore necessarily, what falls outside of the definition of beauty. The transgender beauty pageant, then, challenges traditional aesthetic values while normalizing other forms of beauty. As a result, the value of transgender beauty pageants as a theoretically viable means through which to develop normalization of transgender people within society in practice is a subpar solution.

Historically, beauty pageants have often served as a way for society to determine who is considered to be part of the "in-group" as that society changes and develops. This was mostly tied to the fact that beauty pageants judge what is considered to be a de facto determination of what is the ideal of morality and health (Cohen, Wilk, and Stoelje 1996). In turn, these are functions of what is "healthy," as beauty pageants were tied to the rise of public bathing and only came about after the initial acceptance of degrees of this from spas and the like.

This process, however outside of the ideal, continues to move any individuals who partake in the pageant into the public sphere and toward normalization. Initial modeling appearances and other beauty pageants participated in the normalization of Cubans in 1930s America by bringing them into the public eye (Besnier 2002). This trend has repeated itself time and time again, each time starting with the outside group initially fetishized for their "otherness," only to become normalized over time. As they join the in-group, they are able to work to reclaim their own identities, shifting the way that society at large views them.

This, however, represents a historical but suboptimal method for outsiders to integrate into what is considered beautiful. Many argue that the fetishization and exoticization of transgendered people is not the ideal path to normalization, as this practice is currently resulting in some major problems (Wong 2005). For example, the current normalization of transgendered individuals is most often oriented around their ability to mimic either a realistic or a stereotyped version of a traditional gender type. As a result, they are not normalizing or developing their own personalities, but rather being pressured into developing one that is not true to them.

Further tied to this, the current situation is inexorably one that tests many transgendered persons' ability to mimic traditional gender roles, a factor that still defines them in terms of something outside of themselves by imposing outside norms on them (Wong 2005). Thus, instead of normalizing other ideas of beauty, we are merely rehashing or normalizing a particular existing subset of accepted looks, policing and controlling the way that another gender identity expresses itself.

Within the practice as it stands, through the performance of an exotic otherness (through costumes, names, dances, etc.), the socially marginalized contestants claim to define the local in ways that may oppose the received order, much like the importance of clothing choices as a form of agency, and the specific situations wherein those in higher classes within society are able to dictate the clothing choices of others, further reinforcing their status as "less than" in the public eye (Hansen 2004). However, the difference between locality and nonlocality remains controlled by the privileged (Besnier 2002).

A prime example of this performance of exotic otherness can be seen in Thai transgender pageants, a specific subset that has seen both much media recognition and significant academic inquiry into its dealings. In this particular instance, stereotypes often are used in marketing materials and surrounding media that is considered offensive: see the loud-mouthed, uncouth, pretentious, and always comic *kathoey* from Thai culture (Besnier 2002). Looking back into even our own North American history, we can see the portrayal of cross-dressing in our media, such as in *Friends* and *The Birdcage* where the cross-dresser is played for laughs, and there is a lack of effort made to differentiate between a transgendered individual and a cross-dresser. This is ultimately because most beauty pageants are commercial enterprises, all of which come with baggage such as an undying commitment to the bottom line above all else. The "one true winner" approach of the competition, tied inexorably to the ability to subvert masculinity into femininity (or the alternative) makes the subversion itself a commodity.

This subversion, however, is accomplished through means that require participants to play into a situation that already empowers the traditional binary and that requires transgendered individuals to define themselves solely in relation to that, rather than in a way that is true to themselves (Schacht 2005). The complications of this are further exacerbated by the limited economic options that are often available to members of transgendered beauty pageants, with the tension of trying to define oneself in their own terms, which are directly opposed to the desire to use the pageant as a tool for economic gain. This in turn forces them to pursue the ideal of being "real women," the verbiage that is so often used by those partaking in these pageants. The result is that, in the Thailand example, there is a sense that the participants are epitomizing themselves to a simplified and distorted portrayal for the edification and entertainment of others.

The fact that this has provided a path into the "mainstream" provides little solace for those currently living through this experience; nor does it guarantee a pathway into something more. With transgendered Americans, for example, four times more likely to live in poverty than others (Movement Advancement Project 2016), a variety of problems present themselves for approaching the current situation with this parallel (Besnier 2007). Though normalization is going to have to happen to be able to functionally integrate all those who fall somewhere outside of the two-sex biology approach to gender and sexuality, beauty pageants may present an unfortunately commercialized and subpar approach, even if there is the possibility that they will lead to normalization someday.

Further Reading

Besnier, Niko. 2002. "Transgenderism, Locality, and the Miss Galaxy Beauty Pageant in Tonga." *American Ethnologist* 29, no. 3: 534–66.

Besnier, Niko. 2007. "Language and Gender Research at the Intersection of the Global and the Local." *Gender and Language* 1, no. 1: 67–78.

Cohen, Colleen Ballerino, Richard Wilk, and Beverly Stoelje, eds. 1996. *Beauty Queens on the Global Stage: Gender, Contests, and Power.* New York: Routledge.

Hansen, Karen Tranberg. 2004. "The World in Dress: Anthropological Perspectives on Clothing, Fashion, and Culture" *Annual Review of Anthropology* 33: 369–92.

Movement Advancement Project. 2016. "Paying an Unfair Price: The Financial Penalty for Being Transgender in America." Accessed November 1, 2016. http://www.lgbtmap.org/unfair-price-transgender#sthash.cpnqDeSe.dpuf.

Schacht, Steven P. 2005. "Four Renditions of Doing Female Drag: Feminine Appearing Conceptual Variations of a Masculine Theme." In: *Gendered Sexualities,* edited by Patricia Gagné and Richard Tewkebury, 157–180. Seattle: Emerald Group Publishing.

Wong, Ying Wuen. 2005. "The Making of a Local Queen." International Transsexual Beauty Contest, Sexualities, Genders, and Rights in Asia: 1st International Conference of Asian Queer Studies, July 7–9, 2005. Accessed November 1, 2016. https://openresearch-repository.anu.edu.au/handle/1885/8692?mode=full.

RESPONSE 2
Transgender Pageants: An Occasion for Celebration
By Karen Craigo

We all have a past, and as a feminist today, I cringe a little to admit it, but in 1985, I was in a beauty pageant.

Many are reconsidering the issue of whether pageants are dehumanizing (my view) or empowering for women. Pageant contestant Lani Frazer (2015) writes, "Today's feminism is about allowing people to be whomever they choose to be, whether masculine, feminine, neither, or anywhere in between." She notes that if a woman chooses to participate in a pageant, it is nobody else's business to tell her she is wrong. It's true that self-determination seems like a reasonable feminist ideal.

And Frazer's view of traditional women's pageants offers a useful lens for considering the value of transgender beauty pageants, wherein those who have made a male-to-female gender transition compete for a crown.

The year of my pageant, the Modern Miss Teen Scholarship Pageant, is easy to recall, because from among a hundred pageant contestants, roughly fifty of them performed some version of Whitney Houston's 1985 smash hit, "The Greatest Love of All." Many sang it; some danced to it; one contestant even played it slowly, note by note, on a clarinet. Aside from a source for blackmail material (nipped in the bud by the publication of this article), there was little value to my experience.

Flash forward to today, and internationally, transgender beauty pageants are becoming more and more popular, even in seemingly unlikely places. Just this year, an Israeli pageant was won by an Arab Christian competing against a diverse field that also included Muslims and Orthodox Jews. Haaretz (2016) described the event as an "unconventional show of tolerance and coexistence."

These transgender pageants are a lot like my own traditional female beauty pageant, with evening gown, bathing suit, and talent competitions. Photographs from these pageants show unbelievably gorgeous women—the kind I once tried so hard to be—going through the pageant paces with poise and grace.

Thirty-some years later, I'm here—fully conscious, awake, a feminist. But in high school, I wanted to be the prettiest girl in a ball gown. I wanted a sash declaring me "Miss" something. I wanted a tiara shooting sparks of light from my head.

I made it to the semifinals, largely on the strength of my, ahem, clarinet solo. Finalists get a sash. Semifinalists get to report, years later, that they were semifinalists.

I still remember why I entered. There were scholarships involved, and a lot of people said I was pretty. Just like the similar impulses that got me to belly up to the dance barre or to hit the softball diamond, a "Why not?" attitude took hold, and I figured I'd give it a try.

In my defense—and I think this is about the only defense that realistically holds any water—I was a cis-gender sixteen-year-old girl, and looks mattered.

As an adult, I hold traditional women's beauty pageants in the very lowest regard. To me, they mark the worst in people—an obsession with looks, complicity with a culture that would dare to expect certain ways of standing and walking and sitting (as anything else would be unladylike), a further promotion of unnatural thinness and outsized secondary sex characteristics.

But when it comes to transgender beauty pageants, I'm not entirely opposed, and indeed, as Frazer suggests about her own pageant experience, it really is not my place to be. Transgender pageants appear to be positive celebrations of individuality, choice, and personhood.

In an article in *Broadly*, Diana Tourjee (2016) begins to define the difference, stating, "The honoring of physical beauty may carry special significance for transgender women, who are often punished—both by institutional discrimination as well as street-based and intimate partner violence—for daring to be beautiful, or for embodying their feminine form."

My sixteen-year-old self had her reasons for going for the crown. Beauty got me into the top dozen, but not the top five. Did I need to know that I was statistically in the top 10 percent of people gullible and comfortable enough to pay a pageant entry fee and then travel for a day of competition? Yes. Yes, I did.

The stakes are quite a bit higher for transgender women, who experience a strong correlation between gender conflict and major depression and suicide (Nuttbrock, Bockting, and Rosenblum 2012). The need to be recognized as a woman is almost exactly the same for an adolescent girl and a transgender adult, especially one who has recently transitioned. Just as girls feel they must look pleasing, transgender people feel they must pass as the target gender—and if either fails, the results can be traumatic.

Examine any photo from a transgender beauty pageant, and the physical beauty of the contestants is stunning. The issue of passing or not passing is in the rearview mirror; contestants are plainly beautiful, and a pageant lets them showcase not passing, but surpassing, by miles, the average woman, and even the average beauty queen.

I dearly wish we lived in a world where all people, wherever they are on the gender spectrum, were judged on the basis of their own intrinsic qualities—their intelligence and wit and warmth. Where my sixteen-year-old self and I part ways is that she cared about being beautiful, and I think physical beauty is a very silly thing to judge.

But it must be acknowledged that sometimes a physical transition follows a lifetime of yearning and effort, and the recognition of personal achievement is beautiful to celebrate.

Further Reading

Frazer, Lani. 2015. "In Defense of Beauty Pageants." Accessed November 11, 2016. https://bpr.berkeley.edu/2015/01/30/in-defense-of-beauty-pageants.

Haaretz. "Israeli Arab Ballerina Takes Crown in Israel's First Transgender Beauty Pageant—Culture." Israeli News, May 27, 2016. Accessed October 17, 2016. http://www.haaretz.com/israel-news/culture/1.721880.

Nuttbrock, L., W Bockting and A. Rosenblum. 2012. "Gender Identity Conflict/Affirmation and Major Depression across the Life Course of Transgender Women." *International Journal of Transgenderism*. Accessed October 17, 2016. http://www.tandfonline.com/doi/abs/10.1080/15532739.2011.657979.

Tourjee, D. 2016. "Bold and Beautiful: Behind the Scenes at America's Biggest Trans Beauty Pageant" *Broadly*. October 25, 2016. Accessed November 11, 2016. https://broadly.vice.com/en_us/article/daring-and-beautiful-behind-the-scenes-at-americas-biggest-trans-beauty-queen-pageant.

QUESTION 4
If Beauty Is Only Skin Deep, Why Is It So Important?

A popular cosmetic line in the United States carries the iconic tagline, "Don't hate me because I'm beautiful." Beauty elicits strong emotional responses from people in all places at all times in human history, capable of both elevating and degrading the individual. Depending on the cultural context, beauty may be sanitized or sexualized. Images of beauty can be transformative, causing people to change their behaviors, their relationships, and even their personal morality. Cautionary tales from around the world describe how perceptions of beauty ignite the spirit and compromise the soul.

Children are constantly told by adults that it is "what's inside that counts," but are children receiving mixed messages? Western culture abounds with fairy tales where "beasts" are shown to be worthy of beauty and rewards following trials of character. These stories coax children to see ugly ducklings as swans and to expect humble but beautiful servant girls to win the prince of the land because their moral behaviors match their physical beauty. These stories consistently encourage children to judge others based on actions and not appearances while overwhelmingly reinforcing a logic that assumes "beauty is good." Commonly heard phrases seem to shape what Westerners believe to be fundamental truths about beauty and conventional attractiveness: "beauty is in the eye of the beholder," "never judge a book by its cover," and "beauty is only skin deep." Each of these maxims cautions against making judgments about the worth of an individual based on a single assessment of physical appearance. Empirically, if beauty is only in the eye of the beholder, judgments of attractiveness should do little to influence the conditions of one's life. Similarly, if conventional wisdom urges people to disregard external appearance and to direct attention instead to the behavior or personality of an individual, beauty should not have any effect on the ways people interact, either with their familiars or with strangers.

And yet, paradoxically, study after study conducted by psychologists demonstrates that the effects of attractiveness, especially facial attractiveness, confirm a distinct and biased association in most viewers between beauty and favorable personal qualities. People make important decisions about others based on perceptions of beauty, and these impressions have real-world effects: decades of research in the social sciences show us that those deemed to be more beautiful are treated more positively and are thus more likely to be offered a job, given preferential treatment, or assumed to be morally superior to those judged less attractive. The politics of beauty at the social level also signify difference in powerful and subversive ways, continually reinscribing hardened sets of cultural biases that both produce and reproduce racialized beauty ideals from one generation to the next.

The following writers explore more facets of the cultural norms and experiences that influence social behaviors with regard to beauty.

RESPONSE 1
Beauty and the Law
by Janis L. Prewitt

Since 1964, it has been illegal to discriminate in employment. Title VII of the Civil Rights Act was passed to eliminate discrimination based upon race, color, sex, national origin, and religion. President Johnson signed the Civil Rights Act of 1964. Title VII of the act barred private employers of twenty-five or more workers from discriminating against job applicants and employees on the basis of sex, race, national origin, or religion. The act, however, provided a potential loophole in the "BFOQ" clause, which allowed employers to discriminate in "those certain instances where religion, sex, or national origin is a bona fide occupational qualification [BFOQ] reasonably necessary to the normal operation of that particular business or enterprise."

It is to this law that we look to emphasize that employees should be treated equally. The law in the United States has recognized that beauty should not be a factor in employment; however, not in every case. The courts need to establish clear guidelines that recognize attractiveness is not a qualification for employment.

The Oxford Dictionary defines beauty as "a combination of qualities, such as shape, color, or form, that pleases the aesthetic senses." How do we define beauty: Is it by the amount of makeup we wear? By the size of our bodies? Is it by our age? Is it by our race or national origin? Is it by our wealth? By the clothes that we wear? Is it by our marital status? Every person has their own perception of beauty.

Certain industries have long discriminated based on the attractiveness of the job applicant or employee. The airline industry is one of those industries. In fact, as early as commercial aircraft began flying the companies had standards that the "stewardesses" (now called "flight attendants") must meet certain minimum standards for appearance, and they must be female and not married. They also had a maximum age of 26. The standards also included height and weight restrictions for the females. Because they were not married, obviously pregnancy was not permitted. A violation of any of these standards was grounds for either not hiring or terminating a current employee.

These standards were upheld and recognized as legal up through the 1970s when the U.S. Supreme Court recognized that being thin and attractive was not a BFOQ for serving a soda or protecting the safety of passengers. The court also recognized that being female or not married was not a qualification for that job. The airline industry was forced to change its hiring and employment practices.

So how does Abercrombie and Fitch justify their employment practices? It is not from the lack of the lawsuit—there have been plenty of lawsuits; however, the courts are inconsistent in the results. Some courts recognize that attractiveness is a BFOQ for selling their clothes, believing the idea put forth by the retailer that "sex sells."

Hooters Restaurant has been a defendant in many employment lawsuits. Those cases seem to settle before going to trial, and so they never make it on appeals to see how the judges react to the argument that one must have a certain body type to serve wings and beer. Victoria's Secret may have the best argument for only hiring females; however, they could find certain positions for males. The argument that the salespeople need to be attractive should fail, as those salespeople are not "modeling" their apparel in the store.

Although the Supreme Court was clear that they would not stand for employment qualifications that have an impact on the classes of individuals that Title VII protects, such as the airline industry did with its flight attendants, we clearly need to have more direction in other industries. Dress codes are one modern method of discrimination. Requiring women to wear certain items while not requiring it of men has a disparate impact on females. For example, requiring women to wear pantyhose while not requiring the men to wear them is unfair. Requiring women to wear closed-toed shoes while not requiring everyone to wear closed-toes shoe is illegal.

The law has moved a long way in favor of nondiscrimination because of the way a person looks or what she wears; however, more improvement is needed to achieve total equality in the workplace. The only legal way to create new law is for employment applicants and current employees to point out when a policy or employment rule unfairly affects a class of individuals meant to be protected by Title VII signed into law many years ago. It is not acceptable to use beauty as a standard by which to hire and employ, and the law needs to consistently reflect this principle through enforcement by the courts.

RESPONSE 2
Language Is Skin Deep—A Glance at Metaphorical Beauty
by Marina Manoukian

In a literal sense, sight is one of our most immediate senses; nothing travels faster than light, so information will often hit our eyes before anything else. As a result, it seems fair to say that most of what we as humans understand initially comes from the information we gather by looking. Even most of our science initially stemmed from experience that involved seeing if there were any changes. But then how does this immediacy of sight affect our understanding of other humans, who are much more complex than what is seen at a cursory glance?

In recent years, with science taking the forefront in explaining causes and effects, we try to uphold a purely biological justification. Outward beauty, which often includes highly symmetrical features, is seen as a representation of good genes and good health, which we cannot help but be attracted to as a result of our biological tendencies. We attribute lust to pheromones and fall back on a fatalistic tendency; we can't help ourselves. There are even "sex addicts" who displace the element of choice into predisposed addiction. But although science and biology have been enormously helpful in understanding and trying to explain the world around us, they both fall short in entirely describing humanity and our relationships with one another. It's difficult to observe an experiment while simultaneously being a significant part of it. This is why we can turn to stories and our language in an attempt to understand our behavior, as our thoughts and words are our own attempts to articulate it.

Fairy tales and myths are often the first stories told in an attempt to explain. Growing children are told fantastical stories to describe morals and underline justifications. Early civilizations come up with epics and legends of heroes and monsters in their first attempts to characterize and understand the world around them. At this current time I will refer to only Western tales and language, though this phenomenon is widespread among various cultures. Our setup often includes a beautiful young maiden, whose inner beauty will prevail against others, though her outer beauty would often be a big help too. Cinderella's outer and inner beauty charmed Prince Charming, but doesn't it matter that her stepsisters were ugly on the inside? Isn't that the lesson we should learn? I hesitate to mention The Ugly Duckling, because the story is an example of the reality that although we like to say the outside doesn't matter and that you shouldn't let others belittle you for your appearance, it sure is lucky that the "ugly" duckling gets to grow up to be a beautiful swan. We hear these words and stories while growing up in the contemporary United States, and the metaphors and aphorisms end up following us around the rest of our lives in the form of motivational posters or bumper stickers. But how much of these metaphors about beauty are we merely taking at face value?

Everyone has heard the aphorism that "beauty is in the eye of the beholder." Essentially, beauty is taken out of essence; there is no intrinsic beauty that objectively exists. It is up to the viewer to valuate that beauty of a subject/object, and different viewers and beholders may hold different standards of beauty. This metaphor opens up a subjective relationship of beauty; beauty doesn't exist within the object—it only exists once there is a beholder to determine beauty, similar to the sentiment of whether or not a fallen tree makes a sound if there is no one to hear it. It is up to a relationship between two subjects or object/subject to establish the beauty of something. With regard to underlining the subjective nature of beauty, this is a useful metaphor. But it still pins beauty down to the surface, to appearance, because what can the eye see but appearance, even if it is a beholder's eye? If the beholder is to care instead about what is inside rather than outside, why does beauty then exist in his or her eye? Shouldn't beauty be in the conversation with the beholder? In the time spent getting to know beauty's personality? It also brings up the question of which beholder we should take into account: an other's or our own beholding in a mirror? Does it matter what others behold?

We've also heard the aphorism that "beauty is only skin deep"—the idea that despite any physical perfections and glorifications, any physicality is limited to the literal surface of a person. The amount that beauty makes up in a person's being is literally skin deep. Although what is inside may have been affected and altered based on how this person was treated as a result of their looks, their outside beauty has no bearing on what kind of person they are. In a sense, beauty should be taken for granted (by the beholder) because it has no bearing on what truly matters in a person. But if this is the case, what does it mean when someone says, "Oh, they're beautiful on the inside"? If beauty is only skin deep, then whatever they are inside, does it make sense to refer to these qualities as beauty as well? In these cases, beauty often means appealing, attractive, good, kind—a lot of positive adjectives that come hand in hand with the importance of appearances. There's even the saying that someone is "easy on the eyes," as though unattractive people are literally difficult to look at.

How does this compare to the idea that beauty is only within the beholder? If it's skin deep, that means it's within the skin before the beholder ever got the chance to behold it. Is the statement "beauty is only skin deep" a metaphor as well? It rings similarly to "don't judge a book by its cover." It's the idea that outward appearances don't count, that they shouldn't be used to form value judgments, that it's what's inside that counts. But in this case, beauty is found on the inside, in substance, in personality. But then is this beauty also in the eye of the beholder? Is there any quantifiable substance of beauty that may be determined? An essence of beauty, one might say, that exists outside of the existence and actions of a person? Or is beauty created through those very actions? Can these actions be called beautiful in the same way that we call an actress beautiful?

If beauty is truly only skin deep, is irrelevant, and is outside of our own determinations, then why do we encourage self-beauty? Why do we encourage styles and the use of fashion to display one's personality? Can we display accurately whatever it is we are on the inside? Why not dress in uniform and allow for actions to speak for themselves? Perhaps Shakespeare's line, "Beauty is bought by judgment of the eye," may now reflect more about the marketing interests of the fashion industry than before. But beauty may be bought, bartered, and sold because we have turned it into a commodity. And like all commodities, its value is whatever we ascribe to it.

QUESTION 5
How is Men's Beauty Increasingly Commodified?

Anyone who has ever taken an art history class knows that the appreciation of male beauty began long before our contemporary era. Sculptures and paintings from the classical world present the viewer with lean, fit, young heroes, chiseled with fine features and plenty of muscle tone. Noble men of Renaissance Europe spent time being fitted for fine clothing, and men of high birth wore wigs well into the 17th century.

The history of the United States, however, seemingly changed the imperative for men to cultivate standards of male beauty, instead demanding that "regular Joes" cultivate a rugged and almost deliberate lack of interest in their looks. The masculine ideals of the 18th-century man in the United States reflected landownership and agrarian roots based on production to a marketplace that could yield wealth, power, and status to the right kind of man. In the 20th century, Hollywood legends like John Wayne promoted a scruffy, unpolished vision of hegemonic masculinity ideally suited to a life of action and horseback. "Real men" of this era were expected to present themselves as invulnerable, repressing both emotion and affection. They sought to convey confidence and self-reliance while devaluing traditional female activities, including child care to beauty work. In the United States, ideal masculinity (regardless of race, ethnicity, class, age, or religion) promoted a traditional slate of values for adult manhood that included strength, size, youth, and (hetero)sexual virility.

In the early 21st century, American media sources announced the rise of the "metrosexual." Men, especially those who identified as gay or were living in urban areas, were actively encouraged by a rising wave of grooming and styling products to consume branded products designed to enhance their appearance. Some theorists have speculated that this transformation marks the shift from a modern industrial culture based on production to a "postmodern" culture where identity revolves around the personal consumption of products, ideas, and knowledge. Significantly, these economic and social transformations affected gender roles and gender identity, opening spaces for new expression of the self and personhood that might entail new strategies for "looking good."

Meanings of male beauty are arguably at a critical period of change, with new media representations taking cues directly from the well-rehearsed ways in which the female body has been carved up and offered to the male gaze for approval for decades. The lucrative market of men's magazines offering tips for male readers to look their masculine best has proliferated, with titles including *Men's Health* and *Maxim*. Most feature photographic spreads of male models with well-developed muscles in the arms, pectorals, and the ubiquitous "six-pack" abdomen complete with diet and exercise plans designed to cultivate a "hard" body. Surveys suggest that men think more about their appearance now than ever, and the demand for cosmetic surgery from male customers increased in the past decade.

Are men increasingly being encouraged to care about their looks in a different way than they have in the past? Are male consumers being seduced into spending disproportionate amounts of time and resources on products designed to improve their appearance? Is male beauty synonymous with female beauty in the contemporary United States or in other nations? The following authors offer opinions and perspectives on this timely topic.

RESPONSE 1
Men's Beauty
By Alejandro Arango-Londoño

Beauty has been considered a realm exclusive to women. Even though hygiene and self-care practices (brushing teeth, showering, hair care, skin care) during the 20th century were directed to the society as a whole (Noguera 2003; Quevedo, Borda, and Eslava 2004), beauty products such as weight gainers, perfumes, and cosmetics were created and thought for the female body (Pedraza 1999). In a context such as Latin America with strong race, class, and gender inequalities, dealing with a matter such as beauty might be considered not sufficiently relevant in social research. I will argue that beauty, including male beauty which has often been overlooked in scholarly research, is intertwined with sociocultural dynamics.

In his ethnography of Brazil, Alexander Edmonds argues that beauty is relevant because of the myth of the beautiful Brazilian women. This, according to Edmond's ethnography, translates into a large industry of plastic and cosmetic surgery devoted to correct imperfect bodies. Essentially, being beautiful is a requirement for being a Brazilian woman (Edmonds 2010). The point here is that beauty is contextual. In Colombia, for instance, newspapers from the mid-20th century portrayed fatty female and male bodies as ideals of beauty. These advertisements compared to those from today by Victoria's Secret or Calvin Klein show completely different bodies: more slender, more athletic, less racially mixed.

We could list the features of *the beautiful man* at a global level; but the truth is that beauty acquires more density and meaning when it is narrowed to specific contexts. Beauty is more of a system of classification than a simple descriptive category (beautiful vs. ugly). The Latino man, for instance, might be briefly defined as a muscular voluptuous man, average height, with darker skin, thick hair, big pectorals, big arms, and big buttocks. However, is it just the looks that make the Latino man a true Latino man?

Beauty includes a moral dimension as well. It embodies a set of behaviors, knowledge, and thoughts. Most people would agree that beauty is not only about physical appearance: beauty is a *way of life*. Part of being a beautiful man, at least in Latin

America, has to do with virility and a *strong* masculinity. With "strong" masculinity, I'm referring to the stereotype of machismo that is said to characterize Latin American gender dynamics. This macho-like feature is not necessarily about sexual orientation: it is a body performance. As Carrillo shows, macho-acting homosexuals in Mexico can be considered more attractive (more beautiful) than effeminate gays (Carrillo 2003). The beautiful man must not only be attractive on the outside, but also attractive in the inside. The latter is achieved through certain forms of behaviors.

This means that beauty is gendered. Female aesthetics and male aesthetics work differently. I would not agree with a rampant juxtaposition of the feminine and the masculine in terms of beauty; although it is true that "gender is relational" as Joan Scott states (1985). This same idea applies for beauty. It is not possible to define male beauty without female beauty. An interesting way to explore how beauty is gendered is through the emergence of new markets that address male aesthetics. During the last fifteen years in some Latin American countries, supply of plastic surgery, aesthetic treatments, and cosmetic products exclusive for men have intensified.

From generic products and procedures for beauty, we now find cosmetic interventions *for* men only. These new treatments embody new economic niches rooted in biomedical research that shows why and how men need special interventions because their bodies are different from those of women. Even though some of these procedures mirror some of the most popular among women (i.e., liposuctions and Botox), they are performed differently. For example, liposuctions on men can be more aggressive (extract more fat), whereas liposuctions on women must leave some fat on the tissues for health reasons.

In the same manner, biomedical research has shown that men's skin differs from women's in their pH level; therefore, they need specific products (Revista Imagen 2015). Hence, we see the emergence of cosmetic lines for men: body creams, skin care products, beard and hair care, and waxing products, just to mention some of them. Although body and beauty are more malleable than ever before, they are also a locus for neoliberal capitalism to exploit subjectivity through the idea of being beautiful (or attractive, which might sound "better" among men).

The contents of these "beauties" differ descriptively: women might not care that much about being muscular as men do, whereas men might not care that much about makeup as women do. However, as cultural phenomena, male and female beauty coincide in the idea of being achievable, not inherited. As achievable, they require investment from subjects. This investment takes at least three forms: economic (spend on beautification products), time (make time for beauty: gym and everyday self-care), and moral (learn the regimens of beauty: learning what is/is not beautiful, behaving as a beautiful person). The economic dimension of male beauty implies that those who cannot afford it are automatically excluded from the social benefits of beauty.

So far, I have argued that male beauty is contextual, historic, and gendered. As a cultural phenomenon, it is also part of neoliberal economic dynamics that punish those who cannot afford it and praises those who achieve a beautiful status. The relevance of this is enhanced in contexts such as Colombia or Brazil, in which physical appearance is a crucial aspect of social life. The emergence of a new beauty of male aesthetics not only means a whole new economic niche for capitalism to be exploited, but also a resignification of masculinity (or masculinities). These new emergent masculinities would incorporate male beauty, but this would not necessarily mean a feminization of masculinity. In fact, male beauty narratives reify "traditional" descriptions of manhood: athleticism, virility, strength, discipline, and hard work. Despite the interesting similarities we might find between male and female beauty, the contemporary world encourages us to think in more depth about how male beauty is codified by reproducing gender relations, economic processes, and cultural dynamics.

Further Reading

Carrillo, H. 2003. "Neither Machos nor Maricones. Masculinity and Emerging Male Homosexual Identities in Mexico." In *Changing Men and Masculinities in Latin America*, edited by Matthew Gutmann, 351–369. Durham, NC: Duke University Press.

Eco, Umberto. *History of Beauty*. New York: Rizzoli, 2004.

Edmonds, Alexander. 2010. *Pretty Modern: Beauty, Sex, and Plastic Surgery in Brazil*. Durham, NC: Duke University Press.

Noguera, Carlos. E. 2003. *Medicina y política. Discurso médico y prácticas higiénicas durante la rimera mitad del siglo XX en Colombia*. Medellín, Colombia: Cielos de Arena-Fondo Editorial de la Universidad EAFIT.

Pedraza, Zandra. 1999. *En cuerpo y alma. Visiones del progreso y de la felicidad*. Bogotá, Colombia: Universidad de Los Andes.

Quevedo, Emilio, Catalina Borda and Juan Carlos Eslava. 2004. *Café y gusanos. Mosquitos y petróleo. El tránsito desde la higiene acia la medicina tropical y la salud pública en Colombia 1873–1953*. Bogotá, Colombia: Universidad Nacional de Colombia.

Revista Imagen 2015. No. 172, Dec.—Feb. Accessed January 30 2017. http://www.revistai magen.com.co/

Scott, Joan. 1985. "Gender: A Useful Category for Historical Analysis." *The American Historical Review* 91, no. 5: 1053–75.

RESPONSE 2
Subtle Play by Mr. Gray
by Karen Craigo

The men's grooming industry is booming, and companies producing men's hair care products, shaving supplies, skin care lines, and fragrances saw a 300 percent increase in sales in 2015 alone (Fury, 2016). But outside of the urban centers of the United States, the rise in men's grooming isn't always readily apparent. Those who identify as male and reach for specialized grooming products may be doing so stealthily.

I was raised by an Appalachian father who styled his hair with water—who considered even an old-style pomade, like Brylcreem, to be just a little bit unmanly. His one concession to beauty was a no-frills foamy shave cream. Other than that, and sometimes in place of that, a bar of soap met most of his needs.

Despite what television commercials and magazine ads seem to convey about the keen interest in men's grooming products, I don't always see it in the places where

I've spent most of my life—Appalachia, Midwest farm country, and the Ozarks. In such places, men often present themselves as rather low maintenance; often, their preferred hair treatment is a baseball cap.

There are exceptions, of course. In my city of Springfield, Missouri, some elite men's salons are taking off, like Hudson / Hawk Barber & Shop, which offers a $25 shave. And here in the Ozarks, there is also the Ozark Beard Company, which provides beard oil in scents like Moss Man and Urban Bourbon. Although the men's care industry is surging like never before, locally, at least, it is relying on nostalgia for barbershops and on formulae that seem to align with craft beer and small-batch spirits.

Remember those men's hair color commercials with Walt "Clyde" Frazier and Keith Hernandez? In the most famous of these, pro athletes Frazier and Hernandez are in a bar. They wear suit jackets and hold microphones, and they offer a play-by-play as a handsome man with a grizzled beard approaches a beautiful woman.

The man is shot down in his attempt. "Rejected!" the sports figures say in chorus.

"No play for Mr. Gray," Frazier reports.

In the commercial, Mr. Gray retreats to the bathroom to apply Just for Men Hair Color Gel and then returns, artificially darkened, to snag the woman—or, more accurately, to be snagged by the woman, who yanks him into an embrace.

Obviously, a national, prime-time commercial buy like this Just for Men campaign requires that a product hit everyone—not just the executive, metropolitan men who tend to be depicted in them. And in the broad belly of America, the land between the coasts, a lot of men seem to ignore the supposed revolution in men's grooming—at least, that's what anecdotal evidence suggests.

If the average Midwestern man is to buy into the grooming trend—and the sales figures suggest that they have, quietly—promotions must hit them on one of two levels:

1. Humorously. "No Play for Mr. Gray" has recently made a comeback. Walt and Keith introduce a report from a family's kitchen, where a gray-bearded man breakfasts with his family.

"Hold the show!" says one. "That gray beard is a no-go!" says the other.

At the end of the commercial, the broadcasters are sitting on a bedroom dresser and eating from a bowl of popcorn, mics in hand, as a couple begins to enjoy the benefits of dark facial hair.

Almost any ad for women's hair color will feature slow-motion shots of blazing red or sunny blond locks moving in contrived sunlight, and humor of the broad sort exhibited by Just for Men is eschewed. A comedian may be featured in an ad for women's hair color, but that woman had better lean toward the conventionally beautiful end of the spectrum, like Tina Fey, and the comedy needs to be low-key. Beauty first. Laugh later—but only a little so your face doesn't freeze that way.

2. As sexual enhancement. Men's beauty products, to appeal to an average middle-of-the-United States guy, exist to snare beautiful female partners. But I can't think of a commercial for a grooming product that does this without also including humor, because to be too open about the need for hair color to achieve human connection can

read as kind of sad. And if you're a guy who seeks human connection with other guys through improved self-care, there is almost no chance that you'll see yourself reflected in an advertisement for men's products, even as commercials for everything from insurance companies to cereals to vacation destinations begin to catch up to the rest of society.

I am willing to believe that Midwesterners are just an odd bunch, but as East and West Coast Americans look inward with perplexity, we look right back at them, equally stumped.

One summer I was lucky enough to score an artist's residency in Provincetown, Massachusetts. It was an incredible summer—as different from my life then in Ohio as anything I could have imagined, and I don't mean because Provincetown is considered the nation's "gayest city," at 16.3 percent (Moylan 2011).

It wasn't until I got home after my three months away that I realized what was so different about East Coast people. I realized it at an Ohio bar, all of my friends sitting around in jeans and T-shirts, many of them with ball caps in place. The East Coast vibe meant that people were always very spiffy, from my Midwestern perspective— buying groceries in outfits that I might wear to a job interview, everyone gelled up top, skin smooth with emollient.

The American personal care industry is thriving, and men's grooming products are on the rise, with $4.1 billion sold in 2014, up 19 percent from 2009 (Booth, 2014). Here where I live, though, it appears to me that men who reach for the moisturizer are still doing it on the sly.

Further Reading

Beard Care, Oil, & Men's Grooming Products. 2016. Accessed November 11, 2016. http://www.ozarkbeardcompany.com.

Booth, Barbara. 2014. "Real Men Don't Cry—But They Are Exfoliating." Accessed October 17, 2016. http://www.cnbc.com/2014/12/05/real-men-dont-cry-but-they-are-exfoliating.html.

Fleming, K. 2015. "Keith Hernandez and Clyde Frazier Are Back with Hilarious New 'Just for Men' Ad." *New York Post*, August 3. Accessed October 17, 2016. http://nypost.com/2015/08/03/keith-hernandez-and-clyde-frazier-are-back-with-hilarious-new-just-for-men-ad/.

Fury, A. 2016. "Men's Grooming Is Now a Multi-Billion Pound Worldwide Industry." *The Independent,* January 14. Accessed November 11, 2016. http://www.independent.co.uk/life-style/fashion/features/mens-grooming-is-now-a-multi-billion-pound-worldwide-industry-a6813196.html.

Hudson / Hawk Barber Shop | Springfield and Kansas City. 2016. Accessed November 11, 2016. https://hudsonhawkbarbers.com/.

Moylan, B. 2011. "The U.S. Census Declares the Gayest City in America." *Gawker*, August 22. Accessed October 17, 2016. http://gawker.com/5833349/the-us-census-declares-the-gayest-city-in-america.

Vimeo. "Just For Men 'Play By Play':30." Accessed October 17, 2016. https://vimeo.com/40472851.

Selected Bibliography

Adrian, Bonnie. 2003. *Framing the Bride: Globalizing Beauty and Romance in Taiwan's Bridal Industry.* Berkeley, CA: University of California Press.

Alloula, Malek. 1983. *The Colonial Harem.* Minneapolis: University of Minnesota Press.

Anderson-Frye, E. P. 2012. "Anthropological Perspectives on Physical Appearance and Body Image." In: *The Encyclopedia of Body Image and Human Appearance*, edited by Thomas F. Cook, 15–22. San Diego: Academic Press.

Bailey, Eric. J. 2008. *Black America, Body Beautiful: How the African American Image Is Changing Fashion, Fitness, and Other Industries.* Westport, CT: Praeger.

Barber, Kristin. 2016. *Styling Masculinity: Gender, Class and Inequality in the Men's Grooming Industry.* New Brunswick, NJ: Rutgers University Press.

Barnes, Natasha. 2006. *Cultural Conundrums: Gender, Race, Nation, and the Making of Caribbean Cultural Politics.* Ann Arbor, MI: University of Michigan Press.

Barrig, Maruja. 2001. *El mundo al revés: Imágenes de la mujer indígena.* Buenos Aires: CLASCO.

Becker, Anne E. 1995. *Body, Self, and Society: The View from Fiji.* Philadelphia: University of Pennsylvania Press.

Berry, D. Channsin and Bill Duke. 2011. *Dark Girls.* Film. Directed by D. Channsin Berry and Bill Duke. Duke Media and Urban Winter Entertainment.

Boone, Sylvia Arden. 1986. *Radiance from the Waters.* New Haven, CT: Yale University Press.

Bordo, Susan. 1993. *Unbearable Weight: Feminism, Western Culture, and the Body.* Berkeley, CA: University of California Press.

Butler, Judith. 1990. *Gender Trouble: Feminism and the Subversions of Identity.* New York: New York University Press.

Byrd, Ayana D. and Lori L. Tharps. 2001. *Hair Story: Untangling the Roots of Black Hair in America.* New York: St Martin's Griffin.

Chalfin, Brenda. 2004. *Shea Butter Republic: State Power, Global Markets, and the Making of an Indigenous Commodity.* New York: Routledge.

Chernin, Kim. 1985. *The Hungry Self: Women, Eating and Identity.* New York: Harper Perennial.

Chernin, Kim. 2009. *The Obsession: The Tyranny of Slenderness.* New York: HarperCollins.

Cohen, Colleen Ballerino, Richard Wilk and Beverly Stoeltje, editors. 1996. *Beauty Queens on the Global Stage: Gender, Contests, and Power.* New York: Routledge.

Cordwell, Justine and Ronald A. Schwartz, editors. 1973. *The Fabrics of Culture: The Anthropology of Clothing and Adornment.* Chicago: International Congress of Anthropological and Ethnological Sciences.

Corson, Richard. 1965. *Fashions in Hair: The First Five Thousand Years.* London: Peter Owens Publishing.

Craig, Maxine Leeds. 2002. *Ain't I a Beauty Queen? Black Women, Beauty, and the Politics of Race.* New York: Oxford University Press.

Crais, Clifton C. and Pamela Scully. 2009. *Sarah Baartman and the Hottentot Venus: A Ghost Story and a Biography.* Princeton, NJ: Princeton University Press.

Daley, Caroline. 2003. *Leisure & Pleasure: Reshaping & Revealing the New Zealand Body 1900–1960*. Auckland, NZ: Auckland University Press.

De Garine, Igor and Nancy J. Pollock. 1995. *Social Aspects of Obesity*. Amsterdam: Gordon and Breach Science Publishers.

De Mello, Margo. 2000. *Bodies of Inscription: A Cultural History of the Modern Tattoo Community*. Durham, NC: Duke University Press.

Dopp, Hans-Jurgen. 2011. *In Praise of the Backside*. New York: Parkstone International.

Downing, Sarah Jane. 2012. *Beauty and Cosmetics 1550–1950*. Oxford: Shire Publications.

Du Toit, Herman C. 2009. *Pageants and Processions: Images and Idiom as Spectacle*. Newcastle upon Tyne: Cambridge Scholars Publishing.

Edmonds, Alexander. 2010. *Pretty Modern: Beauty, Sex and Plastic Surgery in Brazil*. Durham, NC: Duke University Press.

Elsaie, Mohamed L. 2013. *Acne: Etiology, Treatment Options and Social Effects*. New York: Nova Science Publishers, Inc.

Etcoff, Nancy. 2000. *Survival of the Prettiest: The Science of Beauty*. New York: Anchor.

Fagan, Garrett G. 1999. *Bathing in Public in the Roman World*. Ann Arbor, MI: University of Michigan Press.

Faludi, Susan. 2009. *Backlash: The Undeclared War Against American Women*. New York: Broadway Books.

Favazza, Amando. 1977. *Bodies Under Siege: Self-Mutilation in Culture and Psychiatry*. Baltimore: The Johns Hopkins University Press.

Foran, Racquel. 2014. *Living with Eating Disorders*. North Mankato, MN: ABDO Publishing.

Foucault, Michel. 1995. *Discipline and Punish: The Birth of the Prison*. Translated by Alan Sheridan. New York: Vintage Books.

Friday, Nancy. 1993. *The Power of Beauty*. New York: HarperCollins Publishers.

Gimlin, Debra L. 2002. *Body Work: Beauty and Self-Image in American Culture*. Berkeley, CA: University of California Press.

González, Raúl. 2007. *Buttocks Reshaping*. Rio de Janeiro: Indexa.

Grogan, Sarah. 2008. *Body Image: Understanding Body Dissatisfaction in Men, Women, and Children*, 2nd edition. London: Routledge.

Haiken, Elizabeth. 1999. *Venus Envy: A History of Cosmetic Surgery*. Baltimore: Johns Hopkins University Press.

Harris, Rachel. 2004. *Singing the Village: Music, Memory, and Ritual Among the Sibe of Xinjiang*. London: Oxford University Press.

Harvey, Jacky Collis. 2015. *Red: A History of the Redhead*. London: Black Dog & Leventhal.

Herzig, Rebecca M. 2014. *Plucked: A History of Hair Removal*. New York: NYU Press.

Hesse-Biber, Sharlene. 2007. *Am I Thin Enough Yet?* New York: Oxford University Press.

Hobson, Janell. 2005. *Venus in the Dark: Blackness and Beauty in Popular Culture*. New York: Routledge.

Hong, Fan. 1997. *Foot Binding, Feminism, and Freedom: The Liberation of Women's Bodies in Modern China*. London: Frank Cass.

Hua, Wen. 2013. *Buying Beauty: Cosmetic Surgery in China*. Hong Kong: Hong Kong University Press.

Jah, Meeta Rani. 2016. *The Global Beauty Industry: Colorism, Racism and the National Body*. New York: Routledge.

Jeffreys, Sheila. 2005. *Beauty and Misogyny: Harmful Cultural Practices in the West*. New York: Routledge.

Jones, Geoffrey. 2010. *Beauty Imagined: A History of the Global Beauty Industry*. Oxford: Oxford University Press.

Jones, Meredith and Cressida Heyes. 2009. *Cosmetic Surgery: A Feminist Primer*. Farnham, England: Ashgate.

Kang, Mailiann. 2010. *The Managed Hand: Race, Gender, and the Body in Beauty Service Work*. Berkeley, CA: University of California Press.

Karp, Ivan and Stephen D. Lavine. 1991. *Exhibiting Cultures*. Washington, D.C.: Smithsonian Press.

Kilbourne, Jean. 1999. *Deadly Persuasion: Why Women and Girls Must Fight the Addictive Power of Advertising*. New York: The Free Press.

Kramer, Laura. 2011. *The Sociology of Gender: A Brief Introduction*, 3rd edition. New York: Oxford University Press.

Kunzle, David. 1982. *Fashion and Fetishism: A Social History of the Corset, Tight-Lacing, and Other Forms of Body Sculpture in the West*. New York: Rowman & Littlefield.

Latzer, Yael, and Daniel Stein. 2012. *Treatment and Recovery of Eating Disorders*. New York: Nova Science Publishers, Inc.

Leigh, Michelle Dominique. 1995. *The New Beauty: East-West Teaching in the Beauty of Body and Soul*. Tokyo: Kodansha American.

Levi, Howard S. 1966. *Chinese Footbinding*. New York: Walton Rawls.

Lobato, Mirta Zaida, editor. 2005. *Cuando las mujeres reinaban: Belleza, virtud y poder en la Argentina del siglo xx*. Buenos Aires: Biblos.

Loftsdóttir, Kristín. 2008. *The Bush Is Sweet: Identity, Power, and Development among WoDaaBe Fulani in Niger*. Uppsala: Nordiska Afrikainstitutet.

Lord, M. G. 1994. *Forever Barbie: The Unauthorized Biography of a Real Doll*. New York: William Morrow and Company.

Louie, Kam. 2002. *Theorizing Chinese Masculinity: Society and Gender in China*. Cambridge, MA: Cambridge University Press.

Lutz, Catherine A. and Jane L. Collins. 1993. *Reading National Geographic*. Chicago: University of Chicago Press.

Manniche, Lise. 1999. *Sacred Luxuries: Fragrance, Aromatherapy, and Cosmetics in Ancient Egypt*. New York: Cornell University Press.

Masi de Casanova, Erynn. 2011. *Making Up the Difference: Women, Beauty and Direct Selling in Ecuador*. Austin, TX: University of Texas Press.

Masi de Casanova, Erynn. 2015. *Buttoned Up: Clothing, Conformity and White Collar Masculinity*. Ithaca, NY: Cornell University Press.

McCracken, Grant. 1995. *Big Hair: A Journey into the Transformation of Self*. Woodstock, NY: Overlook Press.

Mifflin, Margot. 2013. *Bodies of Subversion: A Secret History of Women and Tattoo*. Brooklyn, NY: Powerhouse Books.

Miller, Laura. 2006. *Beauty Up: Exploring Contemporary Japanese Body Aesthetics*. Berkeley, CA: University of California Press.

Mohapatra, Ramesh Prasad. 1992. *Fashion Styles of Ancient India*. Delhi: BR Publishing.

Negrin, Llewellyn. 2008. *Appearance and Identity: Fashioning the Body in Postmodernity*. New York: Palgrave Macmillan.

Newton, Esther. 1972. *Mother Camp: Female Impersonators in America*. Chicago: University of Chicago Press.

Nichols, Elizabeth Gackstetter. 2016. *Beauty, Virtue, Power and Success in Venezuela 1850–2015*. New York: Lexington.

Nichols, Elizabeth Gackstetter. 2014a. "Ultra-Feminine Women of Power: Beauty and the State in Argentina." In: *Women in Politics and Media: Perspectives from Nations in Transition,* edited by Maria Raicheva-Stover and Elza Ibroscheva. London: Bloomsbury.

Nichols, Elizabeth Gackstetter. 2014b. "Virgin Venuses: Beauty and Purity for 'Public' Women in Venezuela." In: *Women in Politics and Media: Perspectives from Nations in Transition,* edited by Maria Raicheva-Stover and Elza Ibroscheva. London: Bloomsbury.

Nichols, Elizabeth Gackstetter and Timothy Robbins. 2015. *Pop Culture in Latin America and the Caribbean.* Santa Barbara, CA: ABC-CLIO.

Ochoa, Marcia. 2014. *Queen for a Day: Transformistas, Beauty Queens and the Performance of Femininity in Venezuela.* Durham, NC: Duke University Press.

Ossman, Susan. 2002. *Three Faces of Beauty: Casablanca, Paris, Cairo.* Durham, NC: Duke University Press.

Peiss, Kathy. 1998. *Hope in a Jar: The Making of America's Beauty Culture.* New York: Henry Holt.

Ping, Wang. 2000. *Aching for Beauty: Foot Binding in China.* Minneapolis: University of Minnesota Press.

Pipher, Mary. 1994. *Reviving Ophelia: Saving the Selves of Adolescent Girls.* New York: Penguin.

Pitts, Victoria. 2003. *In the Flesh: The Cultural Politics of Body Modification.* New York: Palgrave Macmillan.

Prince, Althea. 2009. *The Politics of Black Women's Hair.* London: Insomniac Press.

Rand, Erica. 1995. *Barbie's Queer Accessories.* Durham, NC: Duke University Press.

Rock, Chris. 2009. *Good Hair.* Film. Directed by Chris Rock. HBO Films.

Ross, Becki. 2009. *Burlesque West: Showgirls, Sex and Sin in Postwar Vancouver.* Toronto: University of Toronto Press, Scholarly Publishing Division.

Russo, Mary. 1995. *The Female Grotesque: Risk, Excess, and Modernity.* New York: Routledge.

Said, Edward. 1978. *Orientalism.* New York, Vintage Books.

Saraswati, L. Ayu and Muse Project. 2013. *Seeing Beauty, Sensing Race in Transnational Indonesia.* Honolulu: University of Hawaii Press.

Sault, Nicole, editor. 1994. *Many Mirrors: Body Image and Social Relations.* New Brunswick, NJ: Rutgers University Press.

Savacool, Julia. 2009. *The World Has Curves: The Global Quest for the Perfect Body.* New York: Rodale.

Semmelhack, Elizabeth. 2008. *Heights of Fashion: A History of the Elevated Shoe.* Toronto: Periscope Publishing.

Shapiro, Colleen M. 2011. *Eating Disorders: Causes, Diagnosis and Treatments.* New York: Nova Science Publishers.

Sherrow, Victoria. 2001. *For Appearance' Sake: The Historical Encyclopedia of Good Looks, Beauty, and Grooming.* Westport, CT: Oryx Publishing.

Sherrow, Victoria. 2006. *Encyclopedia of Hair: A Cultural History.* Westport, CT: Greenwood Press.

Siegel, Carol. 2005. *Goth's Dark Empire.* Bloomington, IN: Indiana University Press.

Sobo, Elisa Janine. 1993. *One Blood: The Jamaican Body.* Albany, NY: SUNY Press.

Sommer, Doris. 1991. *Foundational Fictions: The National Romances of Latin America.* Berkeley, CA: University of California Press.

Taylor, Verta and Leila J. Rupp. 2003. *Drag Queens at the 801 Cabaret.* Chicago: University of Chicago Press.

Thomas, Deborah A. 2004. *Modern Blackness: Nationalism, Globalization, and the Politics of Culture in Jamaica.* Durham, NC: Duke University Press.

Thomson, Rosemarie Garland. 1996. *Freakery: Cultural Spectacles of the Extraordinary Body.* New York: New York University Press.

Vale, Vivian and Andrea Juno, editors. 1989. *Modern Primitives: Investigation of Contemporary Adornment Rituals.* San Francisco: Re/Search.

Vartanian, Ivan. 2011. *High Heels: Fashion, Femininity, and Seduction.* London: Thames & Hudson.

Velásquez, Patricia. 2014. *Straight Walk: A Supermodel's Journey to Finding Her Truth.* Franklin, TN: Post Hill Press.

von Fürer-Haimendorf, Christopher. 1962. *The Apa Tanis and Their Neighbors.* New York: Free Press.

Walker, Ida. 2008. *Steroids: Pumped Up and Dangerous.* Broomall, PA: Mason Crest Publishers.

Walker, Susannah. 2007. *Style and Status: Selling Beauty to African American Women, 1920–1975.* Lexington, KY: University of Kentucky Press.

Weiss, Brad. 2009. *Street Dreams and Hip Hop Barbershops: Global Fantasy in Urban Tanzania.* Bloomington, IN: Indiana University Press.

Weitz, Rose and Samantha Kwan, editors. 2014. *The Politics of Women's Bodies: Sexuality, Appearance, and Behavior*, 4th edition. New York: Oxford University Press.

Wingfield, Adia Harvey. 2008. *Doing Business with Beauty; Black Women, Hair Salons, and the Racial Enclave Economy.* Lanham, MD: Rowman & Littlefield.

Wisniewska, Dorota and Agnieszka Lowczanin. 2014. *All That Gothic.* New York: Peter Lang.

Wojcik, Daniel. 1995. *Punk and Neo-Tribal Body Art.* Jackson, MI: University of Mississippi Press.

Wolf, Herbert F. and Thomas M. Hassell. 2006. *Color Atlas of Dental Hygiene.* Stuttgart, Germany: Thieme.

Wolf, Naomi. 1991. *The Beauty Myth: How Images of Beauty are Used Against Women.* New York: William Morrow and Company.

Zuhur, Sherifa. 1992. *Revealing Reveiling: Islamist Gender Ideology in Contemporary Egypt.* Albany, NY: State University Press of New York.

About the Authors
and Contributors

About the Authors

Erin Kenny, PhD, is Associate Professor of Anthropology at Drury University. She also heads the Women and Gender Studies Program. She has conducted ethnographic fieldwork on gender, kinship, and personhood in Guinea, Tanzania, and Jamaica.

Dr. Elizabeth Gackstetter Nichols, PhD, is Professor of Spanish at Drury University. Nichols is a contributing editor for Venezuela and Colombia for the Library of Congress and the author of an introduction to Venezuela, a cultural encyclopedia of popular culture in Latin America, and the recently published *Beauty, Virtue, Power and Success in Venezuela: 1850–2015*.

About the Contributors

Alejandro Arango-Londoño is a PhD student of Cultural Anthropology at the University at Albany–SUNY working on masculinities, gender, critical medical anthropology, and political economy.

Karen Craigo teaches writing in Springfield, Missouri. She is the author of the poetry collection *No More Milk* and blogs at Better View of the Moon (betterviewofthemoon.blogspot.com).

Ashley Cyr, MA, is a Publisher's Representative with Broadview Publishing and is the Editor-in-Chief at Bushmead Publishing.

Shara Johnson is a writer and photographer who logs many of her experiences abroad on a narrative travel blog, SKJtravel.net.

Marina Manoukian is currently working toward a Masters in English Studies at Freie University in Berlin. Find more of her work at marinamanoukian.wordpress.com.

Leah Mueller is the author of a poetry chapbook and two books, and was featured at the 2015 New York Poetry Festival.

Tyler Omichinski, JD, is a freelance writer and policy consultant from Canada.

Janis L. Prewitt, JD, PhD, is an Associate Professor of Management at Drury University and practices law with an emphasis in the field of employment discrimination.

Zaira Reveron, PhD, is a Professor at the Universidad Simón Bolívar (Venezuela) and received her Doctorate in Political Science at the University of Connecticut.

Aimee Ross is a nationally award-winning Ohio educator who's been teaching high school English for the past 24 years. Her memoir, published by KiCam Projects, comes out in 2018.

Index

Page numbers in **bold** indicate the main entries in the encyclopedia.